Surgical Anatomy of the Lateral Transpsoas Approach to the Lumbar Spine

Surgical Anatomy of the Lateral Transpsoas Approach to the Lumbar Spine

Edited by

R. SHANE TUBBS, MS, PA-C, PHD
Professor
Department of Neurosurgery
Department of structural and cellular Biology
Tulane University School of Medicine
New Orleans, LA, United States

JOE IWANAGA
Associate Professor
Department of Neurosurgery
Tulane University School of Medicine
New Orleans, LA, United States

ROD J. OSKOUIAN
Swedish Neuroscience Institute
Seattle, Washington, United States

MARC MOISI
Assistant Professor
Department of Neurosurgery
Detroit Medical Center
Detroit, MI, United States

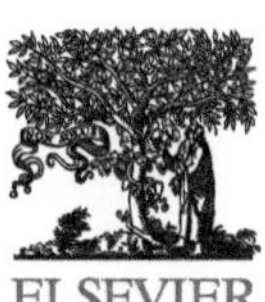

ELSEVIER

Surgical Anatomy of the Lateral Transpsoas Approach to the Lumbar Spine ISBN: 978-0-323-67376-1

Notices

Practitioners and researchers must always rely on their own experience and knowledge in evaluating and using any information, methods, compounds or experiments described herein. Because of rapid advances in the medical sciences, in particular, independent verification of diagnoses and drug dosages should be made. To the fullest extent of the law, no responsibility is assumed by Elsevier, authors, editors or contributors for any injury and/or damage to persons or property as a matter of products liability, negligence or otherwise, or from any use or operation of any methods, products, instructions, or ideas contained in the material herein.

Publisher: Cathleen Sether
Acquisition Editor: Belinda Kuhn
Editorial Project Manager: Megan Ashdown
Production Project Manager: Sreejith Viswanathan
Cover Designer: Mark Rogers

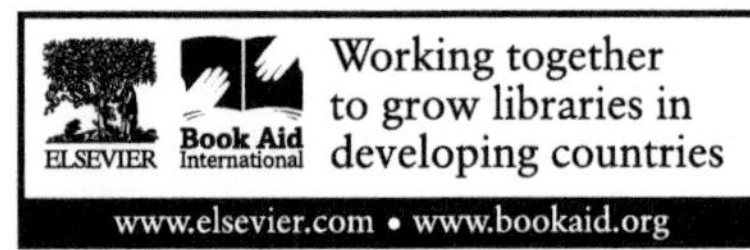

List of Contributors

Darius Ansari, MD
Swedish Neuroscience Institute
Seattle, WA, United States

Stephen J. Bordes, Jr., MD, BA
Research Fellow
Department of Anatomical Sciences
St. George's University School of Medicine
St. George's, Grenada, West Indies

Halle E.K. Burley
Swedish Neuroscience Institute
Seattle WA, United States

Christopher E. Childers, NP-C
Department of Neurosurgery
Detroit Medical Center
Detroit, MI, United States

Beom Sun Chung, MD
Department of Anatomy
Ajou University School of Medicine
Suwon, Republic of Korea

Mary Katherine Cleveland
Auburn University
Auburn, AL, United States

Graham Dupont
Swedish Neuroscience Institute
Seattle, WA, United States

Daniel T. Ginat, MD
Department of Neurosurgery
Detroit Medical Centre
Detroit, MI, United States

Dia R. Halalmeh, MD
Department of Neurosurgery
Detroit Medical Center
Detroit, MI, United States

Shiwei Huang, MD
Department of Neurosurgery
Detroit Medical Center/Wayne State University
Detroit, MI, United States

Joe Iwanaga
Associate Professor
Department of Neurosurgery
Tulane University School of Medicine
New Orleans, LA, United States

Andrew Jack, MD
Swedish Neuroscience Institute
Seattle, WA, United States

Skyler Jenkins, MD
Research Fellow
Department of Anatomical Science
St. George's University
True Blue, Grenada, West Indies

Ari D. Kappel, MD
Department of Neurosurgery
Detroit Medical Center/Wayne State University
Detroit, MI, United States

Bradely Kolb, MD
Department of Neurosurgery
Detroit Medical Center
Detroit, MI, United States

Maxwell T. Laws, MD
Department of Neurosurgery
Detroit Medical Center/Wayne State University
Detroit, MI, United States

Mishan Listmann
Swedish Neuroscience Institute
Seattle, WA, United States

Karishma Mehta
Research Fellow
Department of Anatomical Sciences
St. George's University School of Medicine
St. George's, Grenada, West Indies

Marc D. Moisi, MD
Assistant Professor
Department of Neurosurgery
Detroit Medical Center
Detroit, MI, United States

Seong-Jin Moon, MD
Department of Neurosurgery
Detroit Medical Center
Detroit, MI, United States

Peter Oakes, MD
Department of Surgery
University of South Alabama
Mobile, AL, United States

Rod J. Oskouian, MD
Swedish Neuroscience Institute
Seattle, WA, United States

Felipe H. Sanders, MD
Swedish Neuroscience Institute
Seattle, WA, United States

R. Shane Tubbs, MS, PA-C, PhD
Professor
Department of Neurosurgery
Department of Structural and Cellular Biology
Tulane University School of Medicine
New Orleans, LA, United States

Zane Tymchack, MD
Swedish Neuroscience Institute
Seattle, WA, United States

Alexander von Glinski, MD
Swedish Neuroscience Institute
Seattle, WA, United States

Lauren Wahl
Research Fellow
Swedish Neuroscience Institute
Seattle, WA, United States

Tyler Warner, MD
Research Fellow
Department of Anatomical Science
St. George's University
St. George's, Genada, West Indies

Preface

Originally intended to address lumbar spinal pathology, lateral transpsoas approaches (Figs. 1 and 2) to the lumbar spine have grown in popularity and have been adapted to allow access to the thoracic and thoracolumbar spine from approximately T4 to L5. However, even though considered minimally invasive, this approach has a steep learning curve and demands a command of regional anatomy, specifically, the retroperitoneum (Figs. 3–5). Structures here, most not as well known to the spine surgeon, include the kidneys, ureters, great vessels, and lumbar plexus and its branches.

Therefore, this impetus for this text was to provide the modern spine surgeon who performs such procedures with a resource dedicated to the anatomy as seen via a lateral vantage point. This anatomy can be complex, varied, and much of it is hidden deep to the psoas major, e.g., lumbar plexus (Figs. 6 and 7). Chapters in this textbook include anatomy of the anterolateral and posterior abdominal muscles,

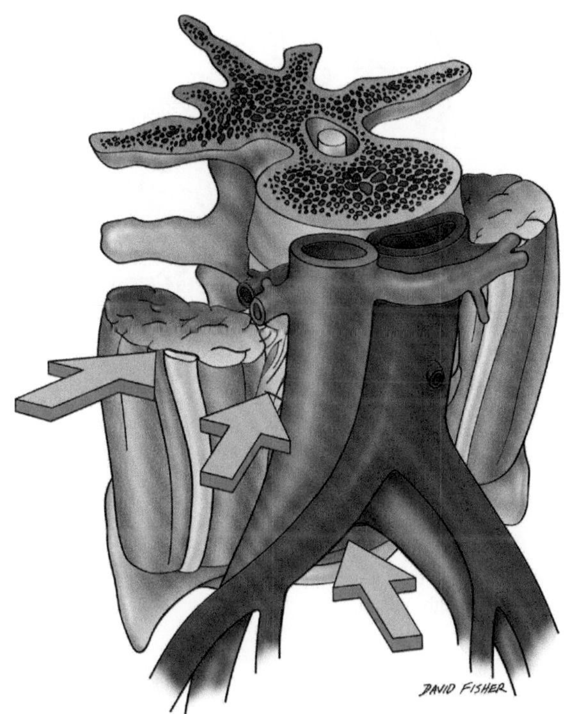

FIG. 1 Surgery for the lumbar vertebral bodies includes anterior, anterolateral, and lateral approaches.

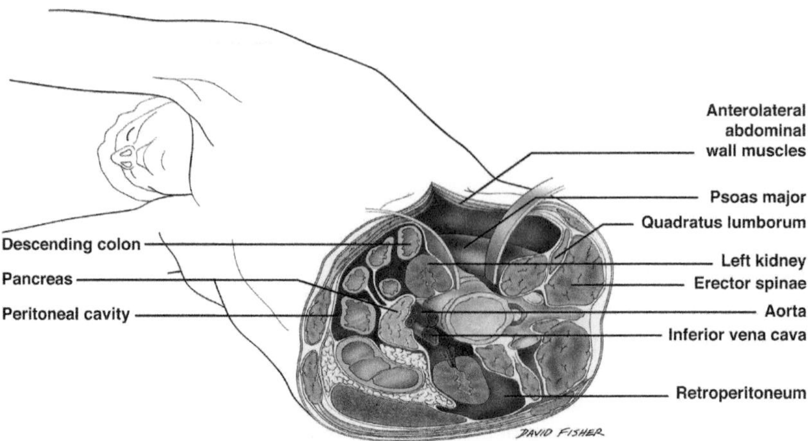

FIG. 2 Schematic drawing of the lateral approach and the unique anatomy encountered.

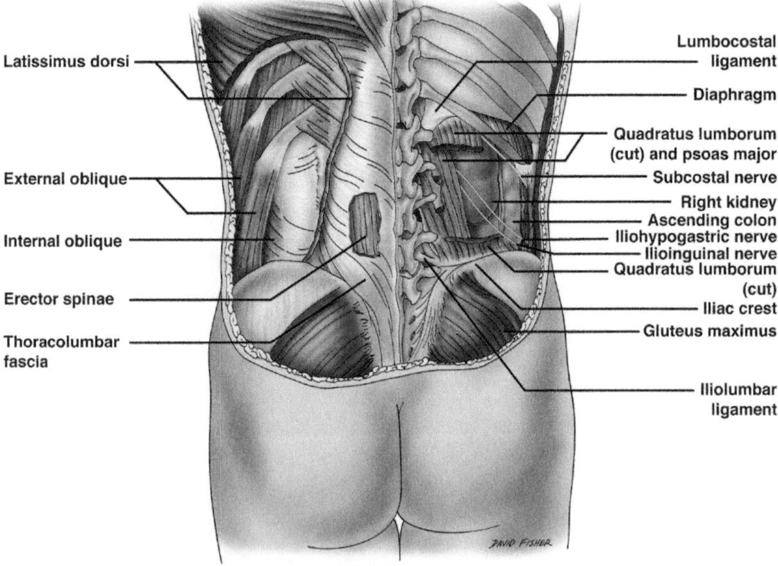

FIG. 3 Posterior view of the narrow corridor of the lateral approach necessitating a course anterior to quadratus lumborum and posterior to the kidneys, ureter, and left and right colon.

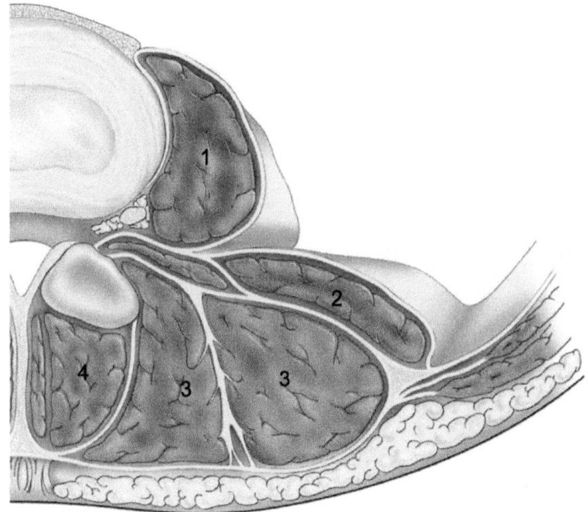

FIG. 4 Axial view of the narrow corridor to the psoas major (1) from a lateral approach just anterior to quadratus lumborum (2). For reference, note the erector spinae (3) and multifidus (4).

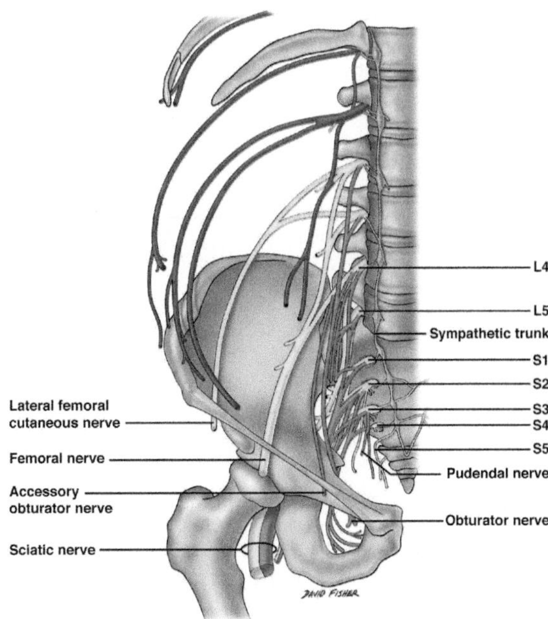

FIG. 6 Nerves of the lumbosacral region as typically illustrated.

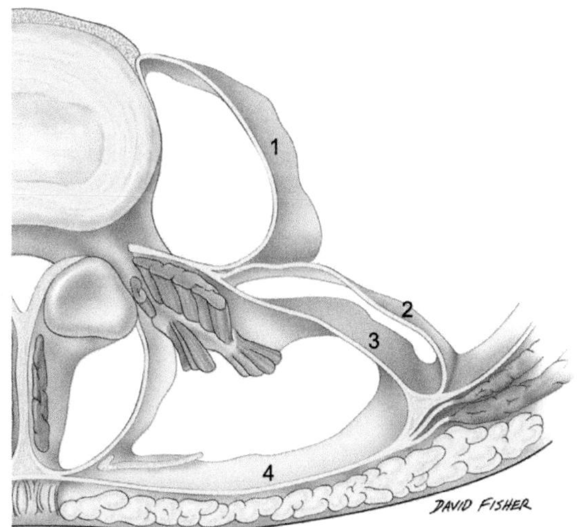

FIG. 5 Fascial layers encountered per the axial view seen in Fig. 4. Psoas fascia (1), and anterior (2), middle (3), and posterior (4) layers of the thoracolumbar fascia.

diaphragm, the retroperitoneum in general, and nerves such as those first encountered with superficial muscle dissection for the lateral approach to the deeper nerves buried within the psoas major. Chapters on the autonomic nerves and sympathetic trunk, often overlooked when discussing the lateral approach, are also found here. Obviously, the anatomy of the lumbar spine and its parts, e.g., discs, ligaments, bone, is included. A chapter dedicated to the sectional anatomy of the retroperitoneum will surely be of interest to the lateral transpsoas surgeon. Anatomical variations are sprinkled among the various chapters and in addition, a chapter has been dedicated to them as incomplete knowledge of such can lead to catastrophic operative complications. The great vessels of the abdomen have their own chapters. Finally, chapters regarding the

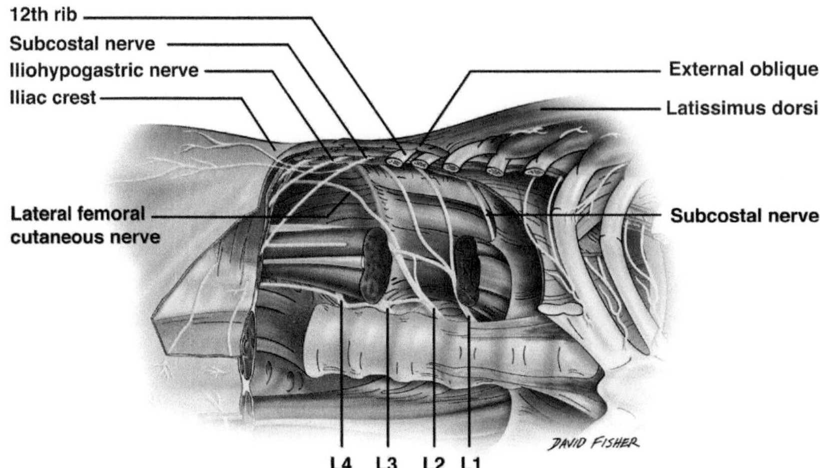

FIG. 7 Nerves of the lumbar plexus as encountered by the lateral transpsoas surgeon.

various surgical nuances of the lateral approach round out the book and are designed to give the reader an overview of the techniques used.

In the end, we hope that this collection of knowledge will improve patient outcomes and decrease surgical morbidity and complications associated with the lateral transpsoas approach to the spine.

R. Shane Tubbs, MS, PA-C, PHD
August 1, 2019

Contents

CHAPTER 1

Superficial Nerves of the Anterolateral Abdominal Wall and the Lateral Transpsoas Approach to the Lumbar Spine

MARY KATHERINE CLEVELAND • JOE IWANAGA • R. SHANE TUBBS

INTRODUCTION

The lateral transpsoas approach to the lumbar spine is increasingly being used to treat degenerative changes requiring fusion (Arnold et al., 2012). In contrast to conventional posterior spinal fusion techniques, this minimally invasive approach spares extensive posterior tissue dissection and resection and decreases operative time, blood loss, postoperative pain, and tissue trauma. Although minimally invasive, this procedure has the approach-related risk to cause lumbar plexus nerve injuries secondary to the insertion and dilation of dilatators or retractors. Plexus injuries are reported in up to approximately 30% of patients, often presenting as neuropathic pain and motor or sensory deficits (Arnold et al., 2012; Pumberger et al., 2012; Rodgers et al., 2011).

Several anatomical studies on plexus nerve anatomy for lateral approaches have been published (Uribe et al., 2010; Benglis et al., 2009); however, few have systematically documented the types of injury typically observed at each spinal level after such procedures. In our earlier study, approximately 50% of all operated-upon segments had plexus nerve injuries occurring at segments L1–L4 and involving nerve roots as well as motor and sensory nerves (Grunert et al., 2017).

Moro and Uribe et al. subdivided each lumbar vertebral segment into four quarters (zone I to zone IV) from the anterior to the posterior border of the vertebral body (Fig. 1.1) (Uribe et al., 2010; Moro et al., 2003). Although describing the relationship of the plexus nerves to the lateral vertebral body surface helps in determining ideal docking points, it oversimplifies the complex plexus anatomy, as the nerves run in anteroposterior, superolateral, and mediolateral directions. As shown in the study of Grunert et al., injuries can occur throughout the entire trajectory of the lateral transpsoas approach to the lumbar spine. Over 50% of the nerve injuries occurred either at the lateral aspect of the psoas major muscle, within the outer abdominal muscles, or in the subcutaneous tissue of the abdominal wall, predominantly affecting the subcostal, ilioinguinal, iliohypogastric, and lateral femoral cutaneous nerves (Grunert et al., 2017).

As the superficial nerves of the region between the iliac crest and 12th rib are so concentrated (Fig. 1.2) and important to avoid with the lateral transpsoas approach to the lumbar spine, this chapter focuses on these structures and their detailed anatomy.

Segmental Lateral Cutaneous Branches

The skin and muscles of the anterolateral abdominal wall are innervated by the ventral rami of T7–T12. The muscles here also receive fibers from at least L1 ventral ramus and, as we have reported, as inferior as an L4 contribution. The lower thoracic and L1 nerves and their branches travel into the abdominal wall between the transversus abdominis and internal abdominal oblique muscles. Distally, they pierce the rectus sheath. Along their course, the nerves supply not only the skin and adjacent musculature but also the parietal peritoneum. These nerves give rise to lateral and anterior cutaneous branches (Figs. 1.3 and 1.4). The former arise at about the anterior axillary line and pierce the anterolateral muscles of the abdominal wall near the midaxillary line. As the lateral cutaneous branches of these nerves reach the skin, they split into anterior and posterior branches. The anterior cutaneous

Surgical anatomy of the lateral transpsoas approach to the lumbar spine. https://doi.org/10.1016/B978-0-323-67376-1.00001-X

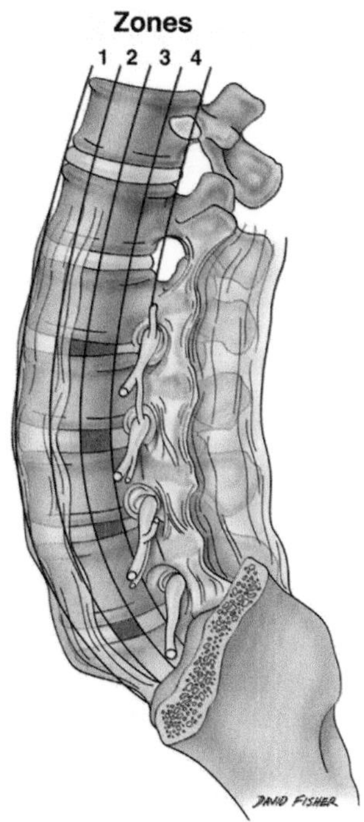

FIG. 1.1 Schematic drawing of the lateral lumbar spine illustrating the zones as developed by Uribe et al.

branches are the terminal branches of each of these segmental nerves and exit the rectus sheath anteriorly to reach the overlying skin where they too split into branches, medial and lateral.

Superior Cluneal Nerves

The superior cluneal nerves (SCNs) (Figs. 1.5–1.8) are the posterior cutaneous branches (from the lateral branch) of the dorsal rami usually described as arising from the upper three lumbar spinal nerves. Historically, it has been believed that the origin of the SCN is the dorsal rami of the L1, L2, and L3 spinal nerves. The SCN is usually depicted as having three branches: medial, intermediate, and lateral SCN.

Out of 20 sides, we previously reported the vertebral level of the origin of the SCN was T12 on 2 sides (10%), L1 on 15 sides (75%), L2 on 18 sides (90%), L3 on 19 sides (95%), L4 on 9 sides (45%) (Fig. 1.9), and L5 on 2 sides (10%), respectively (Iwanaga et al., 2018). The SCN originating from the L5 vertebral level pierced the iliolumbar ligament. Of 10 specimens, 5 (50%) had the same vertebral levels on the right and left sides as the origin of the SCNs. The total number of the vertebral levels of origin of the SCNs on each side was two on two sides (10%), three on eleven sides (55%), four on six sides (30%), and five on one side (5%). The total number of SCN that pierced the thoracolumbar fascia on each side was two on four sides (20%), three on nine sides (45%), four on four sides (20%), and five on three sides (15%). SCNs originating from L1, L2, and L3 were observed on eight sides (40%). On one side (5%), dorsal rami of the L2 and L3 joined and formed a common trunk, and on another side (5%), the dorsal rami of the L1 and L2 merged to form a common trunk. On two sides (10%), the dorsal ramus of L3 divided into two branches proximal to the exit from the

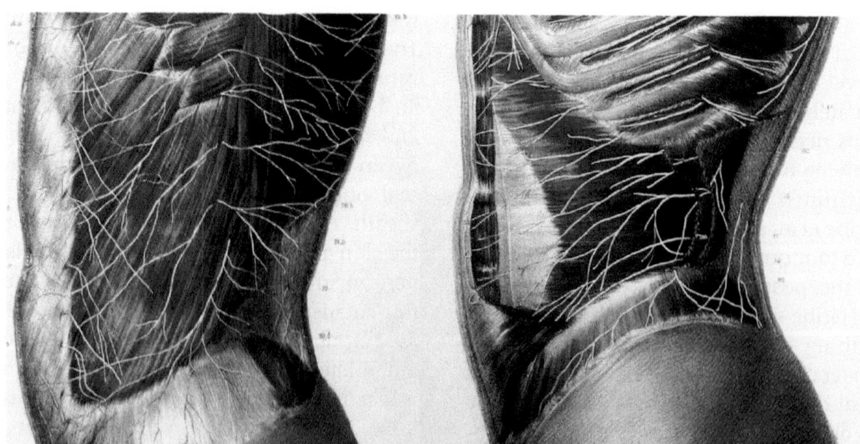

FIG. 1.2 Lateral views of the nerves traversing the anterolateral abdominal wall. The image to the left illustrates the nerves superficially, and the image to the right shows these at a deeper level. (From Bourgery's 19th century Traité complet de l'anatomie de l'homme comprenant la médecine operatoire.)

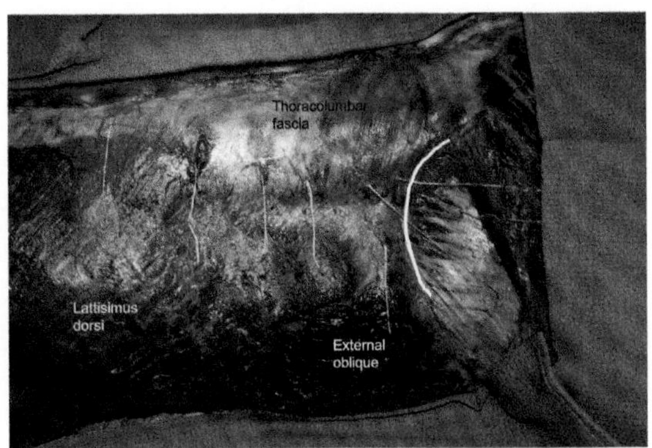

FIG. 1.3 Left posterolateral cadaveric view of segmental nerves (yellow) and their relationship to regional muscles and the iliac crest (white curved line). Note the superior cluneal nerves are crossing the iliac crest at a more vertical angle.

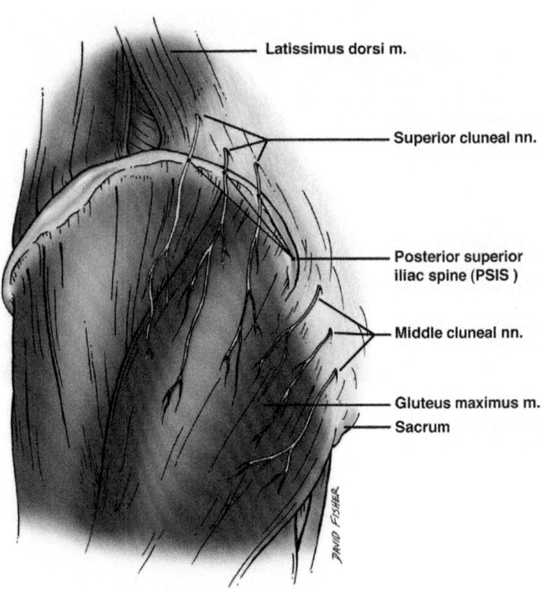

FIG. 1.5 Schematic drawing of the superior cluneal nerves.

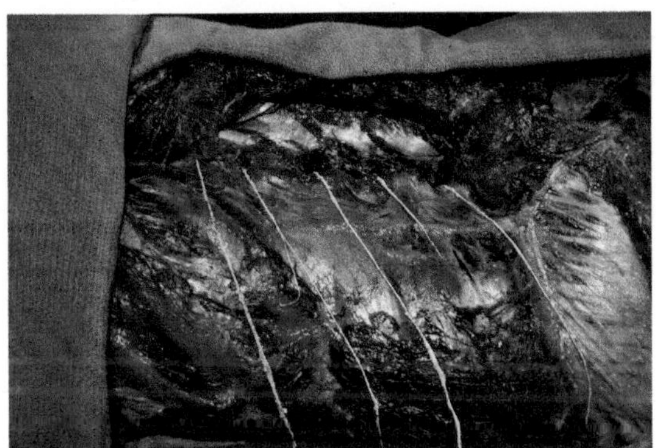

FIG. 1.4 Deeper dissection of Fig. 1.3.

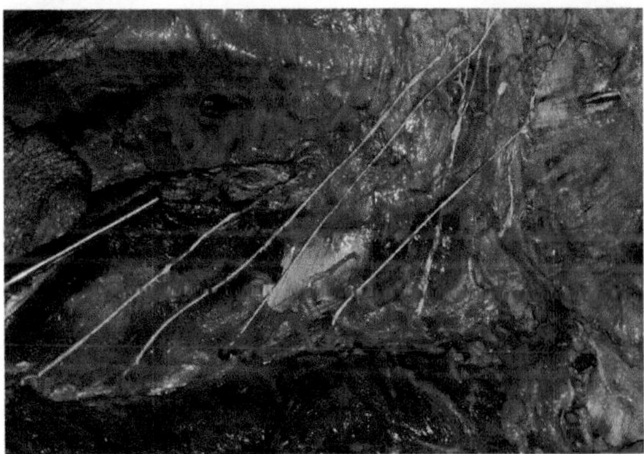

FIG. 1.6 Right-sided cadaveric dissection of superior cluneal nerves crossing the iliac crest to the right. Note the paraspinal muscles are retracted from the spine so that the origin of the nerves is seen.

thoracolumbar fascia, which innervated the superior gluteal region as two separated branches.

In another study of ours (Iwanaga et al. 2018), we found that dorsal rami of L1, L2, and L3 passed lateral to the multifidus muscle and pierced the erector spinae muscle. On five sides (41.7%) with an origin from L1 and on three sides (25.0%) with an origin from L2, the nerve ran between the iliocostalis lumborum and longissimus muscles (course C). On seven sides (58.3%), nerves derived from L1, seven (58.3%) from L2, and ten (83.3%) from L3, the nerves pierced the iliocostalis muscle (course B). On one side derived from L2 (8.3%) and one from L3 (8.3%), the nerves ran lateral to the iliocostalis (course A). On one side (8.3%), L1 and L2 nerves joined and pierced the iliocostalis. On one side (8.3%), L2 and L3 joined and pierced the iliocostalis. On one side (8.3%), L2 had no cutaneous branch but innervated the iliocostalis. On one side (8.3%), L3 had no cutaneous branch but innervated the longissimus muscle.

Subcostal Nerve

The subcostal nerve is the ventral ramus of the T12 spinal nerve and runs along the inferior border of the 12th rib before it travels in the anterolateral abdominal muscles (Figs. 1.10–1.13). At L1/L2, it is only encountered within the outer abdominal muscles (zone III) and the

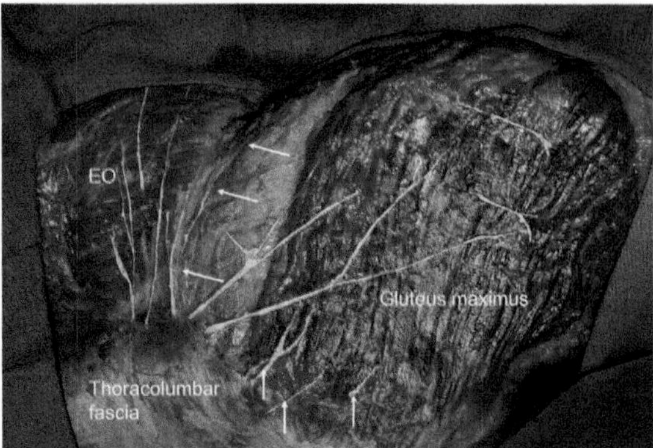

FIG. 1.7 Right-sided cadaveric dissection noting segmental cutaneous branches (far left) coursing over the external oblique muscle (EO), superior cluneal nerves crossing the iliac crest (upper arrows), and middle cluneal nerves (lower arrows) spreading out over the gluteus maximus.

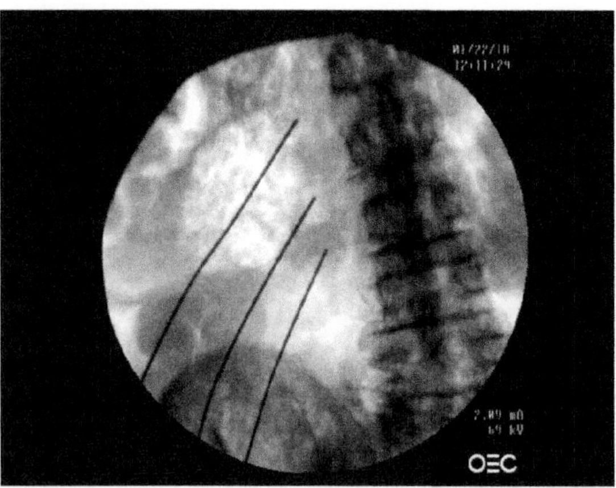

FIG. 1.8 Fluoroscopy of the superior cluneal nerves with metal wires laid over them.

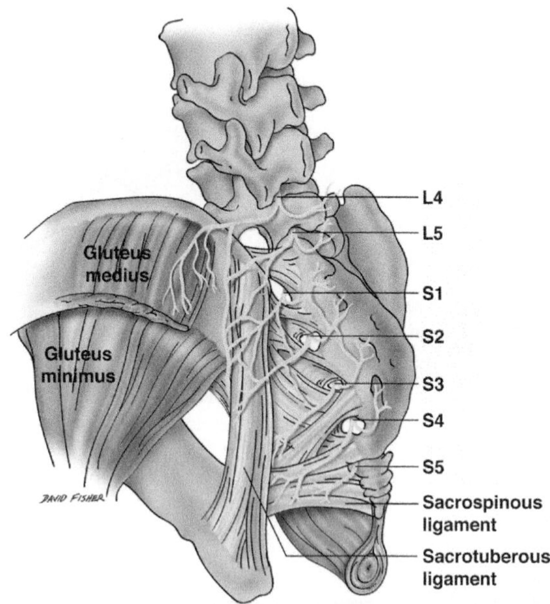

FIG. 1.9 Schematic drawing of a superior cluneal nerve arising from L4.

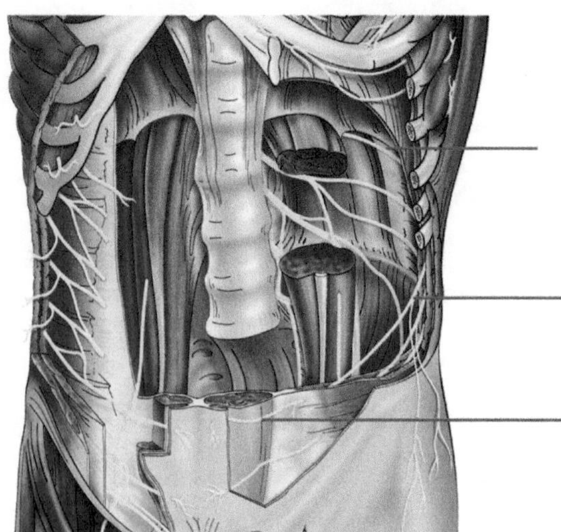

FIG. 1.10 Schematic drawing illustrating the course of branches of the lumbar plexus. Here, the course of the left subcostal nerve is indicated by the blue lines from its origin posteriorly (upper blue line), course in the abdominal wall musculature (middle blue line), and termination anteriorly (lower blue line). On the right side, note the lateral cutaneous branches of other segmental nerves.

subcutaneous tissue (zone IV). This nerve was injured in zones III and IV (Grunert et al., 2017). Careful blunt dissection through the subcutaneous and muscle tissues, without excessive monopolar coagulation, could avoid such injuries. The fasciae of the abdominal muscles should be opened bluntly. In our earlier study of this nerve, in the interval between the iliac crest and last rib, it is the largest nerve with the greatest distribution.

Ilioinguinal and Iliohypogastric Nerves

Emerging from the T12/L1 nerves, the iliohypogastric and ilioinguinal nerves (Figs. 1.14–1.21) run posterior to or within the psoas major muscle (zone I). Leaving the psoas major, both nerves continue their oblique descent on the anterior surface of the quadratus lumborum, along the posterior abdominal wall (zone II). As it reaches the outer abdominal muscles (zone III), small branches pierce the surrounding abdominal muscles

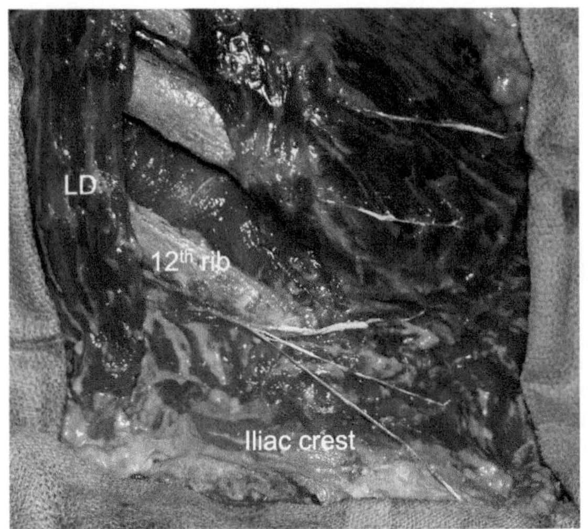

FIG. 1.11 Right cadaveric dissection noting the subcostal nerve coursing below the 12th rib and its iliac branch crossing the iliac crest. For reference, note the latissimus dorsi muscle (LD).

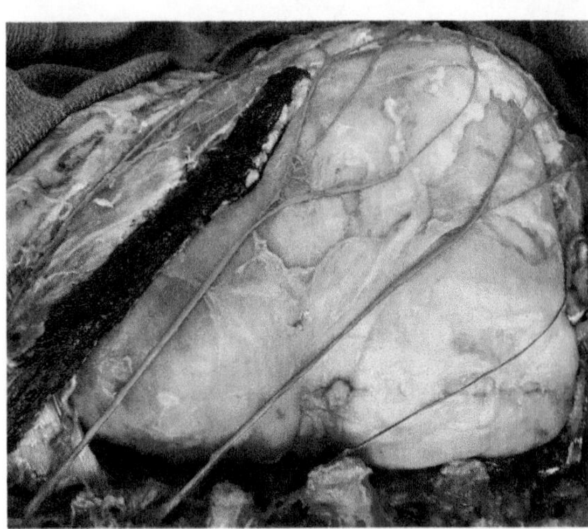

FIG. 1.13 Lateral cadaveric view of the right 12th rib (blue) and from left to right in green, the subcostal, iliohypogastric, and ilioinguinal nerves. Note the relationship of the proximal subcostal nerve to the lumbocostal ligament seen in the lower left corner.

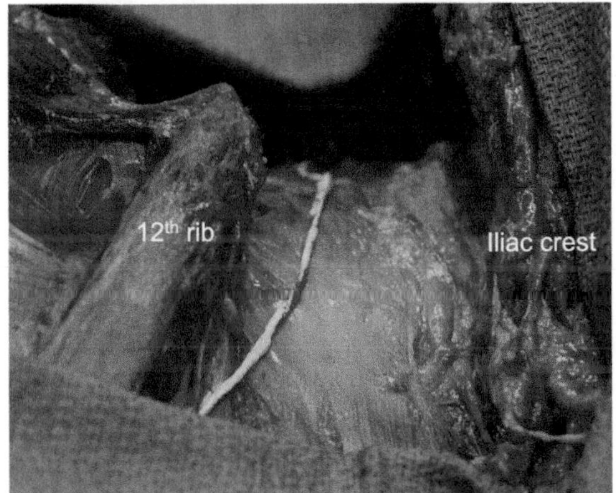

FIG. 1.12 Direct lateral view of the subcostal nerve on the right side of a cadaveric specimen. Note the narrow corridor between the 12th rib and iliac crest.

until they reach the subcutaneous tissue (zone IV). At the L1/L2 level, these nerves can potentially be injured in all anatomical zones (Grunert et al., 2017).

Careful blunt dissection (Fig. 1.16) should be performed as described for the subcostal nerve. The retroperitoneal space is typically not dissected under direct visualization, making both nerves vulnerable. The quadratus lumborum can be located by finger palpation prior to tube insertion, and this could help preclude retractor placement.

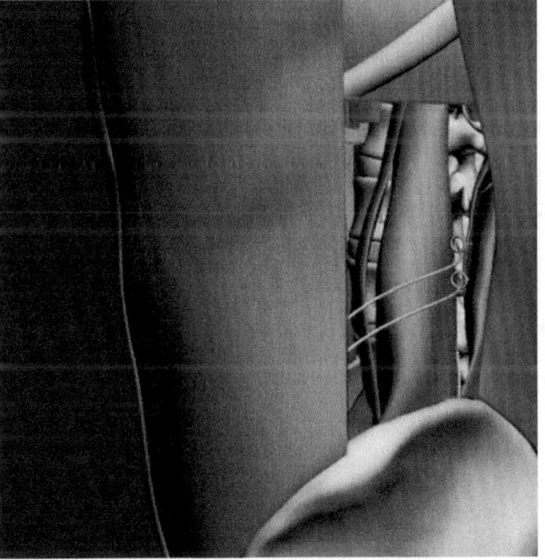

FIG. 1.14 Schematic drawing of the left lateral approach to the lumbar spine. Note the relative position of the iliohypogastric (upper) and ilioinguinal nerves (lower) as they course between the psoas major anteriorly and quadratus lumborum posteriorly. Note the interval between the 12th rib and iliac crest is enlarged in this drawing.

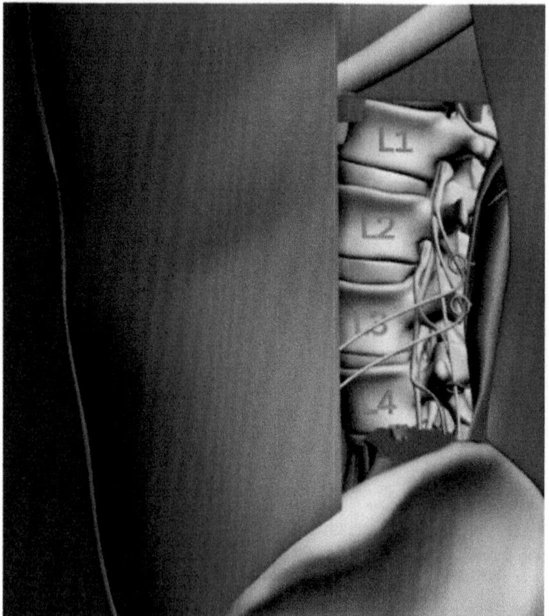

FIG. 1.15 Fig. 1.14 with psoas major removed.

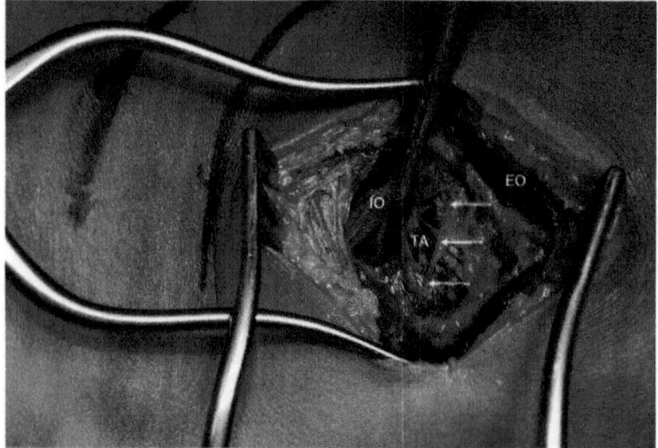

FIG. 1.16 Dissection for a left-sided lateral transpsoas approach to the lumbar spine. The 11th and 12th ribs are marked on the skin in purple ink. Note the external (EO) and internal (IO) muscles and transversus abdominus (TA). Here, the iliohypogastric nerve (arrows) is seen coursing between the internal oblique and transversus abdominus muscles. Blunt dissection avoids damage to nerves during this dissection.

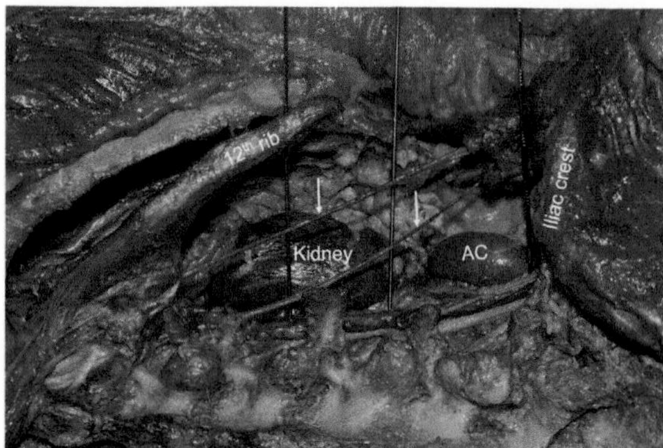

FIG. 1.17 Deeper dissection of Fig. 1.16 noting the relationship of the iliohypogastric nerve (left arrow) and ilioinguinal nerve (right arrow) to the kidney and ascending colon (AC).

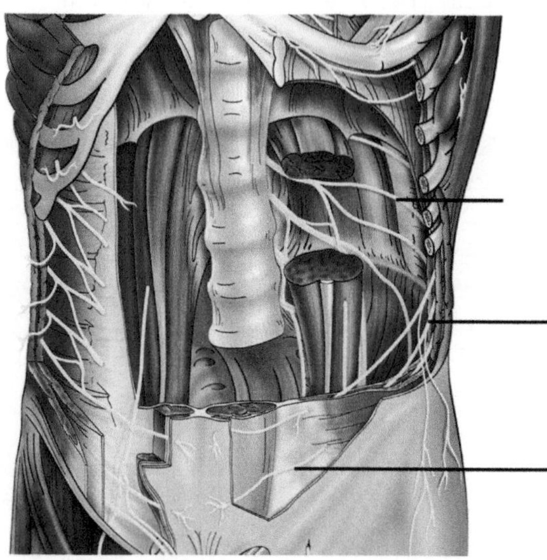

FIG. 1.18 Drawing of the deep to superficial course of the iliohypogastric nerve. The upper black arrow marks its deep course over quadratus lumborum, the middle black arrow its course in the anterolateral wall musculature, and the lower black arrow its course in the anterior abdominal wall.

Surgeons tend to choose a more posterior docking point or overretract at L1/L2, as it is considered a "safe level," since there are no lower extremity motor fibers in this area and is, therefore, usually "silent" on EMG monitoring. This practice should be avoided as both L1 and sometimes L2 nerve roots carry motor fibers for the anterolateral abdominal muscles, and denervation with potential anterolateral abdominal wall hernia can result from injuries to these nerves. The authors therefore recommend "safe zone" retractor placement as described by Uribe et al. (2010): limited retraction, and avoidance of quadratus lumborum muscle compression while the retractor is being placed and dilated (Grunert et al., 2017).

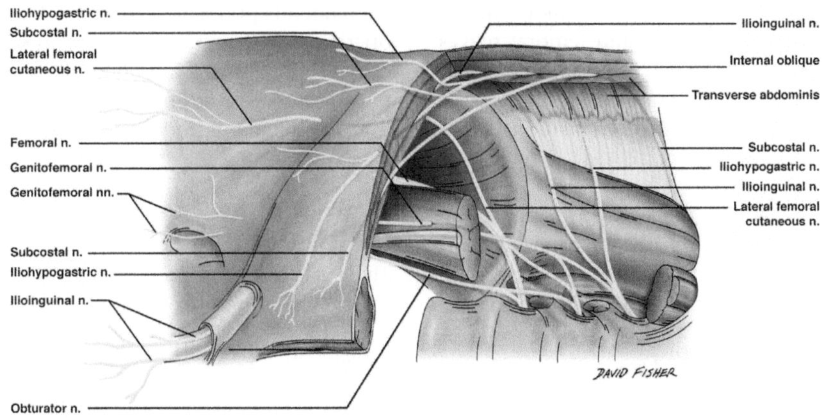

FIG. 1.19 The iliohypogastric and ilioinguinal nerves and their course in the anterolateral abdominal wall as likely encountered by the lateral transpsoas spine surgeon.

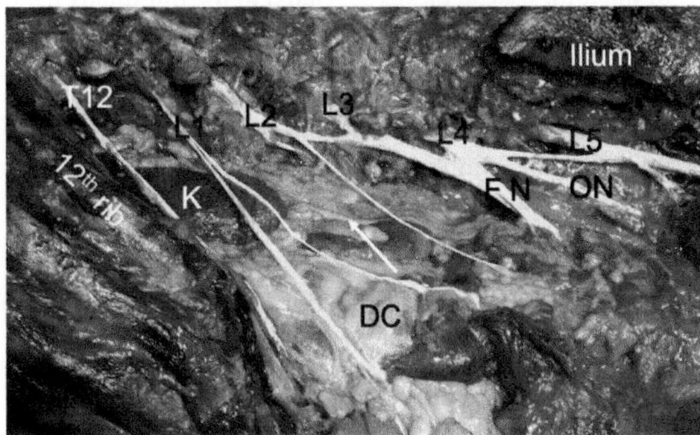

FIG. 1.20 Left posterolateral cadaveric dissection noting the superficial branches of the lumbar plexus. The subcostal nerve (ventral ramus of T12) is seen below the 12th rib and the ventral ramus of L1 is shown branching into the iliohypogastric (left) and ilioinguinal nerves (right). Note the relationship of the subcostal, iliohypogastric and ilioinguinal nerves to the kidney (K) and descending colon (DC). Also note the deeper femoral (FN) and obturator nerves (ON). Much of the iliac crest has been removed.

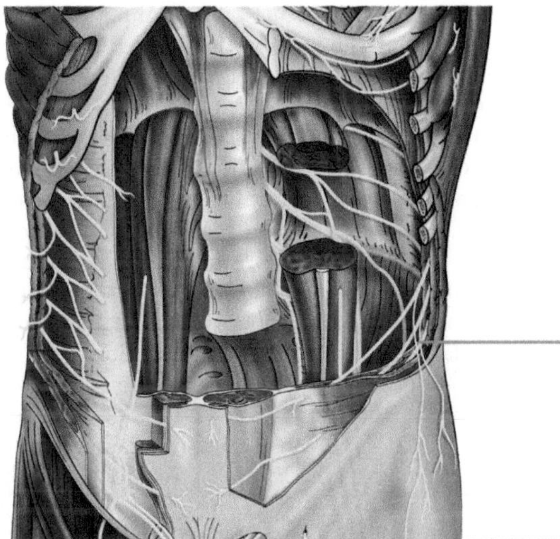

FIG. 1.21 Drawing of the course of the ilioinguinal nerve. Its course in the anterolateral abdominal wall is shown at the upper green line, and its termination as an anterior scrotal/labial branch is shown at the lower green line.

Cutaneous Nerve Injuries in General

Clinical outcome studies have demonstrated that sensory nerve deficits or alterations are common status post lateral approaches (Pumberger et al., 2012; Ahmadian et al., 2013). However, it has been difficult to assess which sensory nerves are affected since many sensory fields, specific to the iliohypogastric, ilioinguinal, genitofemoral, and subcostal nerves, overlap and are therefore difficult to distinguish clinically (Ahmadian et al., 2013). However, Ahmadian et al. summarized the sensory fields of these nerves into sensory cutaneous zones in the proximal anterior and lateral thigh (Ahmadian et al., 2013). Grunert et al. suggests that, at least in a cadaver spine model, all the aforementioned nerves are prone to injury during these procedures, with most injuries occurring at the level of L1/L2 (Grunert et al., 2017).

Monitoring

Intraoperative EMG-based neuromonitoring allows for geographic "mapping" of the lumbar plexus, which improves the safety of lateral approaches (Uribe et al., 2010; Ozgur et al., 2006). Current monitoring techniques use insulated tubes with an isolated stimulation source at the tip (Uribe et al., 2010). This allows for focused stimulation within the psoas major muscle. Given the course of the obturator and femoral nerves and the largest portion of the nerve roots, these monitoring techniques can detect those nerves intraoperatively. The disadvantage of focused stimulation is that motor fibers lateral to the psoas muscle (zones II–IV) are not detected. Although not routinely monitored, motor fibers of the ilioinguinal and iliohypogastric nerves could only be stimulated within their relatively short course in the psoas muscle at the L1/L2 level, and not in their distal course, where injuries were observed.

Type and Mechanism of Nerve Injuries

Despite extensive studies, the types and mechanisms of nerve injury occurring after lateral approaches remains unknown. Most types of injury proposed in the literature are injuries without structural changes to the nerve, such as nerve compression, traction, transient irritation (Pumberger et al., 2012), or ischemic injuries (Ahmadian et al., 2013). These types of injury can be classified as Sunderland grade I: impaired nerve conduction without detectable histological change (Sunderland, 1990; Menorca et al., 2013). However, studies have suggested that structural nerve injuries can occur. In the study of Grunert et al., partial as well as complete transections were observed (Grunert et al., 2017). Partial transections can be rated as Sunderland grades IV–V; complete transections are all rated as Sunderland grade V (Sunderland, 1990; Menorca et al., 2013). The Sunderland grade positively correlates with the time of nerve function recovery. Over 90% of neurological deficits after lateral fusion resolve (Pumberger et al., 2012; Rodgers et al., 2011; Lykissas et al., 2014). However, the time required for significant improvement ranges from 6 weeks to 24 months (Pumberger et al., 2012; Rodgers et al., 2011). Given the differing lengths of recovery time exhibited, it is plausible that various Sunderland grades can result from these approaches. Permanent deficits are likely to be related to complete or partial transection injuries, as they seldom recover without surgical repair (Sunderland, 1990). In this regard, surgical repair of long-term motor deficits after lateral approaches could be suggested. Intraoperative crush injuries typically result from acute traumatic compression by a blunt object (such as retractor blades or cages) causing partial or complete nerve transections (Sunderland, 1990).

CONCLUSION

Lumbar plexus nerve injuries can occur with lateral transpsoas approaches to the lumbar spine. Structural nerve injuries (Sunderland grades IV–V) can also occur from lateral approaches. These can be classified as intraoperative crush injuries from blunt objects. Awareness of the topographic anatomy of the superficial branches of the lumbar plexus nerves can help reduce the risk of injuries in patients undergoing lateral approaches to the lumbar spine.

REFERENCES

Ahmadian, A., Deukmedjian, A.R., Abel, N., Dakwar, E., Uribe, J.S., 2013. Analysis of lumbar plexopathies and nerve injury after lateral retroperitoneal transpsoas approach: diagnostic standardization. J. Neurosurg. Spine 18, 289–297.

Arnold, P.M., Anderson, K.K., McGuire Jr., R.A., 2012. The lateral transpsoas approach to the lumbar and thoracic spine: a review. Surg. Neurol. Int. 3, S198–S215.

Benglis, D.M., Vanni, S., Levi, A.D., 2009. An anatomical study of the lumbosacral plexus as related to the minimally invasive transpsoas approach to the lumbar spine. J. Neurosurg. Spine 10, 139–144.

Grunert, P., Drazin, D., Iwanaga, J., Schmidt, C., Alonso, F., Moisi, M., Chapman, J., Oskouian, R.J., Tubbs, R.S., 2017. Injury to the lumbar plexus and its branches following lateral fusion procedures: a cadaver study. World Neurosurg. 105, 519–525.

Iwanaga, J., Simonds, E., Patel, M., Oskouian, R.J., Tubbs, R.S., 2018. Anatomic study of superior cluneal nerves: application to low back pain and surgical approaches to lumbar vertebrae. World Neurosurg. 116, e766–e768.

Lykissas, M.G., Aichmair, A., Hughes, A.P., et al., 2014. Nerve injury after lateral lumbar interbody fusion: a review of 919 treated levels with identification of risk factors. Spine J. 14, 749–758.

Menorca, R.M., Fussell, T.S., Elfar, J.C., 2013. Nerve physiology: mechanisms of injury and recovery. Hand Clin. 29, 317–330.

Moro, T., Kikuchi, S., Konno, S., Yaginuma, H., 2003. An anatomic study of the lumbar plexus with respect to retroperitoneal endoscopic surgery. Spine 28, 423–428.

Ozgur, B.M., Aryan, H.E., Pimenta, L., Taylor, W.R., 2006. Extreme Lateral Interbody Fusion (XLIF): a novel surgical technique for anterior lumbar interbody fusion. Spine J. 6, 435–443.

Pumberger, M., Hughes, A.P., Huang, R.R., Sama, A.A., Cammisa, F.P., 2012. Neurologic deficit following lateral lumbar interbody fusion. Eur. Spine J. 21, 1192–1199.

Rodgers, W.B., Gerber, E.J., Patterson, J., 2011. Intraoperative and early postoperative complications in extreme lateral interbody fusion: an analysis of 600 cases. Spine 36, 26–32.

Sunderland, S., 1990. The anatomy and physiology of nerve injury. Muscle Nerve 13, 771–784.

Uribe, J., Vale, F., Dakwar, E., 2010. Electromyographic monitoring and its anatomical implications in minimally invasive spine surgery. Spine 35, 368–S374.

Uribe, J.S., Arredondo, N., Dakwar, E., Vale, F.L., 2010. Defining the safe working zones using the minimally invasive lateral retroperitoneal transpsoas approach: an anatomical study. J. Neurosurg. Spine 13, 260–266.

FURTHER READING

Acosta Jr., F.L., Drazin, D., Liu, J.C., 2013. Supra-psoas shallow docking in lateral interbody fusion. Neurosurgery 73, 48–51.

Banagan, K., Gelb, D., Poelstra, K., Ludwig, S., 2011. Anatomic mapping of lumbar nerve roots during a direct lateral transpsoas approach to the spine: a cadaveric study. Spine 36, 687–691.

Cahill, K.S., Martinez, J.L., Wang, M.Y., Vanni, S., Levi, A.D., 2012. Motor nerve injuries following the minimally invasive lateral transpsoas approach. J. Neurosurg. Spine 17, 227–231.

Dakwar, E., Vale, F.L., Uribe, J.S., 2011. Trajectory of the main sensory and motor branches of the lumbar plexus outside the psoas muscle related to the lateral retroperitoneal transpsoas approach. J. Neurosurg. Spine 14, 290–295.

Davis, T.T., Bae, H.W., Mok, J.M., Rasouli, A., Delamarter, R.B., 2011. Lumbar plexus anatomy within the psoas muscle: implications for the transpsoas lateral approach to the L4-L5 disc. J. Bone Jt. Surg. Am. 93, 1482–1487.

Tender, G.C., Serban, D., 2013. Genitofemoral nerve protection during the lateral retroperitoneal transpsoas approach. Neurosurgery 73, 192–196.

CHAPTER 2

Muscles of the Anterolateral Abdominal Wall

LAUREN WAHL • HALLE E.K. BURLEY • R. SHANE TUBBS

INTRODUCTION

The anterolateral abdominal wall musculature of the human abdomen is composed of a thick sheath of flat muscles that act collectively to perform a broad spectrum of functions. These three muscles are layered one atop the other with their respective muscle fibers aligned perpendicularly to strengthen the abdominal wall and provide support to the abdominal viscera, generate positive pressure within the abdomen to perform actions such as expiration, defecation, and micturition, and reduce the risk of herniation ultimately. Their elastic nature allows the abdomen to contract and relax to adjust for the varying volumes of abdominal contents (Standring, 2016; Shafik et al., 2007; Floch, 2005).

The external oblique (Figs. 2.1 and 2.2) is the most superficial anterolateral abdominal muscle and also is the largest of this muscle group. The internal oblique muscle (Figs. 2.3 and 2.4) is deep to the external oblique. It is a relatively thinner and smaller muscle than the external oblique, with muscle fibers that run perpendicular to it. The deepest anterolateral abdominal muscle, the transversus abdominis (Figs. 2.3 and 2.4), whose fibers run in a transverse direction, lays beneath these two muscles (Standring, 2016). This muscle interweaves its aponeurotic fibers medially into the tendinous raphe referred to as the linea alba.

This chapter reviews these muscles' embryology extensively and provides a detailed anatomical overview of each muscle, as well as associated pathologies and other relevant information that may be useful to surgeon. Spine surgeons performing lateral transpsoas approaches to the lumbar spine need a good working knowledge of the relationship of these muscles to the underlying peritoneum and retroperitoneum (Fig. 2.5).

EMBRYOLOGY

In the third and fourth weeks of embryogenesis, the embryo begins to fold in on itself caudally, cranially, and bilaterally, and the latter folds lead to the formation of the anterolateral abdominal muscles and midgut. The muscles' formation begins in Carnegie Stage (CS) 18 at the end of the sixth week of gestation. At this stage, the hypaxial muscle band separates into the three layers that correspond to the anterolateral abdominal wall muscles: the outer layer becomes the external oblique, the middle the internal oblique, and the inner the transversus abdominis. These muscles stem from the fifth, seventh, and second ribs to the level of the first lumbar vertebra, respectively. Between the sixth and eighth weeks of gestation (CS 18–CS 23), the anterolateral abdominal muscles' cranial and caudal connections descend several vertebral segments (Mekonen et al., 2015). Thereafter, the three muscles secure their permanent attachments cranially to the sixth, ninth, and eighth ribs, respectively, and their ventral boundaries migrate more medially during approximately the ninth week of gestation.

EXTERNAL OBLIQUE

The external oblique, a roughly rectangular-shaped muscle, originates from the lower eight ribs' external surfaces and inferior borders, curves around the abdomen's lateral and anterior portions, and inserts into the linea alba, the pubic crest, the pubic tubercle, the anterior superior iliac spine, and the iliac crest's anterior half (Standring, 2016). The attachments on the lower eight ribs intertwine with the serratus anterior and the latissimus dorsi muscles' lower fibers along a rough oblique line that proceeds inferiorly and posteriorly. The external oblique's more superior attachments on

Surgical anatomy of the lateral transpsoas approach to the lumbar spine. https://doi.org/10.1016/B978-0-323-67376-1.00002-1

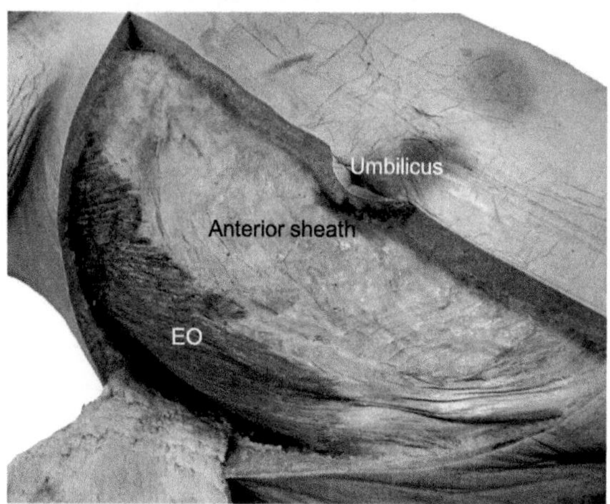

FIG. 2.1 Cadaveric dissection of the external oblique muscle (EO) and the anterior rectus sheath.

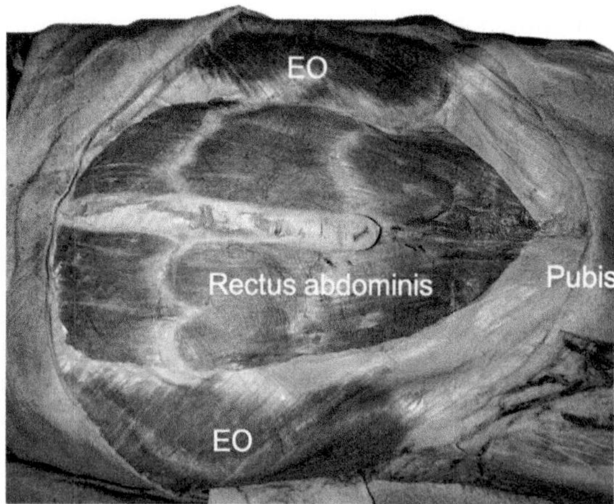

FIG. 2.2 Cadaveric dissection of the external oblique muscle (EO) and the rectus abdominis.

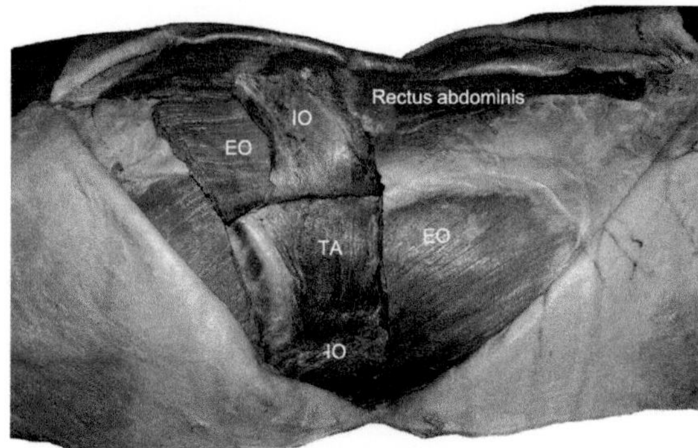

FIG. 2.3 Lateral view of the right-sided external oblique (EO), internal oblique (IO), and transversus abdominus (TA) muscles. The head is to the left and the feet to the right.

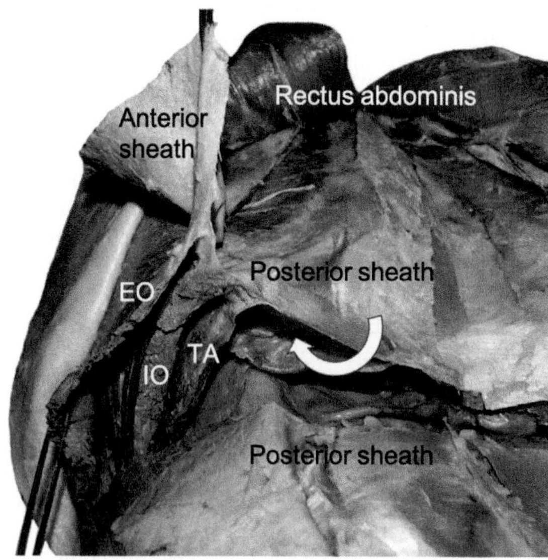

FIG. 2.4 Superior view of the left-sided external oblique (EO), internal oblique (IO), and transversus abdominus (TA) muscles. The peritoneal cavity is indicated at the arrow.

the ribs are relatively close to the respective ribs' costal cartilage, whereas the middle attachments affix to the ribs with a relatively large amount of space between the attachments and costal cartilages. These upper and middle attachments may be absent in some individuals but are most often present. The lowest attachments are to the cartilaginous apexes of the 12th ribs. The fibers of the external oblique that attach to the 11th and 12th ribs extend almost completely vertically and insert into the iliac crest's anterior portion, including the anterior superior iliac spine, pubic tubercle, and pubic crest, whereas its remaining fibers traverse anteriorly and inferiorly and continue as aponeurotic fibers that join to contribute to the formation of the linea alba at the abdomen's midline. The posterior muscle border is not enclosed or attached to any structure and is considered a "free" border (Standring, 2016). The inferior border of the aponeurotic portion of the external oblique forms the inguinal ligament between the pubic tubercle and the anterior superior iliac spine. The aponeurotic external oblique and the inguinal ligament's fibers do not run parallel; the external oblique's fibers travel toward the ligament at an angle of approximately 10–20degrees (Standring, 2016).

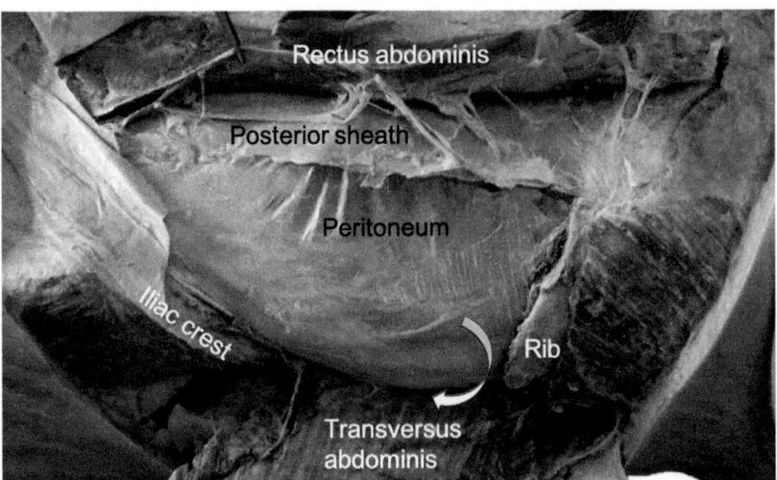

FIG. 2.5 Left dissection through the anterolateral abdominal wall with an intact peritoneum. The retroperitoneum is indicated at the arrow.

The external oblique's arterial supply derives primarily from the subcostal and lower posterior intercostal arteries' branches, as well as the deep circumflex iliac artery, with several smaller contributions, and the lower five intercostal nerves and subcostal nerve from the ventral rami of the lower six thoracic spinal nerves innervate it. While all three muscles serve to maintain abdominal tone and increase intraabdominal pressure, the external oblique also flexes the trunk, both in the sagittal and in the coronal planes. When both external oblique muscles are flexed, flexion occurs in the sagittal plane, and when one flexes unilaterally, the trunk flexes laterally in the coronal plane (Standring, 2016).

Variations

The external abdominal oblique muscle typically originates from the ribs, but the number of ribs from which it originates is highly variable. Generally, it arises from seven to nine ribs total, with the 4th rib being the most superior and the 12th rib being the most inferior. However, many variants of the highest or lowest rib of origin are documented in the literature. The aponeurosis of the external abdominal oblique at its inferior border forms the inguinal ligament and anterior layer of the sheath of rectus abdominis.

Macalister (1875) reviewed many anatomic variations of the external abdominal oblique muscle. He described 12 distinct variants, including differences in the superior extent and the numbers of ribs of origin, partial absence of the origin from some ribs, a double origin from the same rib, and an accessory muscle deep to the external abdominal oblique or between the external and internal abdominal obliques.

Mori (1964) reported that the furthest superior origin of the external abdominal oblique muscle was the fourth rib in 0.6% of cases, fifth rib in 83.1% of cases, and sixth rib in 16.3% of cases in their study of 166 Japanese adults (332 cases, right and left side). Miyauchi et al. (1986) reported similar findings. In contrast to adult, two different studies of fetal musculature found that the most superior origin of the external abdominal oblique was the fifth or sixth ribs. Yonekura (1954) found 77.0% at the fifth rib and 23.0% at the sixth rib, and Kikuchi (1986) found 87.5% at the fifth rib and 12.5% at the sixth rib. The most inferior rib of origin of the external abdominal oblique muscle is the 12th rib in adults, whereas in the fetus, the origin reaches only as far inferiorly as the 11th rib, with no fibers from the 12th rib in 34.0% of cases (Yonekura, 1954). The superior segment of the external abdominal oblique's origin interdigitates with the segments of the serratus anterior muscle that arise from the same region. The inferior portion of its origin crosses the latissimus dorsi muscle to form Gerdy's line. The level of the intersection of the serratus anterior and external abdominal oblique muscles was reported by Murata et al. (1971), who found that they crossed at the 5th rib in 85.0%, 6th rib in 100%, 7th rib in 100%, 8th rib in 98.8%, 9th rib in 71.6%, 10th rib in 14.8%, and 11th rib in 0.3% of cases.

Occasionally, accessory muscle bundles associated with the external and internal abdominal oblique muscles will arise from the ribs. These surplus muscle bundles have been dubbed "M. obliquus externus secundus s. accessorius" (Gruber, 1875), "Federkiel-dicker Muskel" (Weitbrecht, 1735, in Sugiura, 1935), "M. obliquus externus profundus s. minor" (Knott, 1881), "M. rectus lateralis abdominis" (Kelch, 1813, in Knott, 1883), or "M. obliquus externus abdominis minor s. secundus" (Knott, 1883). Old reports by Knott (1881, 1883) and Macalister (1875) briefly mention several forms of musculus obliquus abdominis externus profundus. Knott (1883) described the muscle as arising from the ninth and tenth ribs at the costochondral junction and inserting on the inguinal ligament, approximately one-third of the way from its lateral attachment. Macalister (1875) describes a case in which the musculus obliquus abdominis externus profundus existed in duplicate on the left side, with the deeper muscle traveling from ribs 9 through 11 to the iliac crest, exactly parallel to the normal muscle and separated from it by a fascial sheet. Nakayama and Okuda (1952) presented detailed figures of the obliquus abdominis externus profundus and described two cases occurring in Japanese adults. In one case, a 36-year-old male, the muscle originated from 11th rib and traveled between the internal and external abdominal obliques (length 13 cm and width 1 cm) before inserting at the anterior margin of the iliac crest near the anterior superior iliac spine. In the other case, in an 84-year-old female, the muscle began with two heads at its origin, fascia of the internal abdominal oblique muscle just below the 11th rib. The two heads then merged into one muscle (length 9.5 cm and width 0.5 cm) and inserted at the inner surface of the aponeurosis of the external abdominal oblique muscle near the iliac crest. A similar anatomic arrangement was found bilaterally in one Japanese adult (Shimazaki, 1959).

Miyauchi et al. (1986) reviewed the prevalence of obliquus abdominis externus profundus and described the inconsistencies regarding its frequency of occurrence in the literature. Loth (1912, 1931) found the obliquus abdominis externus profundus in 7% of Caucasians and 3.8% of those of African descent. Nakayama and Okuda, (1952), Yonekura (1954), and Kudo and Otobe, 1952 found it in 1.9%, 2%, and 3% of their study populations, respectively. In contrast to these relatively low figures, Kodama (1986) reported a prevalence of 36.5% in the cases studied. Based on his findings, Kodama (1986) suggested that this surplus muscle should be subclassified based on its innervation.

Other uncommon accessory muscles associated with the external abdominal oblique include the saphenous muscle, which loops around the saphenous vein on its course from one end of the inguinal ligament to the other (Tyrie, 1894), and the interfoveolar muscle, which consists of muscle fibers within the interfoveolar ligament. The interfoveolar muscle has been observed in 46% of Chinese people (Kudo and Otobe, 1952). A tiny slip of muscle extending from the pubic bone to the transversalis fascia and crossing anterior to the interfoveloar ligament/muscle at nearly a right angle was dubbed the pubotransversalis muscle by Luschka (1879).

INTERNAL OBLIQUE

The internal oblique muscle lays directly below the external oblique and is smaller and thinner than its superficial neighbor. This haphazardly four-sided muscle originates from a larger portion of the iliopectineal arch, which is a fascial band that stretches from the anterior superior iliac spine to the pelvis' iliopectineal eminence, as well as the iliac crest's anterior two-thirds, just beneath the external oblique's origin on this structure. It also originates posteriorly from the thoracolumbar fascia. These more posterior fibers travel superiorly and anteriorly to insert into the lower three ribs and their respective cartilaginous extensions, and coalesce into the internal intercostal muscles. Fibers that originate from the iliac crest migrate superiorly across the anterior abdomen, run perpendicular to the superficial external oblique's fibers, and become an anterior aponeurosis that inserts into the seventh, eighth, and ninth rib cartilages. The remaining fibers that lay contiguous with the inguinal ligament proceed inferiorly and anteriorly over the spermatic cord in males and the uterus's round ligament in females and develop into a tendinous band that becomes a part of the transversus abdominis muscle's aponeurosis, and insert ultimately into the pubic crest as well as the pectineal line to form the conjoint tendon, which serves to strengthen and support the inguinal canal's posterior wall (Standring, 2016).

The internal oblique's blood supply is congruent with that of the external oblique (branches from the subcostal and lower posterior intercostal arteries and deep circumflex iliac artery with several smaller contributions) as well as supply from the inferior hypogastric artery. Much like the blood supply, the internal oblique also shares the same innervations as the external oblique (lower five intercostal nerves, subcostal nerve from the ventral rami of the lower six thoracic spinal nerves) as well as innervations from small contributions of the iliohypogastric and ilioinguinal nerves that originate from the first lumbar spinal nerve's ventral ramus

(Standring, 2016). The internal oblique performs the same functions as the external, maintaining abdominal tone and increasing intraabdominal pressure, and flexing the trunk both in the sagittal plane with bilateral use of the oblique muscle, and laterally in the coronal plane with its unilateral use.

Variations

Macalister (1875) documented many anatomical variations of the internal abdominal oblique muscle. He described six distinct types of variants, including variations in the number of costal attachments, fusion with the transversus abdominis muscle, and the presence of tendinous slips interdigitating with the muscle fibers of the internal abdominal oblique near its costal insertions.

According to Macalister (1875), the internal abdominal oblique may have two to five costal attachments. His findings indicated that most people, about 78%, have three costal attachments, and about 17% have four costal attachments. Loth (1912a,b) found the most superior costal insertion of the internal abdominal oblique at the 8th rib in 1.5%, the 9th in 1.0%, the 10th in 66.5%, and the 11th rib in 31% of cases, based on studies in a Polish population. In 200 Japanese adults, Mori (1964) found that the most superior costal insertion on the left side was the 10th rib in 64% and the 11th rib in 36% of cases, and on the right side was the 10th rib in 56% and the 11th rib in 34% of cases. In a study of 100 fetuses, Yonekura (1954) reported that the most superior costal insertion was the 8th, 9th, 10th, and 11th rib in 2.0%, 40.0%, 55.0%, and 3.0% of cases, respectively, whereas Kikuchi (1986) reported that the 10th rib was the most superior insertion in all of 40 fetuses studied.

Knott (1883) described two cases of an internal abdominal oblique muscle fused with the transversus abdominis. He described the internal abdominal oblique as so closely associated with the transversus abdominis that he could not satisfactorily dissect them apart.

Knott (1883) also described several cases of tendinous inscriptions opposite the apex of the 10th or 11th rib. In another two instances, he observed isolated cartilaginous slips opposite the 10th costal cartilage and referenced similar observations reported by Henle (1871) and Macalister (1875). Macalister (1875) mentioned that where the internal abdominal oblique muscle is continuous with the 10th intercostal muscle, a tendinous inscription containing a thin cartilaginous slip separate from the cartilage of the rib will often extend the line of the 10th rib medially. Macalister (1875) also reported partial deficiencies in the anterior and superior segments of the internal abdominal oblique.

TRANSVERSUS ABDOMINIS

The transversus abdominis is the third and deepest anterolateral abdominal wall muscle. This encompassing muscle originates in the iliopectineal arch beneath the origin of the internal oblique muscle, anterior portion of the iliac crest, thoracolumbar fascia beneath the origin of the internal oblique, and the costal cartilage aspects of the lower six ribs. The transversus abdominis travels around the abdomen to the ventral side with its fibers traveling in a transverse fashion, which then become aponeurotic: the lower fibers proceed inferiorly to insert into the pubic crest, whereas the remaining superior fibers join other fibers from the internal and external oblique muscles to help form the linea alba down the midline of the abdomen (Standring, 2016).

The transversus abdominis' arterial supply derives from contributions from the lower posterior intercostal and subcostal arteries, much like the internal and external oblique muscles, as well as the superior and inferior epigastric arteries, the superficial and deep circumflex iliac arteries, and the posterior lumbar arteries. It has the same innervation pattern as the internal oblique muscle and is innervated by the terminal branches of the lower five intercostal nerves, subcostal nerves, iliohypogastric nerve, and ilioinguinal nerves. Like the other two muscles, the transversus abdominis helps maintain abdominal tone and provides intraabdominal pressure by compressing the ribs and abdominal viscera. This action is important in the Valsalva maneuver during defecation, micturition, and delivery in pregnant women (Shafik et al., 2007).

Variations

Macalister (1875) reviewed multiple anatomic variants of the transversus abdominis, including variation in the number of costal origins, fusion with the internal abdominal oblique, and entire or partial absence of the muscle. In one rare case, the transversus abdominis was absent without any other anatomic anomalies. Macalister reported that although the transversus abdominis typically has five costal origins, it occasionally originates from the six or seven lowest ribs. As mentioned above, Knott described the origin of this muscle 1883. He found that 29/36 cases studied had six costal origins, 4/36 cases had four costal origins, and 3/36 cases had five costal origins. In 40 Japanese fetuses studied by Kikuchi (1986), the transversus abdominis originated from the seven lowest ribs in 36 and from the six lowest ribs in 4. In another variation, described by both Macalister (1875) and Knott (1883), the spermatic cord traveled through the inferior part of the transversus abdominis and the muscle fibers normally associated with the inguinal ligament were absent.

Chandler and Schadewald (1944) observed the inguinohypogastric region of 220 body halves in detail and found that the transversus abdominis muscle rarely arose from the entire inguinal ligament and that its fibers ran parallel or oblique to the trajectory of the ligament. Moreover, they described the inferior edge of the muscle as forming an arch that comprises a section of the roof of the inguinal canal.

Gruber (1873a,b) described a case of a tensor laminae posterioris vaginae musculi rectus that was composed of muscle slips originating at the inferior portion of the transversalis fascia and ascending superiorly to fan out and interdigitate at right angles with the transversus abdominis. This muscle is also known as the puboperitonealis.

In a fairly recent report, Urquhart et al. (2005) described five anatomic variations of the transversus abdominis muscle, each in separate specimens. These included complete or partial detachment of the muscle from the iliac crest with an abrupt change in fascicle orientation, fusion of the lower fascicles with the internal abdominal oblique muscle, absence of fascicles below the iliac crest, and passage of the iliohypogastric and ilioinguinal nerves through the septa.

Other anterolateral wall muscle variations

Another muscle variation worth mentioning is the rectus abdominus lateralis, first described by Kelch as credited by Macalister (1875). When this muscle is present, it originates from the middle and inferior segments of the 10th rib and then travels between the internal and external abdominal oblique muscles to where it inserts at the iliac crest. The literature on this muscle is sparse. The only study examining the prevalence of this inconstantly present muscle is that by Sato (1968), who reported that the rectus abdominis lateralis was present in approximately 9% (50/536) of Japanese cadavers. The distribution was similar between genders, with 9.88% (32/324) of males and 8.49% (18/212) of females having a rectus abdominis lateralis muscle. Prevalence on the left versus right sides was not reported (Sato, 1968).

PATHOLOGY

Prune belly syndrome (PBS), also known as Eagle-Barrett syndrome, is a congenital syndrome in which the abdominal wall musculature fails to develop or develops poorly. Hypotonia and ectasia of the urinary system and intraabdominal testes and other comorbidities involving the cardiopulmonary and gastrointestinal systems also may present with this syndrome (Hassett et al. 2012). More often, the abdomen's deeper and more medial muscles are absent and cause hypoplasia in the rectus abdominis and external oblique muscles. The predominant theory in this syndrome's pathogenesis is that the urinary tract is obstructed during embryogenesis, which causes distension of the bladder that prevents normal development of the abdominal muscles and descent of the testicles in males. PBS is seen more commonly in males than females, who represent less than 5% of PBS cases reported in more than 30,000 live births annually (Seidel et al., 2015). Perinatal morbidity rates for PBS have been reported to be between 10% and 25%, with pulmonary hypoplasia and prematurity the primary causes of death (Seidel et al., 2015). As the muscles of the abdomen function to maintain abdominal tone and provide positive intraabdominal pressure to serve bodily functions such as defecation and micturition, these muscles' absence can alter the functions of their respective body systems, increasing the risk for infection and development of other pathologies (Demisse et al., 2017). Common surgical interventions required for children with PBS include laparoscopic orchiopexy, ureteral reimplantation, appendicovesicostomy, kidney transplants, and abdominoplasties with abdominal wall reconstruction (Seidel et al., 2015). Lesavoy et al. (2012) retrospective review examined cases of 20 patients with PBS who received abdominal wall reconstructive surgery with concurrent urinary tract reconstructions and orchiopexies and were followed for an average of 20.4 years after the surgeries to determine the abdominal wall reconstructions' effectiveness. The technique used in all 20 surgeries was a double-breasted fascia repair to maintain all existing fascial components that were used in the reconstruction to provide two layers of fascia for maximum support in the abdomen. No complications from the reconstruction were reported during the follow-ups, and all patients reported a positive and improved quality of life.

Paresis of the abdominal wall muscles has been noted as a complication that can arise after potential iatrogenic nerve lesions caused during abdominal and pelvic surgeries, as well as a result of nerve root compression from a herniated disc, diabetic neuropathy, and infectious diseases, such as *Herpes zoster* and Lyme disease. Surgically, instances of injury to the subcostal, iliohypogastric, and/or ilioinguinal nerves and their smaller terminal branches have been reported in such cases of lateral transpsoas interbody fusion attributable in part to retroperitoneal dissection and trocar placement, and incisions that sever nerves within the abdominal muscles (Dakwar et al., 2011; van Ramshorst et al., 2009; Korenkov et al., 1999). In instances of *Herpes zoster* infection in the lower thoracic levels where it occurs most commonly, the infection can weaken the nerves that supply the abdominal wall muscles, leading to potential paresis and abdominal protrusions and pseudoherniations (Santiago-Pérez et al., 2012). Conservative approaches to managing and treating paresis in this area have been implemented with good outcomes and very few, if any, sequelae. Complete resolution of paresis in these studies has been shown to require between 6 and 12 months.

CONCLUSIONS

Spine surgeons performing lateral transpsoas approaches to the lumbar spine need a good working knowledge of the anterolateral abdominal wall muscles and their potential variations. This understanding will help minimize complications during surgery.

REFERENCES

Chandler, S.B., Schadewald, M., 1944. Studies on the inguinal region. I. The conjoined aponeurosis versus the conjoined tendon. Anat. Rec. 89, 339–343.

Dakwar, E., Le, T., Baaj, A., Le, A., Smith, W., Akbarnia, B., Uribe, J., 2011. Abdominal wall paresis as a complication of minimally invasive lateral transpsoas interbody fusion. Neurosurg. Focus 31, E18.

Demisse, A., Bernhau, A., Tadesse, T., 2017. Unusual presentation of prune belly syndrome: a case report. J. Med. Case Rep. 11, 337.

Floch, M., 2005. Netter's Gastroenterology. Icon Learning Systems, Carlstadt.

Gruber, W., 1873a. Un cas de muscle oblique interne de l'abdomen, prive completement de sa portion inguinal. Bull. l'Acad. Imp. Sci. St. Petersbourg. 18, 157–158.

Gruber, W., 1873b. Sur quelques muscles surnumeraires de l'abdomen chez l'homme. Bull. l'Acad. Imp. Sci. St. Petersbourg. 18, 142–147.

Gruber, W., 1875. Zwei neue Fälle eines rudimentären Musculus obliquus externus abdominis II. Arch. für Pathol. Anat. Physiol. für Klin. Med. 65, 16–21.

Hassett, S., Smith, G., Holland, A., 2012. Prune belly syndrome. Pediatr. Surg. Int. 28, 219–228.

Henle, J., 1871. Handbuch der Muskellehre des Menschen. In: Handbuch der systematischen Anatomy des Menschen. Verlag von Friedrich Vieweg und Sohn, Braunschweig.

Kelch, W.G., 1813. Beiträge zur pathologischen Anatomie. Salfeild, Berlin.

Kikuchi, Y., 1986. Morphological studies on the muscles of the abdomen in Japanese fetuses. J. Nippon Med. Sch. 53, 280–290.

Knott, J.F., 1881. Journal. Anat. Physiol. 14, 15.

Knott, J.F., 1883. Muscular anomalies, including those of the diaphragm, and subbiaphragmatic regions of the human body. In: Proceeding Science. Royal Irish Acad, vol. 2, 727-641.

Kodama, K., 1986. Morphological significance of the supracostal muscles, and the superficial intercostal nerve – a new definition. Kaibogaku Zasshi 61, 107–129.

Korenkov, M., Rixen, D., Paul, A., Köhler, L., Eypasch, E., Troidl, H., 1999. Combined abdominal wall paresis and incisional hernia after laparoscopic cholecystectomy. Surg. Endosc. 13, 268–269.

Kudo, K., Otobe, I., 1952. Statistics on the anatomy of Northern Chinese. The lateral abdominal muscles and others. Hirosaki Igaku 3, 103–108.

Lesavoy, M., Chang, E., Suliman, A., Taylor, J., Kim, S., Ehrlich, M., 2012. Long-term follow-up of total abdominal wall reconstruction for prune belly syndrome. Plast. Reconstr. Surg. 129, 104e–109e.

Loth, E., 1912a. Beiträge zur Anthropologie der Negerweichteile. Strecker & Schröder.

Loth, E., 1912b. Beiträge zur Anthropologie der Negerweichteile (Muskelsystem), vols. 84–87. Strecker & Schröder, Stuttgart.

Loth, E., 1931. Anthropologie des parties molles, vol. 138. Masson & Cie, Paris.

Luschka, H., 1879. Der musc. Pubo-transversalis des Menschen. Arch Anat Physiol Wissen Med 12, 227–231.

Macalister, A., 1875. Additional observations on muscular anomalies in human anatomy. (Third series) with a catalogue of the principal muscular variations Hitherto published. Trans Royal Irish Acad 25, 1–134.

Mekonen, H., Hikspoors, J., Mommen, G., Köhler, S., Lamers, W., 2015. Development of the ventral body wall in the human embryo. J. Anat. 227, 673–685.

Miyauchi, R., Kurihara, K., Tachibana, G., 1986. On the human obliquus abdominis externus profundus. Acta Med. Nagasaki. 31, 59–75.

Mori, M., 1964. Statistics on the musculature of the Japanese. Okajimas Folia Anat. Jpn. 40, 195–300.

Murata, K., Abe, K., Honma, T., 1971. M. serratus anterior of Japanese. 2. The area of its origin and its interdigitation with the M. obliquus externus abdominis. Anat. Sci. Int. 46, 193–196.

Nakayama, T., Okuda, S., 1952. On the M. obliquus abdominis externus profundus. Kaibogaku Zasshi 27, 89–94.

Santiago-Pérez, S., Nevado-Estévez, R., Pérez-Conde, M., 2012. Herpes zoster-induced abdominal wall paresis: neurophysiological examination in this unusual complication. J. Neurol. Sci. 321, 177–179.

Sato, S., 1968. Statistical studies on the anomalous muscles of the Kyushu Japanese. 3. The muscles of the back, breast and abdomen. Kurume Med. J. 15 (4), 209.

Seidel, N., Arlen, A., Smith, E., Kirsch, A., 2015. Clinical manifestations and management of prune-belly syndrome in a large contemporary pediatric population. Urology 85, 211–215.

Shafik, A., Sibai, O., Shafik, I., Shafik, A., 2007. Electromyographic activity of the anterolateral abdominal wall muscles during rectal filling and evacuation. J. Surg. Res. 143, 364–367.
Shimazaki, H., 1959. A case of M. obliquus abdominis externus profundus. Shinshu Igakukai Zasshi 8 (7), 1436–1438.
Standring, S., 2016. Gray's Anatomy. Elsevier, Philadelphia.
Sugiura, R., 1935. On a superfluous pair of muscles accompanying the M. obliquus externus abdominis sinister. Nagoya J. Med. Sci. 8, 139–143.
Tyrie, C.C.B., 1894. Musculus saphenous. J. Anat. Physiol. 28, 288–290.
Urquhart, D.M., Barker, P.J., Hodges, P.W., Story, I.H., Briggs, C.A., 2005. Regional morphology of the transversus abdominis and obliquus internus and externus abdominis muscles. Clin. Biomech. 20, 233–241.
van Ramshorst, G., Kleinrensink, G., Hermans, J., Terkivatan, T., Lange, J., 2009. Abdominal wall paresis as a complication of laparoscopic surgery. Hernia 13, 539–543.
Yonekura, S., 1954. A study of the muscles of the neck, chest, abdomen and back in Japanese fetuses. Igaku Kenkyu 24, 1604–1700.

FURTHER READING

Henle, J., 1873. Sinnesapparte. In: Handbuch der systematischen Anatomie des Menschen. Verlag von Friedrich Vieweg und Sohn, Braunschweig.

CHAPTER 3

The Posterior Abdominal Wall and Retroperitoneum

LAUREN WAHL • MARY KATHERINE CLEVELAND • HALLE E.K. BURLEY • R. SHANE TUBBS

INTRODUCTION

As its name suggests, the posterior abdominal wall forms the posterior boundary of the abdominal cavity. As with the anterior and lateral abdominal walls, it is composed of several layers, including the skin, superficial fascia, muscle, extraperitoneal fat/fascia, and parietal peritoneum. The midline structures of the posterior abdominal wall, the vertebral column and paravertebral muscles, are usually discussed with structures of the back. However, the relationships between the vertebral column and the retroperitoneum/posterior abdominal wall are critical when discussing the lateral transpsoas approach to the spine (Fig. 3.1). The posterior abdominal wall is continuous with the posterior thoracic wall across the posterior attachment of the respiratory diaphragm superiorly, with the posterior wall of the pelvis inferiorly, and with the anterolateral abdominal wall laterally.

The retroperitoneum and its space are termed with the prefix retro-, meaning "backward," which can be interpreted anatomically as "posterior" (Mirilas and Skandalakis, 2010). The retroperitoneal space is demarcated by the parietal peritoneum anteriorly and the transversalis fascia of the abdominal muscles posteriorly (Figs. 3.2–3.6). Note that there is some disagreement in the literature about whether the psoas major and quadratus lumborum muscles should be considered contents or boundaries of this space (Standring, 2016). The retroperitoneal space is bordered laterally by the transversus abdominus muscle. The respiratory diaphragm forms the superior wall of the space, and the pelvic extraperitoneal structures form its inferior wall (Anderson et al., 2007). It is continuous with the extraperitoneal connective tissues of the pelvis inferiorly and the anterolateral abdominal wall laterally. Advances in cross-sectional imaging techniques have improved our understanding of the anatomy of the retroperitoneum, but terminology regarding its components has yet to be standardized. Terms such as spaces, compartments, subcompartments, recesses, and domains have all been used to describe the retroperitoneum or regions within it.

The retroperitoneum houses certain organs of the gastrointestinal tract in whole or in part, specifically the duodenum and the ascending and descending colon, as well as their associated vessels and nerves. Organs of the retroperitoneum also include the pancreas, kidneys, ureters, and suprarenal glands with their vessels and nerves. The abdominal aorta and its branches; the inferior vena cava and its tributaries; the origins of the azygos and hemiazygos veins; the pre- and lateral aortic nodes, the cisterna chyli and the origin of the thoracic duct; the diaphragmatic crura; the lumbar plexus and lumbosacral trunk; and the autonomic plexuses of the abdomen are all contained within the retroperitoneum. The mesenteries of the small intestine, transverse, and sigmoid colon and the ligaments of the liver and spleen all arise from reflections of the posterior parietal peritoneum.

Primary retroperitoneal organs include the kidneys, suprarenal glands, and ureters (Fig. 3.7) with their respective vessels and nerves, and the abdominal aorta and inferior vena cava with their respective branches. Secondary retroperitoneal organs—organs that began their development within the peritoneum and later migrated into the retroperitoneal space—include the ascending colon, descending colon (Fig. 3.7), pancreas, and the portion of the duodenum following the duodenal bulb (Selçuk et al., 2018).

EMBRYOLOGY

In the sixth and seventh weeks of embryogenesis, the fascia and organs of the retroperitoneal space develop from three layers of embryonic connective tissue. The

Surgical anatomy of the lateral transpsoas approach to the lumbar spine. https://doi.org/10.1016/B978-0-323-67376-1.00003-3

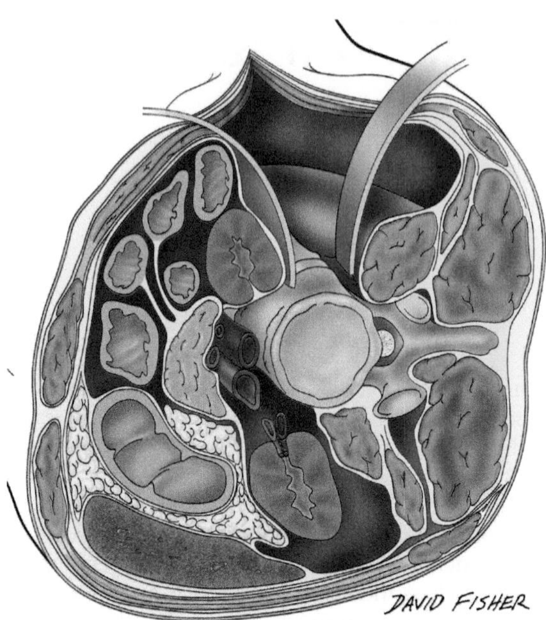

FIG. 3.1 Schematic drawing of a lateral approach to the lumbar spine, which occurs in the retroperitoneum.

outer layer of embryonic tissue becomes the parietal fascia covering the extensor muscles of the vertebral column, internal and external oblique muscles, and transversus abdominus. These are lined by the transversalis fascia and demarcate the posterior boundary of the retroperitoneal space (Mirilas and Skandalakis, 2009). The intermediate layer becomes the extraperitoneal structures (kidneys, suprarenal glands, ureters, and corresponding vessels and nerves) and contributes to the bladder and lower rectum. The perirenal and pararenal spaces, alongside the renal fascia, also develop from this layer. The inner layer becomes the visceral fascia, surrounding the intraperitoneal organs and their vessels and nerves as well as forming the mesentery for these organs. The duodenum, pancreas, ascending colon, and descending colon all begin development intraperitoneally, but ultimately they attach to the posterior abdominal wall, becoming secondary retroperitoneal (Mirilas and Skandalakis, 2009).

SOFT TISSUES

The skin superficial to the posterior abdominal wall is supplied by musculocutaneous branches of the lumbar arteries and veins. It is generally agreed to be innervated by the dorsal rami of the lower thoracic and lumbar spinal nerves, but the exact cutaneous distribution of the dorsal rami of the fourth and fifth lumbar spinal nerves is variable and controversial (Lee et al., 2008). Deep to the skin, the thoracolumbar fascia consists of a multilayered arrangement of fascial planes and aponeurotic sheets that divides the paraspinal muscles from the muscles of the posterior abdominal wall (quadratus lumborum and psoas major).

FASCIAE

Fascial layers have proven to be an unreliable framework for conceptualizing the organization of the retroperitoneum (Dodds et al., 1986). The fasciae of this region are variable and difficult to visualize on cross-sectional imaging, and clinical observations of the spread of pathological fluids and air often do not match anatomically defined fascial boundaries. Naming of fascial layers in the literature is also largely unstandardized. Various authors have used the same eponym for different fasciae as well as different eponyms for the same fascia. For example, "Gerota's fascia" may refer to the entire renal fascia or to its anterior or posterior layers individually (Chesbrough et al., 1989). "Zuckerkandl's fascia" has been used to denote either the posterior or anterior layers of renal fascia (Chesbrough et al., 1989). "Toldt's fascia" has been used to indicate multiple different structures, including the fusion fascia posterior to the ascending or descending colon (Culligan et al., 2013), or the posterior layer of renal fascia, or the fusion fascia posterior to the tail of the pancreas (Kimura et al., 2010). Separate from the fusion fascia at the tail of the pancreas, "Treitz's fascia" has been used to describe the fusion fascia posterior the head of the pancreas (Kimura et al., 2010). As an aside, the term "fusion fascia" describes a retroperitoneal fascial layer created by the fusion of an embryonic mesentery with the anterior wall of the embryonic retroperitoneum (Hikspoors et al., 2018).

Renal Fascia

Traditionally, the retroperitoneum is divided into the anterior and posterior pararenal spaces and the perirenal space (Standring, 2016). The anterior pararenal space lies between the parietal peritoneum lining the posterior abdominal wall and the anterior layer of renal fascia. However, this oversimplification fails to explain all patterns of disease containment or spread (Dodds et al., 1986).

Psoas Fascia

A relatively dense layer of fascia encloses the anterior surface of psoas major and the lumbar plexus within

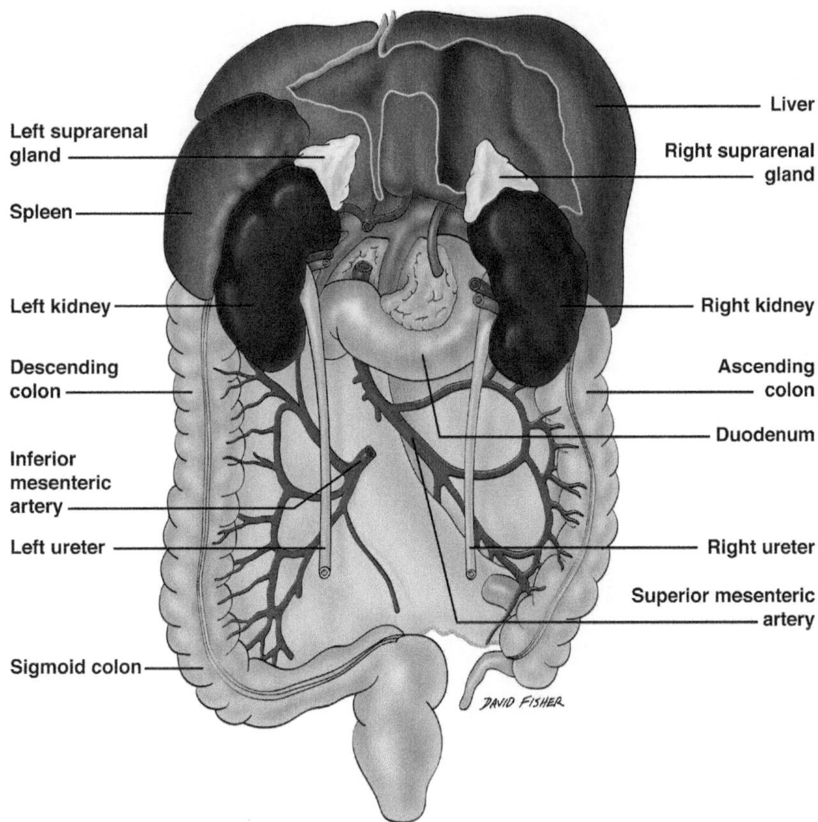

FIG. 3.2 Posterior view from within the retroperitoneum. Many of these structures, e.g., kidneys and ureters are at risk of damage during lateral transpsoas approaches to the lumbar spine.

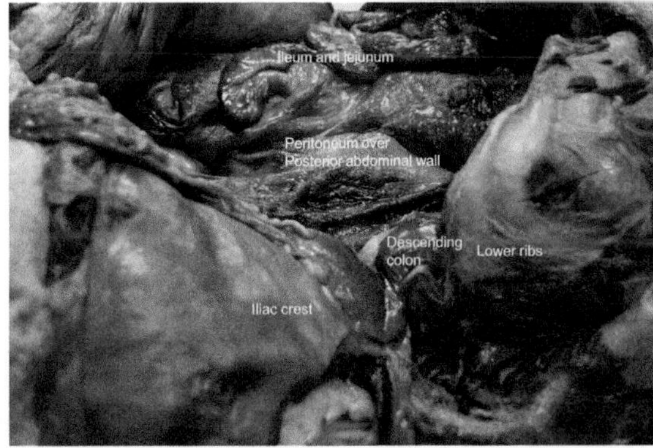

FIG. 3.3 Left lateral view between the lower ribs and iliac crest with the peritoneum over the posterior abdominal wall still intact.

it. At its medial edge, this fascia is continuous with the attachments of the muscle to the transverse processes and bodies of the lumbar vertebrae. Laterally, it blends with the fascia covering the quadratus lumborum superiorly and the iliac fascia inferiorly (Standring, 2016). Superiorly, it merges with the medial arcuate ligament of the respiratory diaphragm. Inferiorly, it continues into the thigh as a sheath around the iliopsoas tendon. The psoas fascia divides the psoas major muscle and lumbar plexus from the retroperitoneal organs.

Iliac Fascia

The iliac fascia covers the anterior surface of the iliacus. It attaches superiorly and laterally to the inner margin of the iliac crest and then blends medially both with the anterior layer of the thoracolumbar fascia over quadratus lumborum and with the psoas fascia. Inferiorly and laterally, it extends into the thigh to fuse with the femoral sheath. At its medial border, it attaches to the periosteum of the ilium and iliopubic eminence near the linea terminalis (Standring, 2016). Both the femoral nerve and the lateral femoral cutaneous nerve pass beneath the iliac fascia in the pelvis, where they

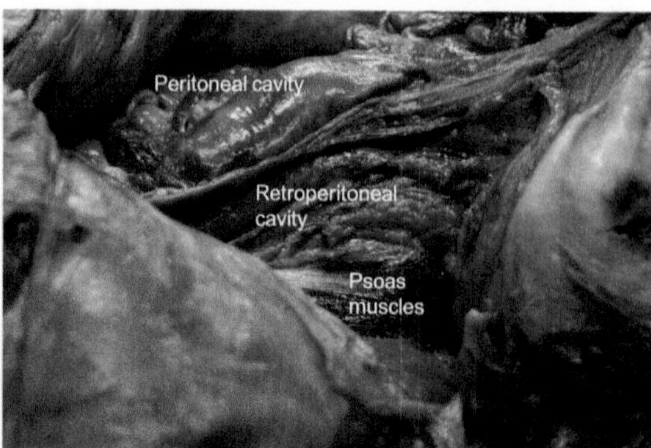

FIG. 3.4 Fig. 3.3 after opening of the peritoneum over the posterior abdominal wall.

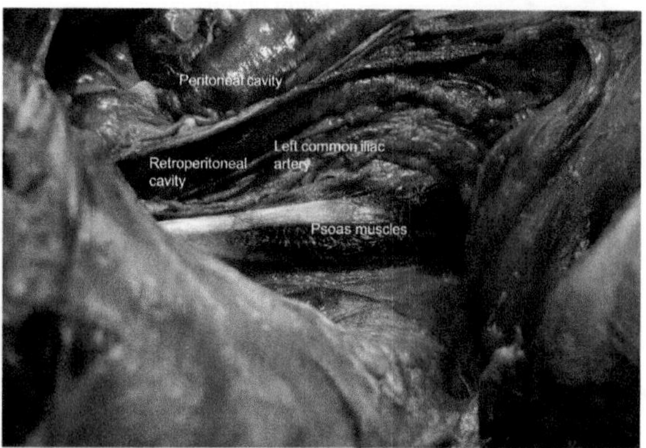

FIG. 3.5 Continued dissection of Fig. 3.4 illustrating the psoas muscles at the posterior abdominal wall.

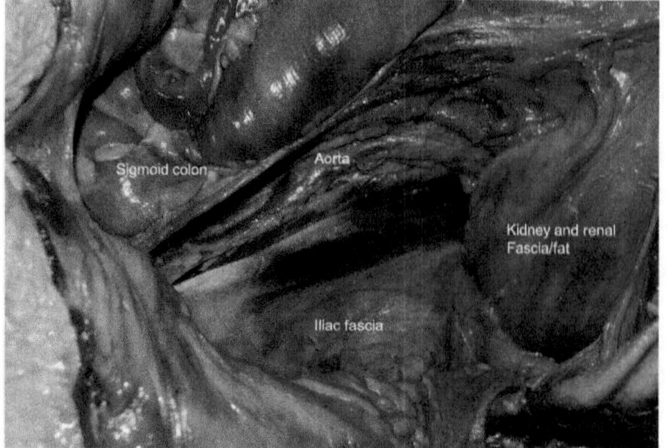

FIG. 3.6 Anterior view of Fig. 3.5 noting the kidney and its fat and fasciae retracted superiorly.

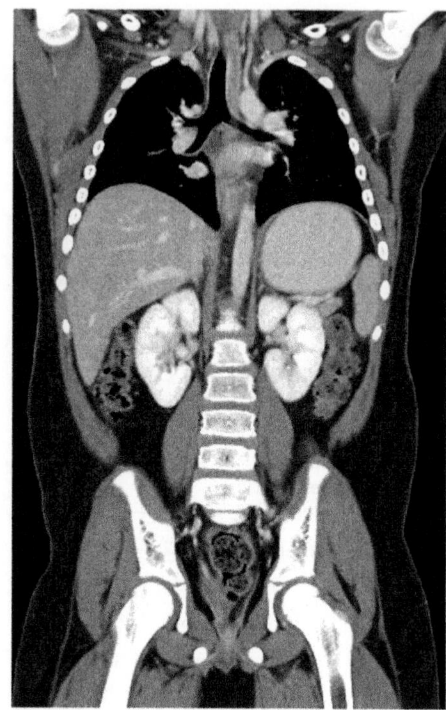

FIG. 3.7 CT of the thorax and abdomen noting several structures of the retroperitoneum such as the psoas major muscles and kidneys.

are accessible for image-guided anesthetic nerve block (Hebbard et al., 2011).

Lateroconal Fascia

Originally, the lateroconal fascia was defined as the fascial layer extending from the parietal peritoneum in the paracolic gutter to the junction of the anterior and posterior sheets of renal fascia (Congdon and Edson, 1941). In common usage, it refers to the lateral projection of the retrocolic fusion fascia that merges with the parietal peritoneum (Standring, 2016).

SPACES

Peripancreatic Space

The peripancreatic space contains the pancreas and duodenum; the retroperitoneal segments of the hepatic artery, hepatic portal vein, and bile duct; and the origins of the superior mesenteric vessels (Standring, 2016). The space is bounded posteriorly by the fusion fascia of the embryonic duodenal mesentery and the anterior wall of the embryonic retroperitoneum (Dodds et al., 1986). In imaging literature, this fusion fascia is dubbed the "retropancreatic" or "retropancreaticoduodenal" fascia, and in surgical literature the "fusion fascia of Treitz" (Kimura et al., 2010).

The lateral extent of the peripancreatic space varies; it stretches as far laterally as the ascending and descending colon and the perirenal space, which bound it anteriorly and posteriorly, respectively (Standring, 2016). At the tail of the pancreas, the peripancreatic space runs along the splenorenal ligament. Anteriorly, it extends to the transverse mesocolon and mesentery of the small intestine. As a result, peripancreatic fluid collections can extend into both mesenteries and posterior to the ascending and descending colon, but they usually do not cross into the perirenal and pericolic spaces (Standring, 2016).

Pericolic Spaces

The ascending and descending pericolic spaces extend from the mesocolons of the ascending and descending colon out laterally to the body wall (Standring, 2016). These narrow, longitudinal spaces contain a variable amount of fat. They are enclosed anteriorly, laterally, and superiorly by the serosa of the colon. Inferiorly, they continue as the retroperitoneum of the iliac fossae. A fusion fascia formed by the joining of the right leaf of the embryonic mesocolon to the left leaf of the embryonic duodenal mesentery and anterior wall of the embryonic retroperitoneum bounds the pericolic spaces posteriorly (Dodds et al., 1986). When conducting a hemicolectomy, this retrocolic fascia (of Toldt) (Culligan et al 2013, 2014) provides an avascular plane of dissection. Lateral to the duodenum and pancreas, the retrocolic fascia and the anterior layer of renal fascia may be indistinguishable on radiological studies (Standring, 2016).

Perirenal Space

The perirenal spaces are a pair of inverted cone-shaped pockets formed by the anterior and posterior renal fascia (Bechtold et al., 1996). They are situated anterior to the posterior pararenal space and lateral to the lumbar spine. This space contains the kidneys, suprarenal glands, renal vasculature, proximal ureters, and perirenal fat (Standring, 2016). The left and right perirenal spaces connect across the midline anterior to the abdominal aorta and inferior vena cava.

Anterior Pararenal Space

The ascending colon and its mesentery, descending colon and its mesentery, duodenum distal to the duodenal bulb, and pancreas occupy the anterior pararenal space (Standring, 2016). The posterior parietal peritoneum forms its anterior boundary, and the anterior renal fascia forms its posterior boundary. Although the anterior pararenal space extends across the midline, diseases tend to remain confined to their laterality of origin (Bechtold et al., 1996). Inflammatory fluid from pancreatitis may descend from the anterior pararenal space into the extraperitoneal pelvic spaces or ascend into the mediastinum, damaging nearby organs as it travels.

Posterior Pararenal Space

The posterior pararenal space lays posterior to the perirenal space, enclosed by the transversalis fascia posteriorly and both the posterior renal fascia and lateroconal fascia anteriorly (Standring, 2016). This region is bounded laterally by the psoas muscle (Bechtold et al., 1996). This space does not house any organs, just variable amounts of fat that extends laterally to merge with the fat of the anterolateral abdominal wall and inferiorly to merge with fat on the iliacus and pelvic wall (Standring, 2016).

CONCLUSIONS

The anatomy of the retroperitoneum must be well understood by the spine surgeon, performing lateral transpsoas approaches to the lumbar spine.

REFERENCES

Anderson, J., Kabalin, J., Cadeddu, J., 2007. Surgical anatomy of the retroperitoneum, adrenals, kidneys, and ureters. In: Wein, A.J. (Ed.), Campbell-Walsh Urology, ninth ed. Elsevier Saunders, Philadelphia, pp. 3–19.

Bechtold, R., Dyer, R., Zagoria, R., Chen, M., 1996. The perirenal space: relationship of pathologic processes to normal retroperitoneal anatomy. Radiographics 16, 841–854.

Chesbrough, R.M., Burkhard, T.K., Martinez, A.J., et al., 1989. Gerota versus Zuckerkandl: the renal fascia revisited. Radiology 173, 845–846.

Congdon, E.D., Edson, J.N., 1941. The cone of renal fascia in the adult white male. Anat. Rec. 80, 289–313.

Culligan, K., Remzi, F.H., Soop, M., et al., 2013. Review of nomenclature in colonic surgery – proposal of a standardised nomenclature based on mesocolic anatomy. Surgeon 11, 1–5.

Culligan, K., Walsh, S., Dunne, C., et al., 2014. The mesocolon: a histological and electron microscopic characterization of the mesenteric attachment of the colon prior to and after surgical mobilization. Ann. Surg. 260, 1048–1056.

Dodds, W.J., Darweesh, R.M., Lawson, T.L., et al., 1986. The retroperitoneal spaces revisited. Am. J. Roentgenol. 147, 1155–1161.

Hebbard, P., Ivanusic, J., Sha, S., 2011. Ultrasound-guided supra-inguinal fascia iliaca block: a cadaveric evaluation of a novel approach. Anaesthesia 66, 300–305.

Kimura, W., Yano, M., Sugawara, S., et al., 2010. Spleen-preserving distal pancreatectomy with conservation of the splenic artery and vein: techniques and its significance. J Hepatobiliary Pancreat Sci 17, 813–823.

Mirilas, P., Skandalakis, J., 2009. Surgical anatomy of the retroperitoneal spaces I: embryogenesis and anatomy. Am. Surg. 75, 1091–1097.

Mirilas, P., Skandalakis, J., 2010. Surgical anatomy of the retroperitoneal spaces II: the architecture of the retroperitoneal space. Am. Surg. 76, 33–42.

Selçuk, İ., Ersak, B., Tatar, İ., Güngör, T., Huri, E., 2018. Basic clinical retroperitoneal anatomy for pelvic surgeons. Turk J Obstet Gynecol 15, 259–269.

Standring, S., 2016. Gray's Anatomy. Elsevier, Amsterdam.

FURTHER READING

Coffin, A., Boulay-Coletta, I., Sebbag-Sfez, D., Zins, M., 2015. Radioanatomy of the retroperitoneal space. Diagn Interv Imaging 96, 171–186.

Gore, R., Balfe, D., Aizenstein, R., Silverman, P., 2000. The great escape: interfascial decompression planes of the retroperitoneum. Am. J. Roentgenol. 175, 363–370.

Mindell, H., Mastromatteo, J., Dickey, K., Sturtevant, N., Shuman, W., Oliver, C., Leister, K., Barth, R., 1995. Anatomic communications between the three retroperitoneal spaces: determination by CT-guided injections of contrast material in cadavers. Am. J. Roentgenol. 164, 1173–1178.

Sugimoto, M., Takada, T., Yasuda, H., Nagashima, I., Amano, H., Yoshida, M., Miura, F., Uchida, T., Isaka, T., Toyota, N., Wada, K., Takagi, K., Kato, K., Takeshita, K., 2005. MPR-hCT imaging of the pancreatic fluid pathway to Grey-Turner's and Cullen's sign in acute pancreatitis. Hepatogastroenterology 52, 1613–1616.

CHAPTER 4

Posterior Abdominal Wall Muscles

MARY KATHERINE CLEVELAND • R. SHANE TUBBS

The posterior abdominal muscles are quadratus lumborum, psoas major, psoas minor, and iliacus (Fig. 4.1). Psoas major and iliacus join to form the iliopsoas tendon, which inserts into the lesser trochanter of the femur. Separation or fusion of these muscles, and the presence of variant muscular slips, have been reported. Psoas minor is an inconsistent muscle and is often absent.

QUADRATUS LUMBORUM

The quadratus lumborum (Figs. 4.1–4.5) is an irregularly shaped rectangular muscle. The inferior attachment is from the iliac crest lateral to the distal end of the transverse process of the fourth lumbar vertebra and/or the iliolumbar ligament. Fascicles pass from the iliac crest to be attached superiorly to either the anteroinferior surface of the 12th rib, or the distal ends of the transverse processes of the upper four lumbar vertebrae, or the lateral surface of the 12th thoracic vertebra. Some fascicles may pass from the lumbar transverse processes to the 12th rib. Fascicles vary in number and size but typically are arranged into anterior, middle, and posterior layers (Phillips et al., 2008). Anterior to the quadratus lumborum is the ascending colon on the right and descending colon on the left, kidney, psoas major and minor (when present), and diaphragm. The subcostal, iliohypogastric and ilioinguinal nerves lie on the fascia anterior to the muscle (Fig. 4.6).

The quadratus lumborum is primarily supplied by branches of the lumbar arteries, the iliolumbar artery, and branches of the subcostal artery. The subcostal nerve and upper three or four lumbar spinal nerves innervate this muscle.

Functionally, the iliocostal fascicles of quadratus lumborum fix the 12th rib, helping to stabilize the lower attachments of the respiratory diaphragm during inspiration. The actions of the iliolumbar fascicles are less clear: their contribution to lateral flexion or extension is reported to be weak (Phillips et al., 2008; Park et al., 2012).

Variations

This muscle usually arises from the iliolumbar ligament and iliac crest and inserts into the inferior border of the 12th rib and the transverse processes of the first through fourth lumbar vertebrae via small tendons of insertion, which can vary in number and thickness. The insertions of quadratus lumborum have been found to consist of the bodies of both the 10th and 11th thoracic vertebrae, the body of the 11th thoracic vertebra only, or the 11th rib. Two components of the muscle have been described, fibers extending from the ribs and separate fibers from the transverse processes.

ILIACUS

The iliacus (Figs. 4.1 and 4.2) is a triangular sheet of muscle that arises from the superior two-thirds of the concavity of the iliac fossa, the inner lip of the iliac crest, the ventral sacroiliac and iliolumbar ligaments, and the upper surface of the lateral part of the sacrum. In front, it reaches as far as the anterior superior and anterior inferior iliac spines. It receives a few fibers from the upper part of the capsule of the hip joint, but most of its fibers are converged into the lateral side of the strong tendon of psoas major. The muscles, the iliacus and psoas major, then insert most of their fibers together into the lesser trochanter, but some fibers are attached directly to the femur.

Within the abdomen, the anterior surface of iliacus is related to its fascia, the lateral femoral cutaneous nerve, the caecum, and the descending colon. In the thigh, its anterior surface comes in contact with the fascia lata, rectus femoris, sartorius, and profunda femoris artery, while its posterior surface is in contact with the hip joint, where it is separated by the iliopectineal bursa.

The iliacus is supplied by the same arterial network as psoas major, which creates a mutual overlap of the arterial territories of each muscle. The main supply comes from the iliac branches of the iliolumbar artery, with contributions from the deep circumflex iliac, obturator, and femoral arteries. The iliacus is innervated by

Surgical anatomy of the lateral transpsoas approach to the lumbar spine. https://doi.org/10.1016/B978-0-323-67376-1.00004-5

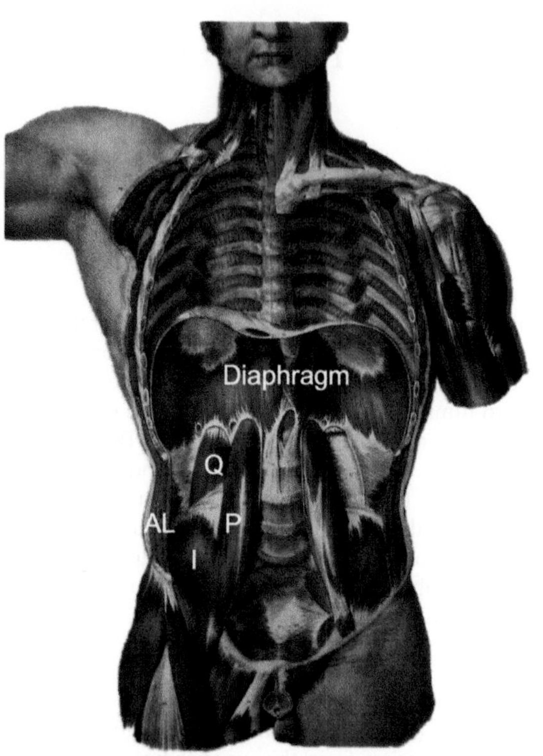

FIG. 4.1 Drawing of the posterior abdominal muscles from Bourgery's 19-th century *Traité complet de l'anatomie de l'homme comprenant la médecine operatoire*.

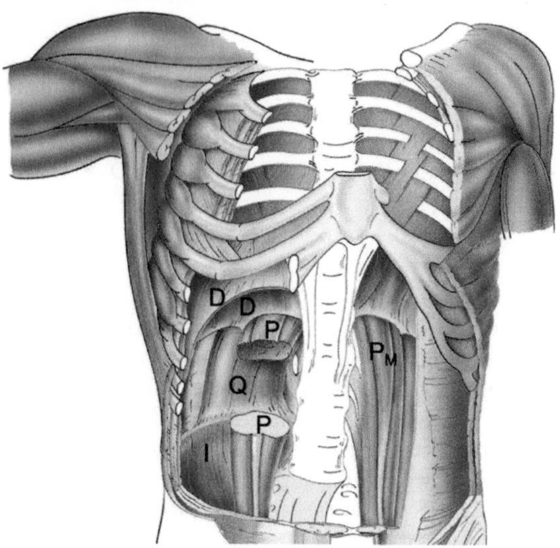

FIG. 4.2 Schematic drawing of the muscles of the posterior abdominal wall. Note that on the right side, a section of the psoas major (P) has been removed to show the deeper lying part of the quadratus lumborum (Q). The iliacus (I), anterior and posterior parts of the diaphragm (D), and left psoas minor (P_M) are also shown.

branches of the femoral nerve. The psoas major acts with the iliacus to flex the thigh.

Variations

The iliacus muscle is one of the muscles that comprise iliopsoas. Anatomical variations of iliacus are rare; however, some variations, such as agenesis, variant muscular slips, and muscular fusion, have been reported. Aleksandrova et al. (2013) reviewed the previous reports and classified the variations into 10 types (A to J) based on criteria that included partial muscular agenesis, the presence of variant muscle slips, the relationship between iliacus and psoas major, and the relationship between variant slips and the femoral nerve.

Type A is partial agenesis of the iliacus. The course of the femoral nerve is basically normal in this classification. To our knowledge, only one case of this type has been reported, and that case was described by Aleksandrova et al. (2013).

Type B is complete separation of iliacus and psoas major, with the femoral nerve following a normal course. This type of variant has been described in older literature. Macalister described the psoas major as perfectly separated from the iliacus.

Type C, in contrast to type B, is complete fusion of the iliacus and psoas major. Fabrizio (2011) reported one case in which the iliacus and psoas major were fused at the level of the superior one-third of the ilium. The femoral nerve ran along the superior margin of the blended muscles at their uppermost connection.

Type D is variant slips of higher origin with the femoral nerve running on the surface of the slip. Aleksandrova et al. (2013) reported one case of this type, in which partial agenesis of the iliacus muscle was combined with variant slips arising from beyond the iliac crest. The psoas quartus muscle, an extremely rare muscle that has only been reported twice in the literature (Clarkson and Rainy, 1889; Tubbs et al., 2006), may belong to this classification. Tubbs et al. (2006) described a case with a psoas quartus muscle (Figs. 4.7 and 4.8) that arose from the transverse process of the L3 vertebra and the anteromedial aspect of the quadratus lumborum and united with the psoas major and iliacus muscles at the level of the inguinal ligament. In Clarkson's case (1889), muscle slips arose from both the anterior surface of the quadratus lumborum and the transverse process of the fifth lumbar vertebra. The psoas tertius was also present in this case (Clarkson and Rainy, 1889) (Fig. 9). This muscle arose from the

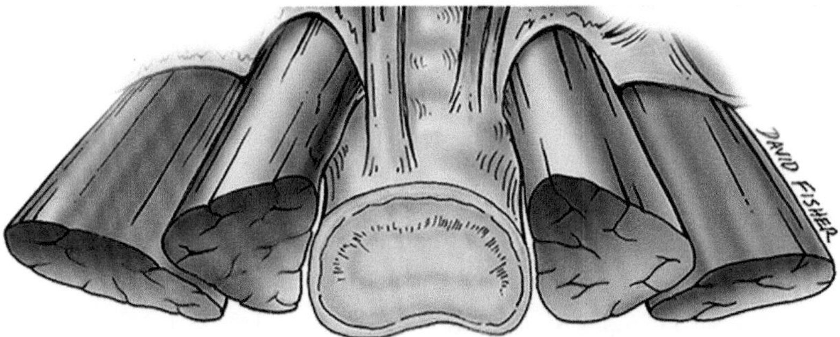

FIG. 4.3 Anterior inferior view of the muscles of the posterior abdominal wall. From medial to lateral, note the diaphragmatic crura, psoas major, and quadratus lumborum.

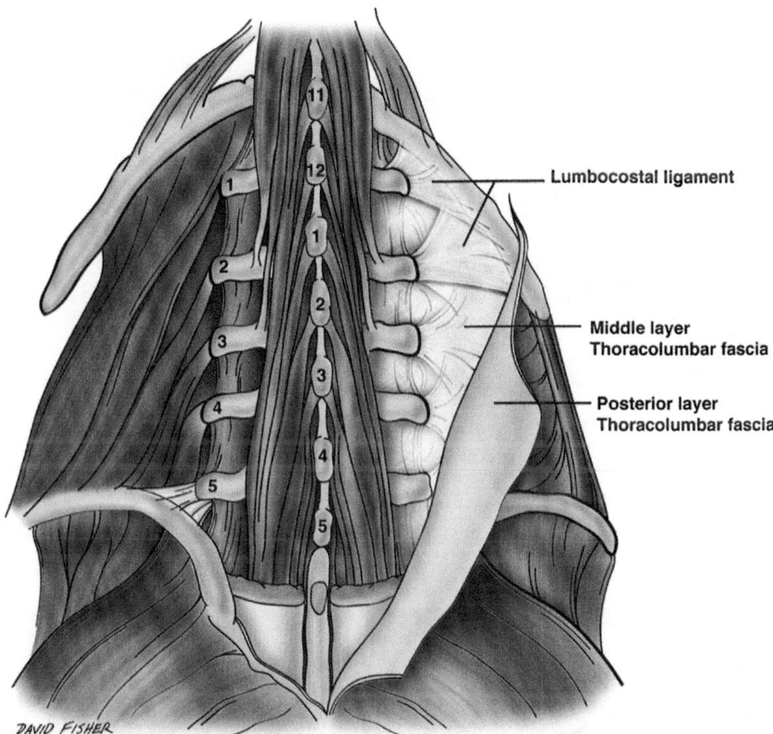

FIG. 4.4 Posterior view of the left quadratus lumborum and its relationship to the deep back muscles and thoracolumbar fascia.

inner surface of the 12th rib and the transverse process of the first through fourth lumbar vertebrae, ran deep to the quadratus lumborum and iliacus muscles, and ended in tendinous fibers that fused with the tendon of the psoas major and psoas quadratus near the level of the inguinal ligament.

Type E is called the iliacus minor muscle or iliocapsularis muscle and not to be confused with iliacus minimus. The femoral nerve runs normally in this classification. According to Macalister (1875), this muscle is a small detached portion of the iliacus, arising from the anterior inferior spine of the ilium and inserting into the anterior intertrochanteric line. Das (1950) described the difference between the iliacus minor, which inserts entirely into the intertrochanteric line, and the iliocapsularis, which inserts entirely into the iliofemoral

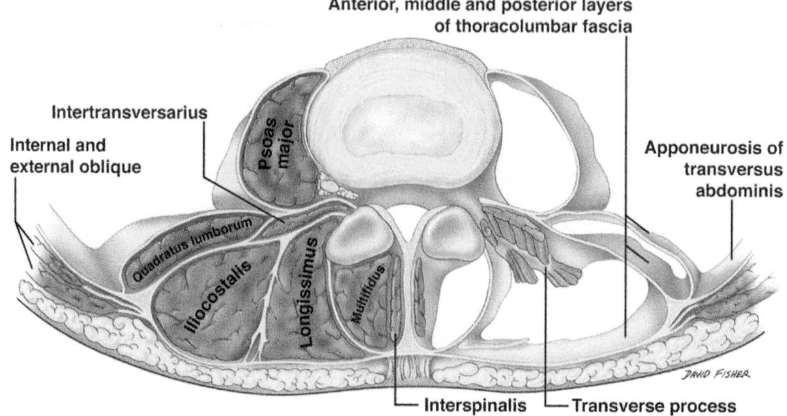

FIG. 4.5 The fasciae and muscles of the posterior abdominal wall as related to the lumbar spine.

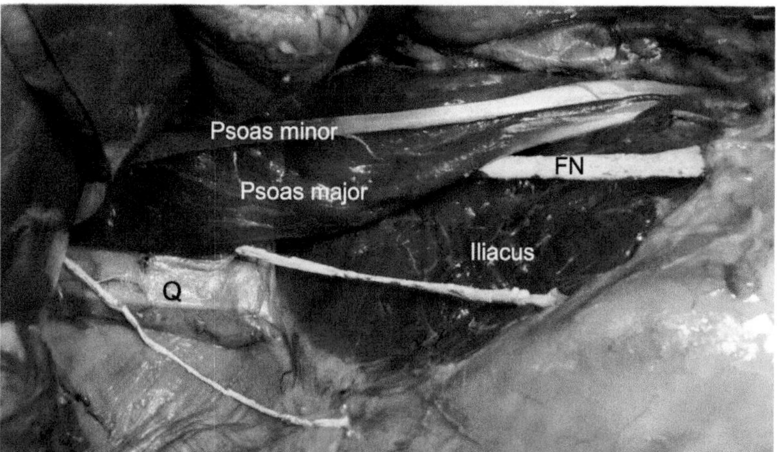

FIG. 4.6 Right cadaveric dissection noting the psoas muscles, iliacus, quadratus lumborum (Q), and femoral nerve (FN). The two nerves to the left are the lateral femoral cutaneous nerve and ilioinguinal nerve.

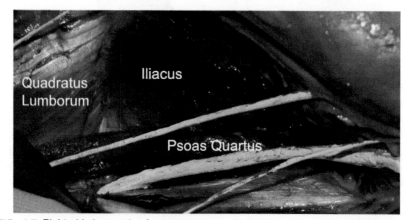

FIG. 4.7 Right-sided example of psoas quartus and related branches of the lumbar plexus.

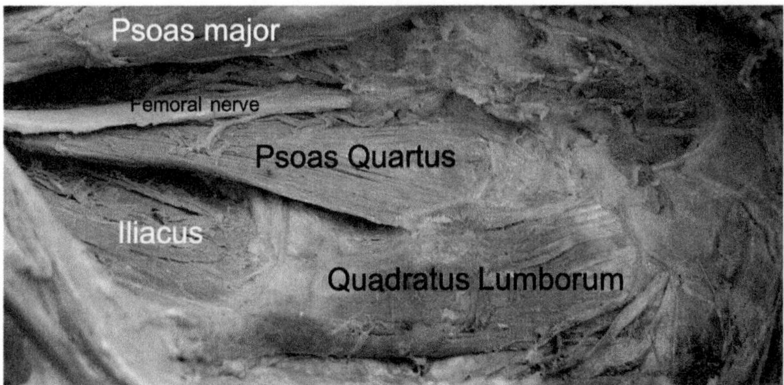

FIG. 4.8 Left-sided example of psoas quartus and its relationship to psoas major and the femoral nerve.

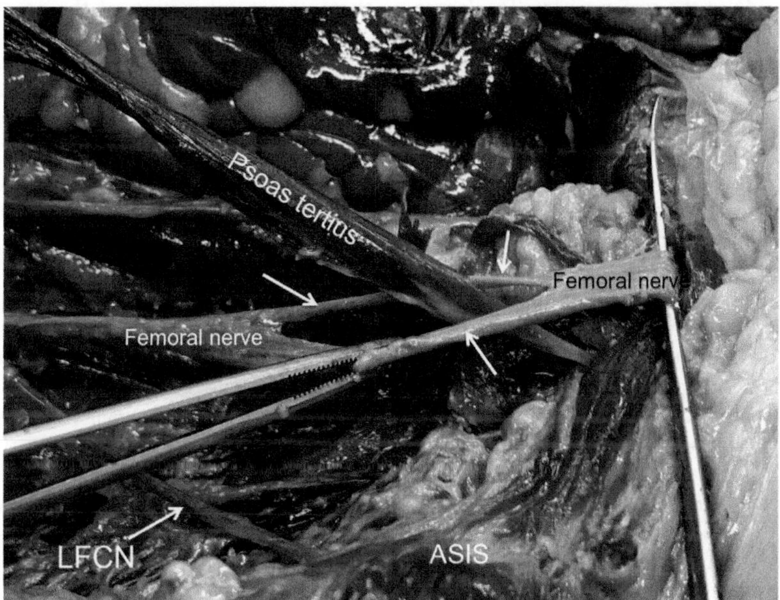

FIG. 4.9 Example of a right-sided psoas tertius that, here, is piercing the femoral nerve. For reference, note the anterior superior iliac spine (ASIS) and lateral femoral cutaneous nerve (LFCN).

ligament. In some recent studies of hip surgery, the authors claimed that iliocapsularis was a constant muscle observed in all cases (Ward et al., 2000; Babst et al., 2011). Babst et al. (2011) suggested that the iliocapsularis muscle was particularly important in dysplastic hips, where contractions of this muscle would help to stabilize the femoral head in a deficient acetabulum. Thus, this muscle may be hypertrophied in dysplastic, and atrophied in stable and well-constrained, hips.

Type F is the condition in which the iliacus muscle is split into deep and superficial layers. The femoral nerve splits in two, with one branch running between the two layers of the iliacus muscle.

Type G is when the iliacus has two large, variant, superficial slips. The femoral nerve is split in two and variant muscle slips run between the two nerve branches. Rao et al. (2008) reported one case of bilateral iliacus variations. On the left side, there were two variant slips on the surface of the iliacus muscle, the iliacus minimus (Fig. 4.10) on the medial side and the accessory iliacus muscle on the lateral side. The femoral nerve was split into two and its branches ran on the

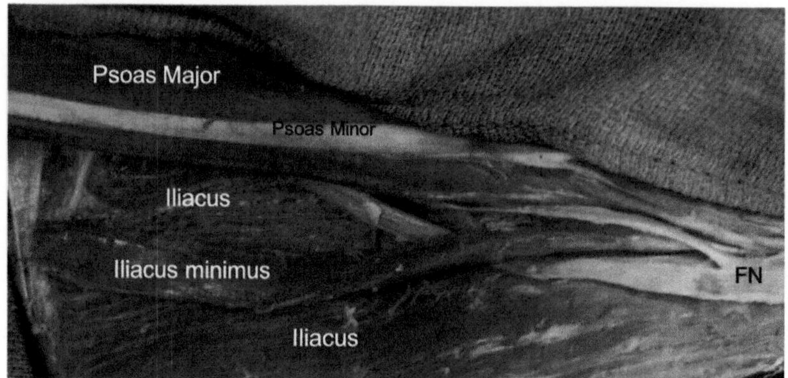

FIG. 4.10 Right-sided example of iliacus minimus piercing the femoral nerve.

medial and lateral side of the two muscles. The larger portion of the nerve ran on the lateral side (between the muscles slips and iliacus) and the smaller portion of the nerve ran superficial to the muscle slips on the medial side.

Type H is a single large variant slip of the iliacus muscle with the main trunk of the femoral nerve running between the variant muscle slip and iliacus. D'costa et al. (2008) reported the muscle slip originating from the middle third of inner lip of the iliac crest and inserting with the iliopsoas complex at the lesser trochanter. The L4 contribution to the femoral nerve ran between the muscle slip and iliacus, whereas the L2 and L3 roots ran superficial to the variant muscle slip. Rao et al. (2008) reported bilaterally abnormal iliacus muscles. On the right side, the iliacus muscle had one additional slip, and the femoral nerve splits into two parts in order to enclose the variant muscle slip and then fused again to form a single trunk.

Type I has two variant muscular slips, and the femoral nerve is split into two portions that run both superficial and deep to these muscle slips, enclosing them. Jelev et al. (2005) reported one case of this type. The medial side of the variant slip was located lateral to the normal psoas major muscle, and originated from the left L3 vertebra and from the intertransverse ligament between L3 and L4, and inserted with a short tendon to the iliopsoas tendon. This muscle has been described as the "accessory psoas major muscle" (Le Double, 1897; Rickenbacker et al., 1985; Jelev et al., 2005). The lateral side of the variant slip arose from the middle third of the iliac crest and inserted into the tendon of the above-mentioned variant slip. The author named this muscular slip the "accessory iliacus muscle" (Jelev et al., 2005). Jelev et al. (2005) named the "accessory iliopsoas muscle," describing them as a combination of the accessory psoas major and accessory iliacus muscles.

Type J has a small muscular slip piercing the femoral nerve. Spratt et al. (1996) first reported this type of variation and named it "iliacus minimus" (Fig. 4.10), which should not be confused with the iliacus minor. Spratt's case (1996) had a variant muscular slip originating from the iliolumbar ligament, piercing the femoral nerve, and splitting into two tendons that went to the lesser trochanter of the femur and the medial thigh. This muscle is presumed to have variations in its insertion. It may insert into the lesser trochanter of the femur or end by joining the iliopsoas muscle. The former insertion was reported by both Spratt et al. (1996) and Aristotle et al. (2003). In 2006, Tubbs et al. reported a similar case of a variant muscle slip that arose from the iliolumbar ligament, traveled on the iliacus, and pierced the femoral nerve. However, it ended by fusing with the iliopsoas muscle at the level of inguinal ligament, and did not reach the lesser trochanter. Aleksandrova et al. (2013) also reported a similar case, in which the muscle slip ended by joining the iliopsoas tendon.

PSOAS MAJOR

The psoas major is a long muscle that lies on either side of the lumbar vertebrate column and the pelvic brim (Fig. 4.1). Its complex proximal attachments include the anterior surfaces and lower borders of the transverse processes of all the lumbar vertebrate. Each of the five digitations come from the bodies of two adjoining vertebrate and their intervertebral disk. The highest arises from the lower margin of the body of the 12th thoracic vertebra, the upper margin of the body of the first lumbar vertebra, and the interposed intervertebral disk, while the lowest arises from the adjacent margins of the bodies of the fourth and fifth lumbar vertebra and the interposed disk. Between these digitations are a series of tendinous arches that extend across the narrow parts of the bodies of the lumbar vertebra. Medial to these arches, the lumbar arteries and veins, and filaments from the sympathetic trunk, pass. The upper four lumbar intervertebral foramina bear important relations to these attachments of the muscle. Anteriorly, the foramina lie to the transverse processes while posteriorly, they lie to the attachments of the vertebral bodies, intervertebral disks, and tendinous arches. Thus, the roots of the lumbar plexus enter the muscles directly, the plexus lodged with in it, and its branches emerge from its borders and surfaces.

The muscle descends down along the pelvic brim then continues posterior to the inguinal ligament, and anterior to the capsule of the hip joint. It then converges to a tendon that, having received on its lateral side nearly all the fibers of the iliacus, becomes attached to the lesser trochanter of the femur. The tendon is separated from the pubis and capsule joint by the large subtendinous iliac bursa, which occasionally communicates with the cavity of the hip joint.

The upper limit of the psoas major is posterior to the diaphragm in the lowest part of the posterior mediastinum, and it may be in contact with the posterior extremity of the pleural sac. In the abdomen, its anterolateral surface is related to the medial arcuate ligament (a linear, arched, thickening in the psoas fascia), extraperitoneal tissue and peritoneum, the kidney, psoas minor, renal vessels, ureter, testicular or ovarian vessels, and the genitofemoral nerve. Anteriorly, on the right the inferior vena cava overlaps, and the terminal part of the ileum crosses the psoas, while on the left it is crossed by the colon. The transverse process of the lumbar vertebrae and the medial edge of the quadratus lumborum are related to the posterior surface of the psoas major. Posteriorly, the lumbar plexus is embedded in the substance of the psoas major, and medially the muscle is related to the bodies of the lumbar vertebrae and lumbar vessels. Along its anteromedial margin is where it comes into contact with the sympathetic trunk, aortic lymph nodes, and along the external bridge of the external iliac artery. On the right side, this margin is covered by the vena, while on the left side, it lies posterior and lateral to the abdominal aorta. In the thigh, the iliopsoas relates anteriorly to the fascia lata and femoral artery and posteriorly to the capsule of the hip joint, which is then separated by a bursa. At the medial border, it is related to the pectineus and the medial circumflex femoral artery. On its lateral border, it is related to the femoral nerve and the iliacus. The femoral nerve then descends down through the fibers of the psoas major and then through the furrow between it and the iliacus.

From the abdominal part of the psoas major emerge branches of the lumbar plexus. From the lateral border emerge the iliohypogastric, ilioinguinal, and the lateral femoral cutaneous and femoral nerves, from above downwards. The genitofemoral nerve emerges from the anterolateral surface, and from the medial border emerge the obturator, accessory obturator nerves (when present), and the upper root of the lumbosacral trunk.

The psoas major is supplied by a rich network of arteries that have been derived from the lumbar, iliolumbar, obturator, external iliac, and femoral arteries. Simply, the upper part of the muscle is supplied by the lumbar arteries; the midpart by the anterior branch of the iliolumbar artery (the main artery to the muscle), with contributions from the deep circumflex and external iliac arteries; and the distal part by the femoral artery and its branches. The psoas sheath has an arterial supply that is independent from the muscle, though some of the same vessels may contribute to both. The psoas major is innervated by the ventral rami of the lumbar spinal nerves. Mahan et al. (2017) found the following: Nerve branches innervating the muscle originated from the ventral rami of L1-L4, with an average of 6.3 branches per muscle. The L1 nerve branch was the least consistently present, whereas L2 and L3 branches were the largest, the most numerous, and always present. The nerve branches to the psoas major commonly crossed the intervertebral disk obliquely; 76%, 80%, and 40% of specimens had a branch to the PMM and cross the midportion of the L2-3, L3-4, and L4-5 disks, respectively.

The psoas major acts with the iliacus to flex the thigh. EMG does not support a medial rotation component of the psoas major. In the upright stance, the iliopsoas has some action from below that helps to maintain the vertebral column in its upright position.

Variations

Both complete separation and complete fusion of the iliacus and psoas major have been reported. Macalister described psoas major as perfectly separated from iliacus. Fabrizio (2011) reported one case in which iliacus and psoas major were blended together at the level of the superior one-third of the ilium. Psoas major may be divided longitudinally into fascicles (Bergman et al., 2012). Jelev et al. (2005) reported one case in which psoas major was split longitudinally into three parts: a superior part arising from the body of the L1 vertebra and the intervertebral disk between L1 and L2; a middle part arising from the L2/L3 intervertebral disc; and an inferior part arising from the lower borders of the L3 to S3 vertebrae. Macalister (1875) also described cases in which psoas major originated from the fifth lumbar vertebra. Bergman et al. (1988) depicted a "variant psoas major fascicle" arising from the L4 body, L5 transverse process, and descending posterior to the psoas major muscle to be inserted just posterior to the psoas minor insertion onto the pubic bone.

PSOAS MINOR

The psoas minor (Figs. 4.1 and 4.11) may or may not be present. It arises from the sides of the bodies from the 12th thoracic and first lumbar vertebrae, along with the intervertebral disks between them. It ends in a long, flat tendon that is attached to the pecten pubis, iliopubic ramus, and, laterally, to the iliac fascia. It is situated on the anterior surface of the psoas major and is comprised mostly of tendon.

The main arterial supply for the psoas minor is derived from the lumbar arteries. There may be minor contributions from other vessels of the network that also supply the psoas major. Psoas minor is innervated by a branch from L1 or, as we have sometimes observed, from the genitofemoral nerve. Psoas minor is probably a weak flexor of the trunk.

Variations

Psoas minor is an inconsistent muscle that is often absent. The frequency of appearance of this muscle differs between races. Ghandhi et al. (2013) reviewed previous reports and found that this muscle had a prevalence of 33.4%–52% in the studied populations. Comparison among races is difficult because the reported prevalences are highly variable, even between researchers studying the same race. For example, Mori (1964) reviewed reports of the prevalence of psoas minor in Japanese populations and found that the prevalence ranged from 35% to 55%. However, Hanson et al. (1999) compared the prevalence of psoas minor between young black and white men and found that psoas minor was absent in 91% of black subjects but in only 13% of white subjects. Psoas minor is consistently absent in those with trisomy 18 (Agichani et al., 2013).

This muscle may be replaced by tendon (Macalister, 1875, Bergman et al., 2012) or may have a remarkably long tendon (Ghandhi et al., 2013). Guerra et al. (2012) reported that the tendon comprised 57% of the total length of the muscle. The average proportion

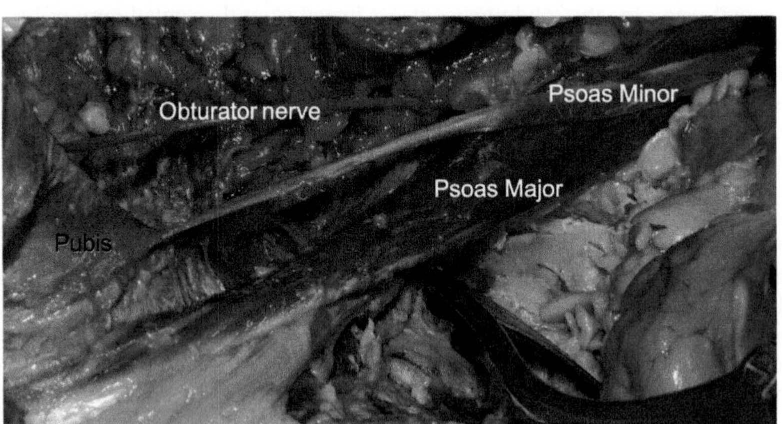

FIG. 4.11 Left-sided example of the psoas minor with its attachment onto the pubic bone.

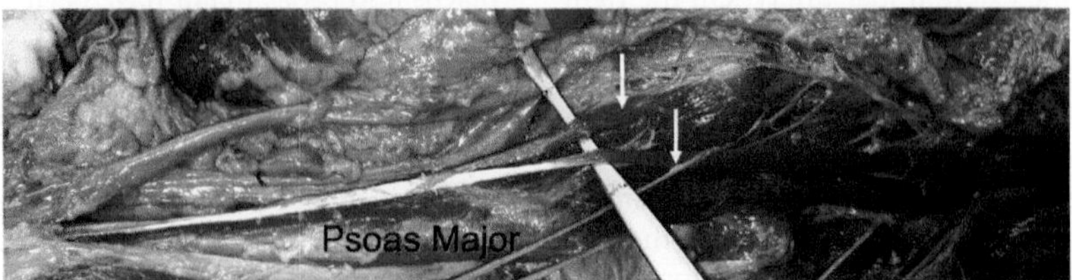

FIG. 4.12 A left-sided, double-headed psoas minor (arrows). Note the relationship of the obturator nerve.

of the total length comprised by the tendon was 60% in females and 54% in males (Guerra et al., 2012). Agichani et al. (2013) found that the average length of the muscle belly of psoas minor was 7.85 cm (right, 7.56 cm; left, 8.14 cm) and the length of the tendon was 13.13 cm (right, 13.56 cm; left, 12.7 cm).

Some variations in the origin and insertion of psoas minor have been reported. The origin of the muscle may consist of two heads (Fig. 4.12), which may split partially or completely prior to insertion (Ghandhi et al., 2013). Part of the split muscle may lie deep to the other part (Macalister, 1875; Bergman). The psoas minor originated as a ramification of the fibers of the psoas major (Macalister, 1875). Although this muscle is generally described as inserting into the iliopectineal eminence, some variations in its insertion have been reported; these include the pectineal line of the femur (Bankart et al., 1869; Guerra et al., 2012), the arched line, the iliac fascia, and the pectineal ligament. Insertion was, in many cases, present at more than one of these points (Muttarak and Peh, 2000; Guerra et al., 2012; Ghandhi et al., 2013).

Ghandhi et al., (2013) describes insertion of psoas minor into the iliac fascia, inguinal ligament, and the neck of the femur or lesser trochanter in unison with psoas major in the cases with two heads at its origin. In a case with a bifurcation in its tendinous insertion, the additional variant band is inserted into the synchondrosis between the fifth lumbar vertebra and the sacrum (Kraychete et al., 2007; Ghandhi et al., 2013). As an additional variation of psoas minor, Joshi et al. (2010) reported psoas accessories arose from the deep surface of the tendon of psoas minor and continued on the superficial surface of the psoas major until its insertion. This variation was observed in 25% of the cases.

REFERENCES

Agichani, S., Sontakke, Y., Joshi, S.S., Joshi, S.D., 2013. Morphology of Psoas Minor Muscle-Reviewed.

Aleksandrova, J.N., Malinova, L., Jelev, L., 2013. Variations of the iliacus muscle: report of two cases and review of the literature. Int J Anat Var 6, 149–152.

Aristotle, S., Sundarapandian, S., Felicia, C., 2013. Accessory iliacus muscle with splitting of the femoral nerve: a case report.

Babst, D., Steppacher, S.D., Ganz, R., Siebenrock, K.A., Tannast, M., 2011. The iliocapsularis muscle: an important stabilizer in the dysplastic hip. Clin. Orthop. Relat. Res. 469, 1728–1734.

Bankart, J., Pye-Smith, P.H., Phillips, J.J., 1869. Notes of abnormalities observed in the dissecting room during the winter sessions of 1866–7 and 1867–8. Guy's Hosp. Rep. 14, 436–455.

Bergman, R.A., Thompson, S.A., Afifi, A.K., Saadeh, F.A., 1988. Compendium of Human Variation. Urban & Schwarzenberg, Baltimore.

Bergman, R.A., Afifi, A.K., Jew, J.J., Reimann, P.C., 2012. Anatomy atlases. Illustrates encyclopedia of Human Anatomic variation: Opus I: Muscular system: Extensor carpi ulnaris. http:/anatomyatlases. org.

Clarkson, R.D., Rainy, H., 1889. Unusual arrangement of the psoas muscle. J. Anat. Physiol. 23 (Pt 3), 504.

Das, 1950. Iliacus minor; a report. Ind. Med. Gaz. 85, 492.

D'costa, S.U.J.A.T.H.A., Ramanathan, L.A., Madhyastha, S., Nayak, S.R., Prabhu, L.V., Rai, R., Prakash, 2008. An accessory iliacus muscle: a case report. Rom. J. Morphol. Embryol. 49 (3), 407–409.

Fabrizio, P.A., 2011. Anatomic variation of the iliacus and psoas major muscles. Int. J. Acoust. Vib. 4.

Gandhi, S., Gupta, N., Thakur, A., Anshu, A., Mehta, V., Suri, R.K., Rath, G., 2013. Anatomical and clinical insight of variation morphologies of psoas minor muscle: a case report. Int J Cur Res Rev 5 (14).

Guerra, D.R., Reis, F.P., Bastos, A.D.A., Brito, C.J., Silva, R.J.D.S., Aragão, J.A., 2012. Estudio Anatómico del Músculo Psoas Menor en Fetos Humanos. Int. J. Morphol. 30 (1), 136–139.

Hanson, P., Magnusson, S.P., Sorensen, H., Simonsen, E.B., 1999. Anatomical differences in the psoas muscles in young black and white men. J. Anat. 194 (2), 303–307.

Jelev, L., Shivarov, V., Surchev, L., 2005. Bilateral variations of the psoas major and the iliacus muscles and presence of an undescribed variant muscle–accessory iliopsoas muscle. Ann. Anat. 187 (3), 281–286.

Joshi, S.D., Joshi, S.S., Dandekar, U.K., Daini, S.R., 2010. Morphology of psoas minor and psoas accessorius. J. Anat. Soc. India 59 (1), 31–34

Kraychete, D.C., Rocha, A.P.C., Castro, P.A.C.R.D., 2007. Psoas muscle abscess after epidural analgesia: case report. Rev. Bras. Anestesiol. 57 (2), 195–198.

Le Double, A.F., 1897. Traite des variations du systeme musculaire de l'homme et de leur signification au point de vue de l'anthropologie, zoologique, vol. 2. Schleicher frères.

Macalister, A., 1875. Additional observations on muscular anomalies in human anatomy. (Third series) with a catalogue of the principal muscular variations hitherto published, 25. The Transactions of the Royal Irish Academy, pp. 1–134.

Mahan, M.A., Sanders, L.E., Guan, J., et al., 2017. Anatomy of psoas muscle innervation: cadaveric study. Clin. Anat. 30, 479–486.

Mori, M., 1964. Statistics on the musculature of the Japanese. Okajimas Folia Anat. Jpn. 40, 195–300.

Muttarak, M., Peh, W.C., 2000. CT of unusual iliopsoas compartment lesions. RadioGraphics 20 (Suppl. 1), S53–S66.

Park, R.J., Tsao, H., Cresswell, A.G., Hodges, P.W., 2012. Differential activity of regions of the psoas major and quadratus lumborum during submaximal isometric trunk efforts. J. Orthop. Res. 30, 311–318.

Phillips, S., Mercer, S., Bogduk, N., 2008. Anatomy and biomechanics of quadratus lumborum. Proc. Inst. Mech. Eng. H 222, 151–159.

Rao, T.R., Vanishree, K.P., Rao, S., 2008. Bilateral variation of iliacus muscle and splitting of femoral nerve. Neuroanatomy 7, 72–75.

Rickenbacker, J., Landholt, A.M., Theiler, K., 1985. Applied Anatomy of the Back. Springer, Heidelberg.

Spratt, J.D., Logan, B.M., Abrahams, P.H., 1996. Variant slips of psoas and iliacus muscles, with splitting of the femoral nerve. Clin. Anat. 9 (6), 401–404.

Tubbs, R.S., Oakes, W.J., Salter, E.G., 2006. The psoas quartus muscle. Clin. Anat. 19 (7), 678–680.

Ward, W.T., Fleisch, I.D., Ganz, R., 2000. Anatomy of the iliocapsularis muscle: relevance to surgery of the hip. Clin. Orthop. Relat. Res. 374, 278–285.

FURTHER READING

Kirchmair, L., Lirk, P., Colvin, J., et al., 2008. Lumbar plexus and psoas major muscle: not always as expected. Reg. Anesth. Pain Med. 33, 109–114.

Willard, F.H., Vleeming, A., Schuenke, M.D., et al., 2012. The thoracolumbar fascia: anatomy, function and clinical considerations. J. Anat. 221, 507–536.

CHAPTER 5

The Diaphragm

PETER OAKES • R. SHANE TUBBS

INTRODUCTION

The diaphragm possesses a domelike shape that serves to separate the thorax and abdomen from one another (Allaix and Patti, 2015; Morton et al., 2019) (Figs. 5.1 and 5.2). The diaphragm is unique in the sense that it is the only skeletal muscle upon which life depends (Gayan-Ramirez and Decramer, 2015). Because of this muscle's importance, this chapter is dedicated to the diaphragm, explains its anatomy, and explores the way knowledge of this anatomy can be applied to thoracolumbar spinal surgery in an attempt to reduce morbidity and mortality associated with diaphragmatic injuries.

EMBRYOLOGY

In Schoenwolf et al. (2008) description, the first step in the diaphragm's formation during approximately the fourth and fifth weeks of gestation is the septum transversum's caudal displacement. The septum's ventral portion then affixes to the anterior body wall at approximately T7, and inserts dorsally into the esophageal mesenchyme at approximately T12. Subsequently, the greater part of the septum transversum becomes the central tendon. At the same time, myoblasts differentiate within the septum and become the diaphragm muscle itself ultimately. Other myoblasts that originated in the septum transversum migrate into the pleuroperitoneum with their nervous branches, which causes deferred pain generated by irritation of this region. Gradually, the forming muscle becomes innervated by C3-5 spinal roots, which combine to create the phrenic nerves.

However, not all of the diaphragmatic muscle fibers form in this manner. The diaphragm's edge is created by body wall mesoderm derived from somatic mesoderm. Myoblasts from somites nearby invade this peripheral area and cause its innervation to originate at the T7-12 levels. The crura also have a unique origin, as they are created by mesoderm that originates from L1-L3, which aggregates and forms the two structures. Taken as a whole, the muscle includes four embryonic origins: the pleuroperitoneal membranes, the mesoderm of the body wall, the esophageal mesenchyme, and the septum transversum (Schoenwolf et al., 2008).

PHYSIOLOGY

The diaphragm is a skeletal muscle similar to those found in the arms and legs, with some important differences. Because it is essential for respiration, it is no surprise that the muscle has become specialized for constant activity. Such adaptations include a higher capacity for oxidative metabolism, increased resistance to fatigue, and a greater number of capillaries (and therefore, increased blood flow). An examination of the specific types of muscle fibers found within the diaphragm demonstrated that approximately 80% are oxidative fibers, which is remarkable, given that most limb muscles in nonathletes peak at approximately 46% oxidative fibers. This also translates into twice the density of mitochondria in the diaphragm when compared to less specialized skeletal muscles. Similarly, the concentration of capillaries in diaphragmatic muscle was found to be approximately twice that in other skeletal muscles, which indicates its strenuous and constant activity throughout life (Gayan-Ramirez and Decramer, 2015).

A unique system regulates the diaphragm's voluntary and involuntary activity. Neurons in the brainstem that control respiration use the phrenic nerve to regulate the mechanical aspects of breathing, including respiratory rate and tidal volume (Morton et al., 2019). When neuromuscular transmission occurs, the diaphragm's excitation and action potentials' spread cause the muscle to contract (Sinderby and Beck, 2013), and several respiratory reflexes in the respiratory center of the brainstem modulate this transmission (Morton et al., 2019). In healthy individuals, the total time the signal for inspiration requires to reach the diaphragm from the respiratory center is 26–28 ms, while the time required for the signal to breathe to propagate from the nerve roots to the diaphragm is between six and eight milliseconds.

Surgical anatomy of the lateral transpsoas approach to the lumbar spine. https://doi.org/10.1016/B978-0-323-67376-1.00005-7

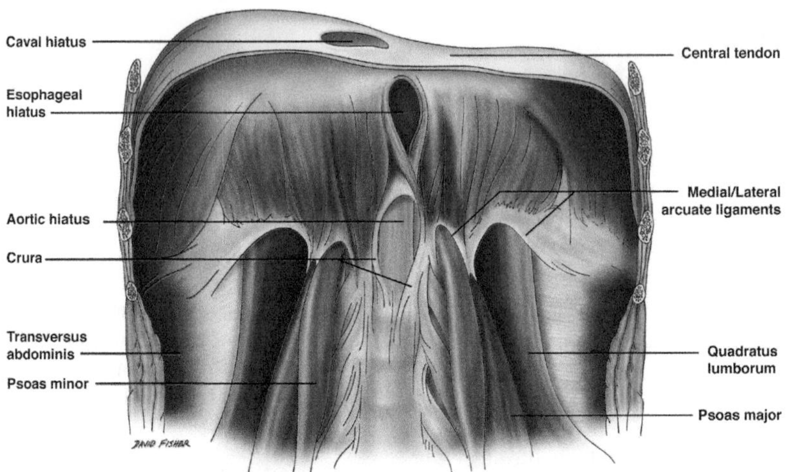

FIG. 5.1 Schematic drawing of the diaphragm and surrounding anatomy.

These times can become prolonged if respiratory workload is increased, the function of the muscles involved in respiration are impaired, or if the signal to inspire decreases in strength (such as during general anesthesia; Sinderby and Beck, 2013).

ANATOMY IN SITU

The diaphragm is a thin, oval-shaped, domed muscle with a fibrous central tendon that runs down the middle (although located more anteriorly than posteriorly) into which the diaphragm's various muscular elements insert (LeBlond et al., 2015). The diaphragm is subdivided into two "hemidiaphragms," each of which possesses its own apex, referred to as a cupula or dome. The diaphragm's points of origin include T12 through L3 vertebrae posteriorly, the lower six ribs' costal arches laterally, and the sternum's xiphoid process anteriorly (Allaix and Patti, 2015; Morton et al., 2019). The right hemidiaphragm is able to ascend to the level of the fourth costal cartilage anteriorly with full, forced expiration, while on the left, the maximum height tends to be approximately the fifth rib (Loukas, 2016). The right portion of the dome overlays the liver, right kidney, and suprarenal gland, while the left sets atop the stomach's fundus, liver's

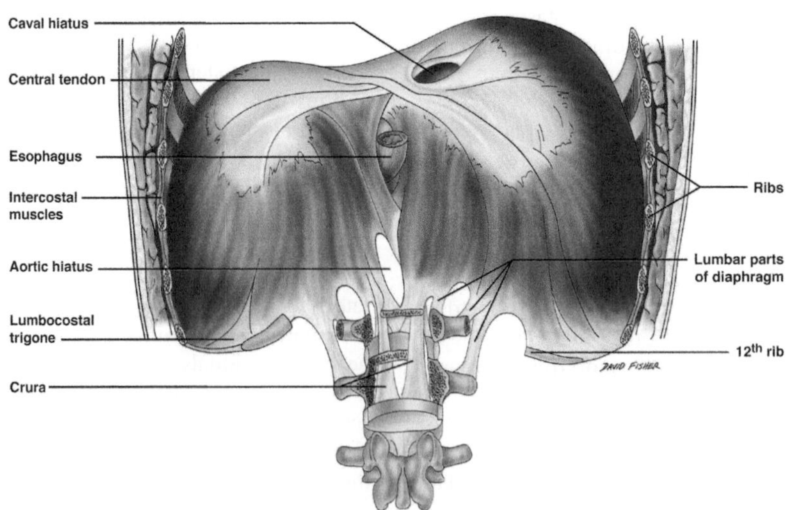

FIG. 5.2 Posterior view of the diaphragm and its attachments.

left lobe, spleen, left kidney, and suprarenal gland (Morton et al., 2019; Loukas, 2016). The center of the diaphragm lays just inferior to the pericardium, and the muscle's cranial surface is associated closely with the pericardium as well as the pleura of each lung. The peritoneum abuts nearly all of the diaphragm's caudal surface (Loukas, 2016). The right side of the diaphragm is positioned more often than not more cranially than is the left (Morton et al., 2019). However, it must be noted that this generality is an oversimplification—height, body habitus, body position, and ventilatory phase all play roles in the diaphragm's configuration at any given time. In pathological states, such as emphysema or other causes of lung hyperinflation, the diaphragm tends to assume a less pronounced dome appearance (Loukas, 2016).

The diaphragm can be subdivided into three distinct portions: sternal, costal, and lumbar. The sternal diaphragm originates from the posterior portion of the xiphoid process, which runs nearly horizontally to attach to the central tendon. The costal portion originates from the six lower ribs' medial aspects and intermingles with the transversus abdominal muscles on the opposite end. Finally, the diaphragm's lumbar portions (Fig. 5.2) originates from the lateral and medial arcuate ligaments (outer and inner arches of Haller, respectively), as well as from the upper lumbar vertebral bodies. This portion has the longest span before it reaches the central tendon (Loukas, 2016).

The lateral arcuate ligaments (Fig. 5.1) cover the quadratus lumborum muscle, attach to the anterior portion of L1 at its transverse process, and insert laterally into the 12th rib's inferior portion. The medial arcuate ligament spans across the psoas major at its superior pole and attaches to the actual body of L1 or L2 (Loukas, 2016).

The diaphragm's crura (Figs. 5.3–5.6) intermingle with the anterior longitudinal ligament upon insertion and possess fibrous characteristics at this junction. The right crus of the diaphragm is longer than is the left, originates from the upper three lumbar vertebrae, and enfolds the esophagus as it enters the abdomen. The left crus originates from L1 and L2. Both meet in the center of the diaphragm and join to form the median arcuate ligament, which lays anterior to the aorta (Loukas, 2016).

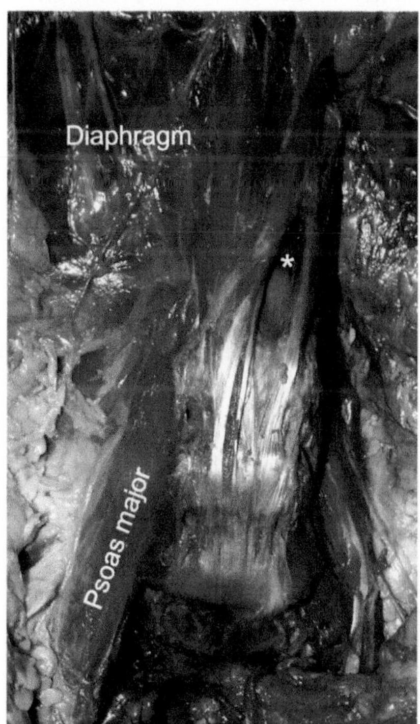

FIG. 5.3 Cadaveric view of the diaphragm and its relationship to the lumbar spine.

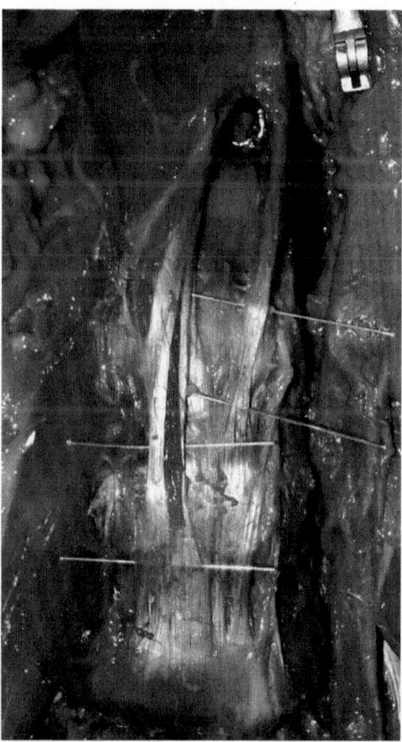
FIG. 5.4 Metal wires are placed under the left and right crura.

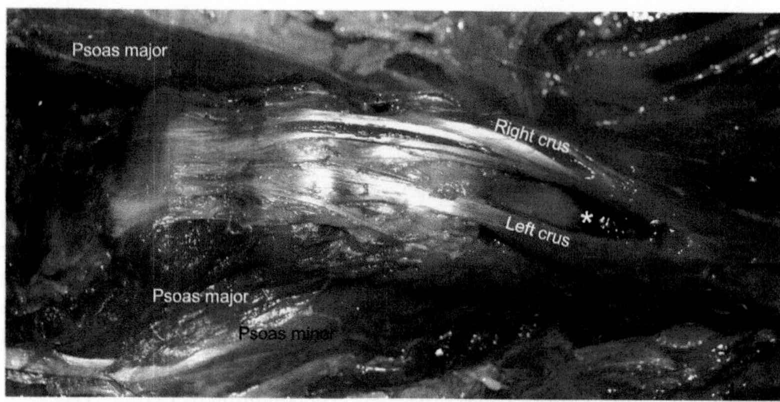

FIG. 5.5 Semilateral view of the diaphragmatic crura.

PASSAGE THROUGH THE DIAPHRAGM

As the diaphragm serves to compartmentalize the thoracoabdominal cavities, it is unsurprising that many important structures pass through it. It is worth examining these structures in detail to avoid their injury in any surgery in the diaphragm's proximity. The aorta (Fig. 5.7) passes through the diaphragm approximately at the level of T12, and the thoracic duct, the sympathetic trunk occasionally, and various lymph nodes that drain the low posterior thoracic wall, and the azygos venous system also pass through this aortic hiatus (Allaix and Patti, 2015; Morton et al., 2019; Loukas, 2016). The two diaphragmatic crura create this hiatus laterally, while the vertebral column abuts it posteriorly, and the median arcuate ligament anteriorly (Fig. 5.3). When defined by these borders, the aorta is in fact posterior to the diaphragm, and therefore, protected from any contraction or relaxation of the muscle although some clinical consequences of this relationship have been reported (Loukas, 2016). The esophagus passes through the diaphragm between T9-11, and its hiatus is located left of the midline, and more anteriorly than is the aortic hiatus (Allaix and Patti, 2015; Loukas, 2016) (Figs. 5.7 and 5.8). As mentioned previously, the diaphragm's right crus serves to enfold the esophagus as it passes through the diaphragm, and separates the aorta and the diaphragm (Allaix and Patti, 2015). In addition to the esophagus, the vagus and gastric nerves, esophageal branches of the left gastric vessels, and various smaller lymphatic vessels also pass through this aperture (Allaix and Patti, 2015; Morton et al., 2019; Loukas, 2016). The inferior vena cava passes through the diaphragm between T8-10, approximately at the level of the intervertebral disc (Allaix and Patti, 2015; Loukas, 2016), and several small branches of the right phrenic nerve pass through the diaphragm in this aperture as well (Allaix and Patti, 2015; Morton et al., 2019) (Figs. 5.7 and 5.8). Furthermore, each crus can be pierced by the greater or lesser splanchnic nerves (Fig. 5.8). In most patients, the sympathetic trunks enter the abdominal cavity posterior to the diaphragm as a whole, and specifically, posterior to the medial arcuate ligaments. Finally, some small regions of areolar tissue have been noted where the sternal and costal portions of the diaphragm meet that allow the superior epigastric artery, together with select lymphatics, to traverse the diaphragm (Loukas, 2016).

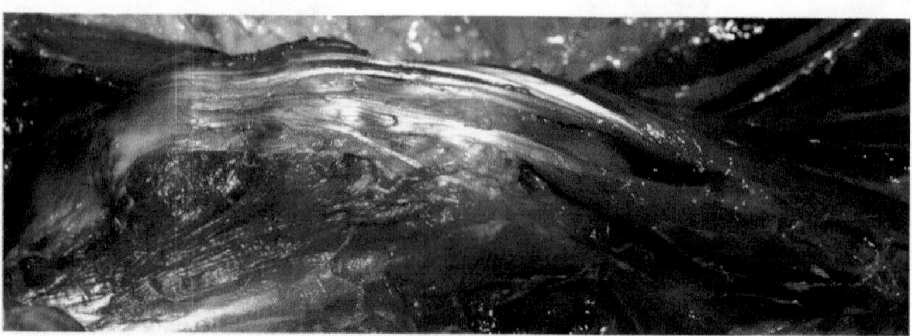

FIG. 5.6 Lateral view of the diaphragmatic crura.

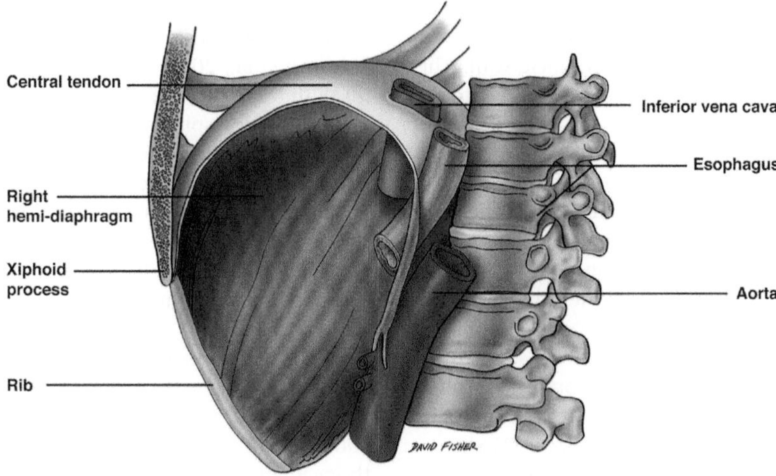

FIG. 5.7 Schematic drawing of the right hemidiaphragm and the relationships of the inferior vena cava, esophagus, and aorta.

VASCULATURE OF THE DIAPHRAGM

The blood supply to the diaphragm derives from many sources: the superior and inferior phrenic arteries, the lower five subcostal and intercostal vessels, and some of the final branches of the internal thoracic arteries (i.e., the pericardiacophrenic and musculophrenic arteries (Allaix and Patti, 2015; Loukas, 2016). While it is important to be aware of all of these sources, the most important are the inferior phrenic arteries (Loukas, 2016) (Fig. 5.8). Usually, the right inferior phrenic artery branches either from the celiac trunk or directly from the aorta itself. Rarely, the artery originates from the left gastric or proper hepatic artery. It tends to course posterior to the inferior vena cava, but then onto the right side of its hiatus. The left inferior phrenic artery can branch from the celiac trunk or directly from the aorta. It runs in a manner similar to its counterpart, posterior to the esophagus, but then anteriorly to the left side of its hiatus. Both arteries subdivide further into lateral and medial branches, which tends to occur at the central tendon's posterior boundary. The median offshoots travel anteriorly and communicate with each other, as well as the terminal branches of the internal thoracic artery, on the opposite side of the central

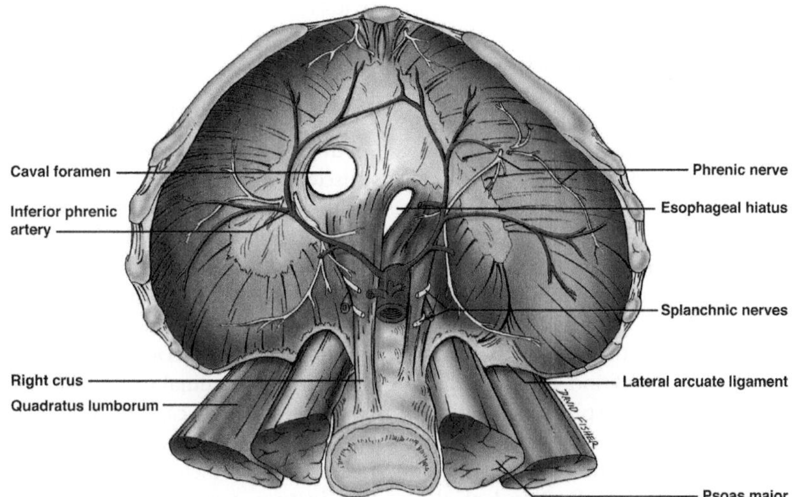

FIG. 5.8 Inferior view of the diaphragm with related neurovascular structures.

tendon. These arteries' lateral branches anastomose with the musculophrenic arteries and inferior posterior intercostal arteries as they near the thoracic wall. The right-sided lateral subdivision supplies the inferior vena cava, while the left supplies the esophagus in part (Loukas, 2016).

In addition to the inferior phrenic arteries, there are several other important vessels that supply the diaphragm, including the superior phrenic arteries, which supply its cranial surface. Both the right and left superior phrenic arteries originate most often directly from the thoracic aorta or the 10th intercostal artery (the proximal more often than distal segment). The intercostal and subcostal arteries' most important contribution is to the costal portion of the diaphragm, of which they are the major supplier (Loukas, 2016).

Similar to the diaphragm's blood supply, its upper and lower surfaces' drainage tends to differ. The pericardiacophrenic and musculophrenic veins drain its cranial portion and course along a similar path as their arterial counterparts. Similarly, the inferior phrenic veins drain its caudal surface, in which the right empties into the inferior vena cava (usually below the diaphragm) or more rarely, the right hepatic vein, while the left also tends to empty into the inferior vena cava below the diaphragm. The lymphatics that drain the diaphragm rest on its convex face and can be separated into three groups: posterior, middle, and anterior. In addition to the diaphragm, these lymphatics also drain part of the liver and the gastroesophageal junction. From their location on the diaphragm, they drain to the anterior mediastinal and parasternal chains, as well as the posterior mediastinal and brachiocephalic nodes (Loukas, 2016).

INNERVATION OF THE DIAPHRAGM

As stated previously, the phrenic nerves, each of which contains both motor and sensory fibers for their respective hemidiaphragm, are the diaphragm's primary source of innervation (Fig. 5.8). The roots of the nerve derive from C3-C5 (although C4 is the principal contributor; Morton et al., 2019; Loukas, 2016), and its motor fibers cause the diaphragm to contract (Morton et al., 2019). In addition to most of the diaphragm (both peritoneal and thoracic surfaces), this nerve also provides some sensation for the parietal pericardium and parietal pleura (diaphragmatic and mediastinal portions; Morton et al., 2019; LeBlond et al., 2015). Because it has its roots in the cervical spine, aggravation or irritation of the phrenic nerve's distribution can cause referred pain to the neck, often worsened by deep inspiration or certain valsalva maneuvers (LeBlond et al., 2015). The fifth and sixth intercostal nerves lead to an additional sensation of pain on the muscle's periphery (Morton et al., 2019; LeBlond et al., 2015).

With respect to its course, the phrenic nerve descends from its cervical spinal roots on the anterior scalene muscle's anterior aspect (between the subclavian artery and vein, together with the pericardiacophrenic artery and vein; Morton et al., 2019). The right phrenic nerve is not as long as the left and tends to follow a path more perpendicular to the diaphragm. The right phrenic descends laterally compared to the brachiocephalic vein and vena cava. The nerve then enters the diaphragm at the central tendon in the vicinity of the inferior vena cava hiatus. On the left, it passes the left subclavian artery anteriorly, but still posterior to the thoracic duct, and continues to run caudally anterior to the left internal thoracic artery. The nerve travels lower in the thoracic cavity, first in the space between the left common carotid artery and the subclavian artery. Anterior to the vagus nerve, but posterior to the brachiocephalic vein, it continues down to innervate the left hemidiaphragm, and then enters the diaphragm more anteriorly than does the right phrenic nerve through the muscle itself (Loukas, 2016). In the chest, both nerves continue to travel with the pericardiacophrenic vessels when they cross anterior to the lung's root to reach the diaphragm in the space between the mediastinal parietal pleura and pericardium (Morton et al., 2019; Loukas, 2016). Upon making contact with the diaphragm, both nerves divide typically into three separate branches (an anterior or sternal, an anterolateral, and a posterior; Loukas, 2016). The first courses toward the sternum, the second runs laterally along the central tendon, and the last has a short posterior course, which divides into a posterolateral ramus that runs posterior to the anterolateral branch, and a posterior ramus that supplies the crura (Loukas, 2016).

FUNCTION OF THE DIAPHRAGM

As discussed previously, the diaphragm is the primary muscle of inspiration (Morton et al., 2019) and accomplishes this goal through several sequelae associated with its contraction. Firstly, its contraction causes an increase in the chest cavity's volume craniocaudally, which decreases its pressure momentarily to create a vacuum effect that allows air to enter the lungs (Morton et al., 2019; Gayan-Ramirez and Decramer, 2015). This descent also causes the abdominal wall to move outward, which expands the lower rib cage and the chest cavity even further. Finally, the descent also exerts direct tension on the lower ribs because of their connection to the diaphragm, and this, in turn, causes these ribs to rotate outward more to increase the chest cavity's volume (Gayan-Ramirez and Decramer, 2015). All of these effects combine to lower the pressure in the pleura and alveoli, causing inspiratory flow via lung distension (Sinderby and Beck, 2013). When it relaxes, the diaphragm ascends within the chest cavity and conversely decreases its volume, which causes a subsequent increase in the pressure in that space, and pushes air out of the lungs (Morton et al., 2019). When expiration is complete, the diaphragm rests higher in the chest, and the thoracic walls are drawn closer together, while at full inspiration, the opposite may be true (LeBlond et al., 2015).

In addition to respiration, the diaphragm performs several other ancillary functions. It contributes to the creation of any Valsalva maneuver by forced exhalation against a closed upper airway, which causes increased pressure in the abdomen that can be used for several purposes, such as "popping" one's ears (attributable to pressure equalization), emesis, defecation, and micturition (Morton et al., 2019). The diaphragm also helps prevent gastroesophageal reflux disease by contributing the crura's pressure on the gastroesophageal junction through constriction during inspiration at this point. This, combined with specialized smooth muscle cells, prevents reflux of gastric contents into the esophagus. The phrenicoesophageal ligament aids in this endeavor, as it links the esophagus to the diaphragm and prevents the esophagus from excessive longitudinal motion into the chest cavity, but allows some leeway for its movement during swallowing and inhalation (Loukas, 2016). Finally, in addition to pressure changes that cause air to flow into and out of the lungs, the diaphragm also cause changes in blood flow, which the body uses to augment the return of venous blood to the heart during inspiration, when the hiatus of the inferior vena cava opens and increases abdominal pressure, which sends blood to the heart (Morton et al., 2019; Loukas, 2016).

APPLICATIONS TO SURGERY

The question may arise, most notably during thoracolumbar spinal surgery: how can the diaphragm be manipulated in a way that allows maximal visualization of the vertebrae desired and also minimizes any morbidity associated with frank diaphragmatic injury following the procedure? In general, an anterior thoracolumbar approach is desirable for any patient with pathology in the spine between T11 and L2 (Schuchert et al., 2014). Many have speculated that the best beginning to any anterior approach to the thoracolumbar spine is with Papin's method because of its simple execution and the options it provides for the surgeon (Mirbaha, 1973). Should the surgeon wish to gain access to a lower level of the spinal column, simple extension of the incision allows for this (Mirbaha, 1973). Often, operations that call for access to the intervertebral disc of T12-L1 require only a simple division of the diaphragm at its point of insertion, which some perform by continuing the incision of the pleura onto the diaphragm, followed by blunt dissection of the diaphragm from the vertebrae (Newton and Perry, 2009) (Fig. 5.9). Operations that require access to the L1 vertebral body itself often necessitate transection of the diaphragm (Hamilton and Trost, 2017). Other authors have suggested that division of the diaphragm is not necessary to visualize the vertebrae desired appropriately, and that, in fact, simple dissection of the diaphragm's attachments off the vertebrae with table fixed retractors allows both supra- and infradiaphragmatic visualization and therefore, the benefit of both. For example, when a transpsoas approach is attempted, it is advisable to take a retropleural approach in which the diaphragm is released from the vertebral body and other spinal elements above L1 (Deukmedjian and Uribe, 2014).

When positioning the patient for a transthoracic approach, they are placed often in the lateral decubitus position, and usually a 10th rib, sometimes a 9th rib, incision is made to reach the T12-L1 space, after which this rib can be resected, as can the 11th or 12th, to allow greater space and visualization of the field (Hamilton and Trost, 2017). One advantage of detaching the 12th rib's medial portion is because it attaches not

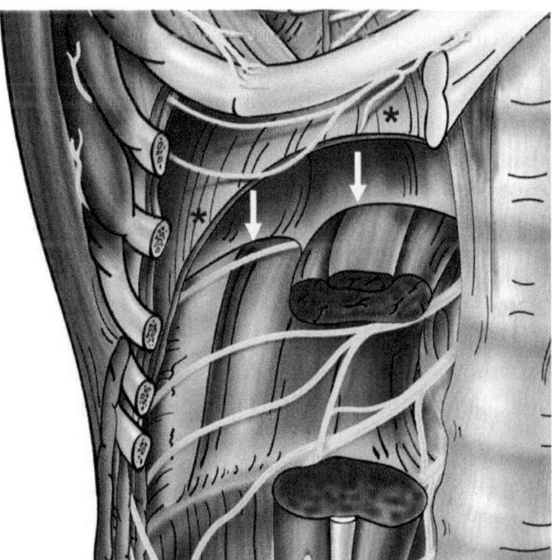

FIG. 5.9 Anteroinferior (asterisk) and posteroinferior parts of the diaphragm. For the posteroinferior parts, note the medial and lateral arcuate ligaments (arrows).

only to the diaphragm but to the quadratus lumborum as well, retraction of which allows access to the retroperitoneal extrapleural space anterior to the vertebral column. Next, a short incision can be made over the lumbar region at the apex of Petit's triangle, followed by retraction of the latissimus dorsi and external oblique muscles, after which the internal oblique's posterior portion is retracted to separate it from the quadratus lumborum. Then, the floor of Grynfeldt's triangle (consisting at this point of the transversus abdominis) is opened, and the retroperitoneal space is accessed (Mirbaha, 1973). A self-retaining thoracotomy retractor is then used before proceeding. The surgeon must be aware of the danger to the spleen on the left side at this level, or to the liver on the right. When approaching the vertebrae from below the diaphragm in the retroperitoneal space, it is helpful often to dissect the crura from their vertebral attachments (Hamilton and Trost, 2017).

When access to the mid-lumbar vertebrae is desired, a slightly different technique is used, one similar to a lumbar sympathectomy. This approach is conducive to visualizing the spinal canal from L2 to the pelvic brim. Additional advantages include its relative familiarity and clear exposure of the vertebrae desired, but unfortunately, the crus of the diaphragm limits the field superiorly and the pelvic girdle inferiorly, in addition to the psoas, which limits accessibility to the neuroforamina. If access only to the L1–L2 disc space is desired, then oftentimes, an extrapleural, subcostal approach with rib resection at T12 is desirable, as it does not require transecting the diaphragm (Hamilton and Trost, 2017) (Fig. 5.10).

Francioli developed a more restrictive alternative to transecting or releasing the diaphragm from its spinal attachments. To gain access to the thoracolumbar sympathetic trunk, dissection is performed both superior and inferior to the diaphragm. However, because the diaphragm is left attached to the spine, this is a much more limited approach than those that release the diaphragm at this point, and likely is suitable only for biopsies or procedures that involve the sympathetic chain rather than the vertebral bodies at this level (Moskovich et al., 1993).

The diaphragm remains a consideration even in spinal surgery at higher levels, as it forms the lower boundary of the field in many surgical procedures. For example, when approaching T4-T10, often anteriorly along a transthoracic pathway, a medial incision through the diaphragm provides access as low as the disc between L2 and L3. Again, having the patient in the lateral decubitus position is preferable when the spine is approached in this manner, and the level of the incision is tailored to the vertebra of interest. The alternative is the subcostal retroperitoneal approach, which, when combined with

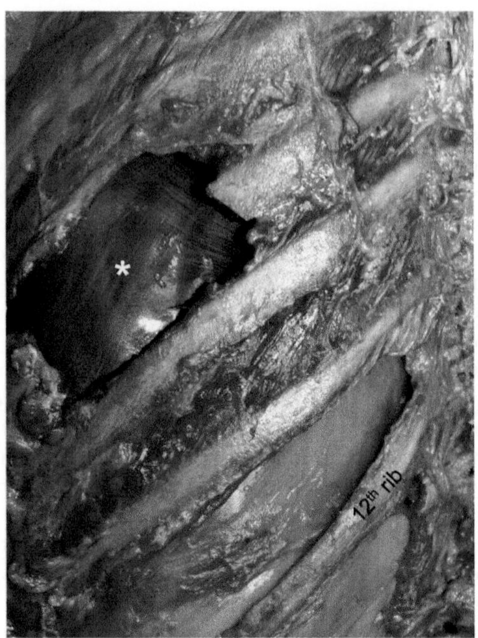

FIG. 5.10 Cadaveric view of the posterior diaphragm covered with pleura (asterisk). The 12th rib is shown with peritoneum just above it and retroperitoneal fat just below it.

medial transection of the diaphragm, has allowed some surgeons to approach as high as T12 (Klekamp and Samii, 2007) (Fig. 5.11).

Several sources of morbidity and mortality are associated with surgery that involves the diaphragm. In general, if the diaphragm is transected, it should be performed on the muscle's periphery, as otherwise, the phrenic nerve is at risk of transection (Hamilton and Trost, 2017). If circumferential division of the hemidiaphragm is deemed necessary, a margin of at least 1 centimeter along the chest wall is recommended for it to remain possible to reattach the diaphragm, and it is recommended to use 0-0 prolene sutures during this step (Schuchert et al., 2014). One source of increased morbidity and mortality when the diaphragm is transected is violation of both the pleural and retroperitoneal cavities (Hamilton and Trost, 2017). This is a greater risk than entering only one body cavity in a retroperitoneal approach, and the advantages and disadvantages should be weighed appropriately. One alternative that has been proposed is making an incision one rib lower (at the 11th rib) to violate only the retroperitoneal cavity. Disadvantages of this approach include decreased exposure of the vertebrae in question, longer operative time, and greater technical difficulty. Furthermore, excessive traction on the patient's left side should be avoided, as splenic injury is a potential consequence

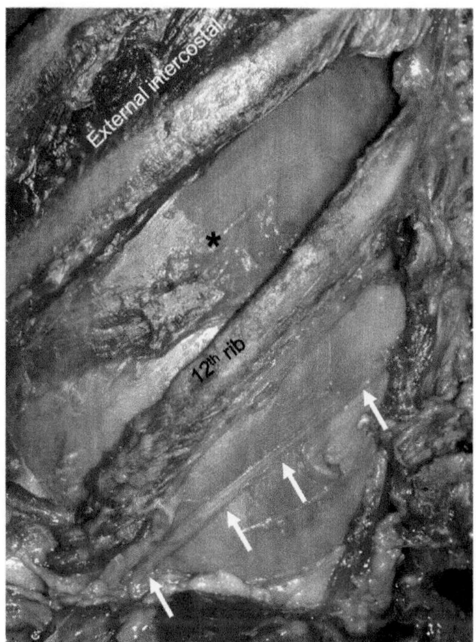

FIG. 5.11 Image shown in Fig. 5.10 with the subcostal nerve indicated at the arrows and peritoneum at the asterisk.

(Hamilton and Trost, 2017). If it is necessary at any point to elevate the insertion of the diaphragm on the vertebrae, postoperative radiography is advised, as there is the potential for a tear in the pleura and subsequent development of pneumothorax (Klekamp and Samii, 2007).

CONCLUSION

The diaphragm is an important muscle, and loss of its function can be a devastating complication. However, surgeons may find it necessary to manipulate the muscle at one point to access the thoracolumbar spinal column. This chapter's goal was to impart pertinent information about both the diaphragm's anatomy, and different approaches to consider when it is involved in surgery.

REFERENCES

Allaix, M., Patti, M., 2015. Chapter 20: Esophagus and diaphragm. In: Doherty, G. (Ed.), Current Diagnosis and Treatment: Surgery, fourteenth ed. McGraw-Hill Education, New York.

Deukmedjian, A., Uribe, J.S., 2014. Chapter 28: Minimally invasive anterior column reconstruction for sagittal plane deformities. In: Wang, M., Lu, Y., Anderson, G., Mummaneni, P. (Eds.), Minimally Invasive Spinal Deformity Surgery: An Evolution of Modern Techniques. Springer, New York, pp. 281–291.

Gayan-Ramirez, G., Decramer, M., 2015. Chapter 3: The respiratory muscles. In: Grippi, M. (Ed.), Fishman's Pulmonary Diseases and Disorders, fifth ed., Minimally Invasive Spinal Deformity Surgery: An Evolution of Modern Techniques. McGraw-Hill Education, New York.

Hamilton, K., Trost, G., 2017. Section 7: Perioperative management. In: Steinmetz, M., Benzel, E. (Eds.), Benzel's Spine Surgery: Techniques, Complication Avoidance, and Management, fourth ed. Elsevier, Inc., Philadelphia, PA, pp. 1739–1741.

Klekamp, J., Samii, M., 2007. Chapter 5: Epidural tumors. In: Schröder, G. (Ed.), Surgery of Spinal Tumors. Springer, Heidelberg, pp. 378–387.

LeBlond, R., Brown, D., Suneja, M., Szot, J., 2015. The chest: chest wall, pulmonary, and cardiovascular systems; the breasts. In: Henry, S., Pancotti, R. (Eds.), DeGowin's Diagnostic Examination, 10e. McGraw-Hill Education, New York.

Loukas, M., 2016. Chapter 55: Diaphragm and phrenic nerves. In: Spratt, J., Standring, S. (Eds.), Gray's Anatomy, 41st ed. Elsevier, Philadelphia, pp. 970–973.

Mirbaha, M., 1973. Anterior approach to the thoracolumbar junction of the spine by a retroperitoneal-extrapleural technique. Clin. Orthop. Relat. Res. 91 (91), 41–47. Available at: https://www.researchgate.net/publication/18463470_Anterior_Approach_to_the_Thoraco-Lumbar_Junction_of_the_Spine_by_a_Retroperitoneal-Extrapleural_Technic.

Morton, D., Foreman, K., Albertine, K., 2019. Chapter 2: Anterior thoracic wall. In: The Big Picture: Gross Anatomy, second ed. McGraw-Hill, New York.

Moskovich, R., Benson, D., Zhang, Z.H., Kabins, M., 1973. Extracoelomic approach to the spine. J. Bone Joint Surg. Br. 75 (6), 886–893.

Newton, P., Perry, A., 2009. Thorascopic deformity correction. In: Ozgur, B., Benzel, B., Garfin, S. (Eds.), Minimally Invasive Spine Surgery: A Practical Guide to Anatomy and Techniques, first ed. Springer, New York, NY, p. 80.

Schoenwolf, G., Bleyl, S., Brauer, P., Francis-West, P., 2008. Development of the respiratory system and body cavities. In: Larseon's Human Embryology, fourth ed. Elsevier, Philadelphia.

Sinderby, C., Beck, J., 2013. Neurally adjusted ventilatory assist. In: Tobin, M. (Ed.), Principles and Practice of Mechanical Ventilation, third ed. McGraw-Hill, New York.

Schuchert, M., McCormick, K., Abbas, G., Pennathur, A., Landreneau, J., Pitanga, A., Gomes, J., Franca, F., El-Kadi, M., Peitzman, A., Ferson, P., Luketich, J., Landreneau, J., 2014. Anterior thoracic surgical approaches in the treatment of spinal infections and neoplasms. Ann. Thorac. Surg. 97 (5), 1750–1757. Available at: www.annalsthoracicsurgery.org/article/S0003-4975(13).

CHAPTER 6

Lumbar Plexus

TYLER WARNER • R. SHANE TUBBS

INTRODUCTION

Lateral transpsoas approaches to the lumbar spine require a detailed knowledge of surrounding neurovascular structures. Of most importance, the spine surgeon who performs such approaches must have a command of the anatomy of the lumbar plexus (Fig. 6.1). Therefore, this chapter is dedicated to the detailed anatomy of this collection of nerves derived from the ventral rami (Fig. 6.2) of the upper four lumbar nerves and often, the T12 ventral ramus.

THE SUBCOSTAL NERVE

Anatomy

The subcostal nerve is the ventral ramus of the 12th thoracic nerve (T12) that travels below the last rib (Fig. 6.3). The first 11 intercostal thoracic nerves run between the ribs and their branches are classified as either collateral, lateral, cutaneous, anterior cutaneous, or muscular nerves (Harman, 1898; Standring, 2015). Each spinal segment gives rise to dorsal and ventral thoracic nerve roots, which will leave the spinal cord to bifurcate into a ventral and dorsal ramus. Postganglionic sympathetic fibers that originate from the sympathy trunk enter the ventral rami after passing through the gray rami. The ventral rami of T6 to L1 emit branches at each segment of the vertebral column (Lykissas et al., 2013; Standring, 2015). The ventral ramus of T12 is larger than the other ventral rami, and gives off a communicating branch to the first lumbar ventral ramus, also referred to as the dorsolumbar nerve. The nerve gives off a collateral branch to innervate the intercostal muscles and the adjacent parietal pleura (Moore et al., 2010; Standring, 2015), while it travels along the inferior border of the 12th rib, accompanied by subcostal vessels. The vein and artery travel superior to the nerve and are hidden within the coastal groove, which leaves the nerve exposed and prone to iatrogenic injury during surgical procedures. The subcostal nerve then courses posterior to the lateral arcuate ligament and kidney, and anterior to the upper region of the quadratus lumborum (Standring, 2015). After it perforates the aponeurosis of the origin of the transversus abdominis, the subcostal nerve continues to course between the transversus abdominis and internal abdominal oblique (Standring, 2015) where it innervates in a similar fashion as the other intercostal nerves (Moore, 2010) distributing muscular branches to the muscles of the anterior abdominal wall (Dakwar et al., 2011; Standring, 2015). The nerve innervates the most inferior part of the external abdominal oblique, the rectus abdominis, and the transversus abdominus ((D'Souza et al., 1994; Fahim et al., 2011; Tokita, 2006), which contributes to its role in respiration. The subcostal nerve then joins with the first spinal nerve of the lumbar plexus, the iliohypogastric nerve, and sends a branch to the pyramidalis (a muscle of the anterior wall that attaches to the pubic symphysis and crest). Innervation by the subcostal nerve allows this muscle to tense the linea alba (Standring, 2015; Tubbs et al., 2015). Similar to the other intercostal nerves, the subcostal nerve has a branch called the lateral cutaneous branch, which pierces the internal and external abdominal oblique muscles supplying the lowest region of the external abdominal oblique. The nerve descends and courses over the iliac crest approximately 5 cm posterior to the anterior superior iliac spine (ASIS) to innervate the anterior gluteal skin, but some filaments may descend as low as the greater trochanter of the femur (Moore et al., 2010; Standring, 2015; Tokita, 2006).

Variations of the Subcostal Nerve

The subcostal nerve does not always contribute to the lumbar plexus (Dakwar et al., 2011; Lovering and Anderson, 2008) with some authors stating that this occurs about half of the time. In addition, studies have highlighted variations in the innervation of the pyramidalis muscle (Tokita, 2006; Williams et al., 2008). One study reported that the anterior rami of T12, L1, and L2 can all give branches to the pyramidalis muscle (Tokita, 2006). D'Souza also found variations in the thickness of the lateral cutaneous branch of the subcostal nerve (D'Souza et al., 1994).

Surgical anatomy of the lateral transpsoas approach to the lumbar spine. https://doi.org/10.1016/B978-0-323-67376-1.00006-9

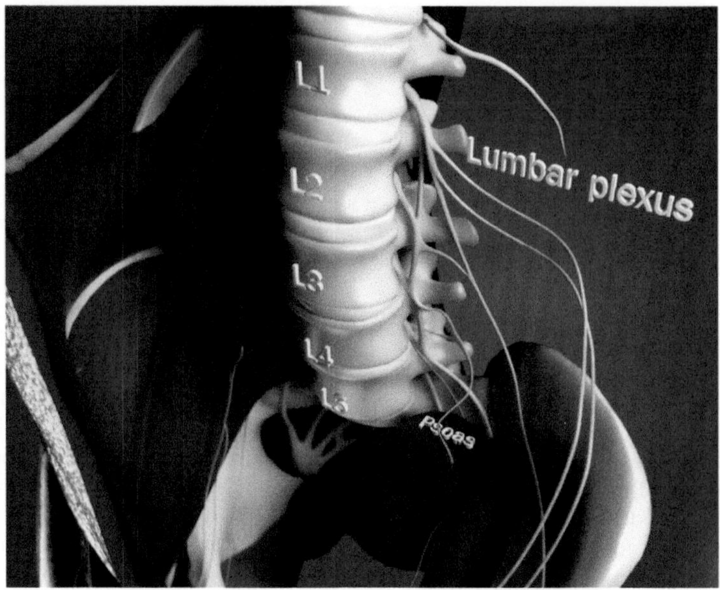

FIG. 6.1 Schematic drawing of the lumbar plexus.

Pathology of the Subcostal Nerve

The subcostal nerve has been implicated in several pathological conditions. One of these is intercostal neuralgia, which is described by literature as a strong, shooting pain over its corresponding dermatome, which can be caused by a nerve entrapment, a tumor, thoracotomy, breast surgery, or conditions like herpes zoster virus (Kim et al., 2015; Nasseh et al., 2013; Ombregt, 2013). Furthermore, Nasseh et al. performed a cross-sectional study on 68 patients who experienced ipsilateral abdominal pain or upper thigh numbness after a percutaneous nephrolithotomy (Nasseh et al., 2013) and found the most commonly affected area was innervated by the subcostal nerve, or T12, dermatome (Ombregt, 2013). In some situations, patients can develop a postoperative neuroma of the subcostal nerve. A retrospective study by Williams et al. reported that a neuroma of the 12th thoracic spinal nerve could occur after an open nephrectomy (Williams et al., 2008). Postoperative abdominal wall bulging (also

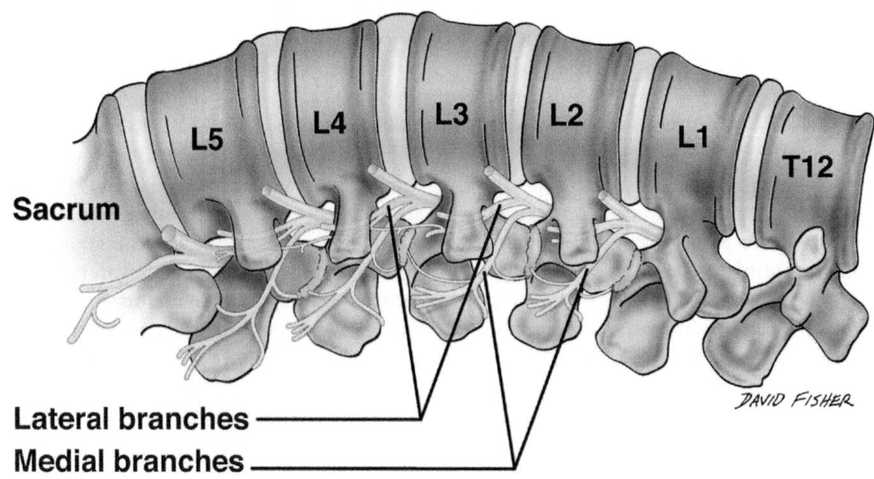

FIG. 6.2 Lateral view of the lumbar spine and its ventral and dorsal rami.

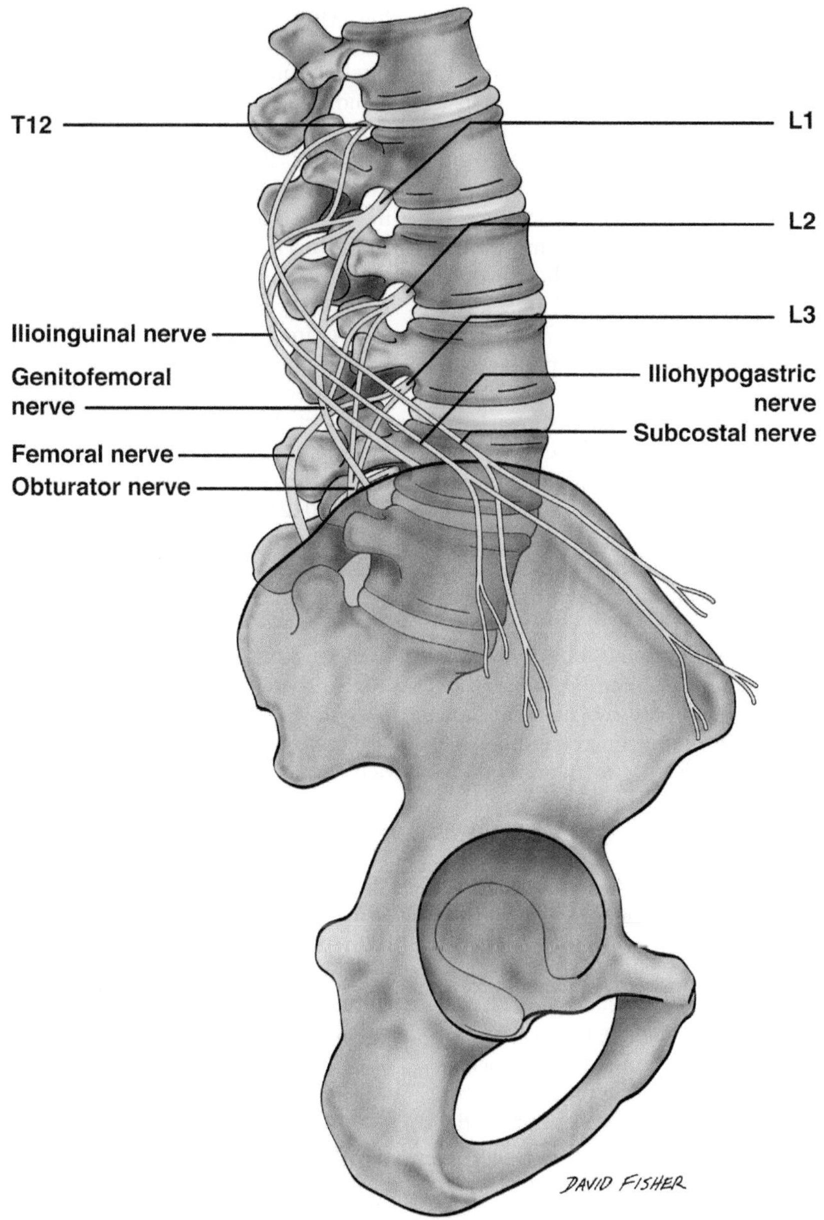

FIG. 6.3 Lateral view of the lumbar plexus and its relationship to the spine and pelvis.

known as a pseudohernia or a flank bulge) can occur if the subcostal nerve has been injured after performing a nephrectomy as well (Tubbs et al., 2015a,b). Flank bulge is also a common complication after lumbotomy for renal surgery. As a result of the initial incision or closing sutures after the procedure, iatrogenic damage to the intercostal and subcostal nerves can develop leading to problems in tissue innervated by the nerve. Damage to these nerves and subsequent denervation results in paralysis, atrophy of its respective muscles, laxity in the muscle, and bulging of the abdominal wall (van der Graaf et al., 2011). Tumors of the subcostal nerve can also compress the conus medullaris of the spinal cord affecting the normal function of the bladder and anus, which presents symptoms similar to saddle anesthesia (Cranfield et al., 1997). Unlike the vein and artery, the subcostal nerve is exposed posteriorly which may leave it susceptible to damage and increase the likelihood of injury when operating on the kidney.

Malposition of the costovertebral joint can cause compression of the intercostal nerve, which can result from a clinical condition with dislocation of the 12th rib, known as slipping rib syndrome. This syndrome, also known as 12th rib syndrome (Machin and Shennan, 1983), is associated with extensive movement of the rib, such that the rib can impinge on the subcostal nerve and cause severe pain (Cranfield et al., 1997). The subcostal nerve can also become entrapped as it pierces the aponeurosis of the rectus sheath, leading to rectus abdominis syndrome (Standring, 2015; Tran et al., 2009). Additionally, some reports have shown that some pain syndromes may be the result of compression of the lateral rami exiting the subcostal and iliohypogastric nerves above the iliac crest (Maigne et al., 1986). Maigne et al. performed an anatomical study of the nerve pathways and pattern of distribution. The rami arising from the subcostal and iliohypogastric nerves cross close together creating a bony groove that is transformed into an osseomembranous tunnel by the aponeurosis of these muscles and can be palpated in thin patients. This region is directly subcutaneous and exposes it to possible friction and microtrauma. As a result, this arrangement can give rise to an entrapment syndrome (Maigne et al., 1986).

Surgical Procedures

The subcostal nerve is involved in different procedures, including ultrasound-guided transversus abdominis nerve blockade which uses the lumbar triangle (of Petit) as a landmark for injections to anesthetize spinal nerves T11-L1 (Chou et al., 2004). Furthermore, reports in the literature show that the subcostal nerve is at risk for iatrogenic injury during certain surgical approaches. D'Souza et al. discovered a variation in the distance between the ASIS and the lateral cutaneous branch of the subcostal nerve while performing an osteotomy (D'Souza et al., 1994). Using the modified Smith-Peterson approach, they found that the lateral cutaneous branch of the subcostal nerve crossed 2–5 cm behind the ASIS, which would be relevant to avoid sensory loss or disturbances while operating in the gluteal region ((D'Souza et al., 1994). Another study by Chou et al. reported that the subcostal nerve was highly likely to be injured while harvesting bone from the iliac crest because the subcostal nerve branches may exist over the iliac crest posterior to the ASIS, where the incision would be made. This study advises surgeons to dissect carefully once reaching 6 cm posterior to the ASIS to avoid injury. It is a general rule that the nerve may be encountered as early as four fingerbreadths behind the ASIS and therefore, surgeons should be extremely cautious when operating in this region. However, if the nerve is accidently cut, it is best to allow the nerve to fall back into healthy tissues and avoid including the nerve during the closing of the fascia (Cahill et al., 2012). The nerve is also at risk for iatrogenic injury during minimally invasive approaches to the lateral spine, specifically during exposure of the upper lumbar vertebrae and can occur while suturing the abdominal wall (Cahill et al., 2012; Tubbs et al., 2015). Authors suggest making an incision parallel to the subcostal nerve to reduce the risk of injury to the subcostal nerve (Cahill et al., 2012).

Although one would naturally assume that injury to the subcostal nerve would impair the function of the muscle it innervates, Standring states that the anterolateral wall of the abdomen is innervated by several branches of segmented spinal nerves (Standring, 2015). Therefore, injury to one spinal nerve is very unlikely to produce any notable loss in muscle tone, unless there was injury to more than one of the spinal nerves that innervate the muscle (Standring, 2015).

THE ILIOHYPOGASTRIC NERVE

The iliohypogastric nerve (Fig. 6.3) is approximately 210 mm in length (Izci et al., 2005) and provides both motor and sensory innervation to numerous structures in the lower abdominopelvic regions. The motor component contributes to the innervation of both the transversus abdominis and internal abdominal oblique muscles that function to maintain abdominal tone, increase intraabdominal pressure, and allow for lateral flexion, particularly for the internal abdominal oblique (Standring, 2016). The sensory component supplies the skin over the hypogastric region, as well as the upper lateral aspect of the thigh and gluteal region (Anloague and Huijbregts, 2009; Griffin, 1891; Klaassen et al., 2011; Papadopoulos and Katritsis, 1981). The nerve is vulnerable during procedures that implicate the peritoneal cavity, pelvis, or perineum, and if damaged intraoperatively, can lead to motor dysfunction of the lower abdominal wall and sensory disturbances in the aforementioned regions.

Anatomy

The iliohypogastric nerve originates in the anterior ramus of the L1 spinal nerve (Klaassen et al., 2011), measuring approximately 4 mm in diameter (Izci et al., 2005). After leaving the L1-L2 intervertebral foramen, the L1 spinal nerve root bifurcates into the iliohypogastric and ilioinguinal nerves, which course posterior to the psoas major (Anloague and Huijbregts, 2009; Standring, 2016). The nerves emerge from the superior lateral margin of the psoas major and posterior to the medial arcuate ligament at the level of L1-L2 (Papadopoulos and Katritsis, 1981). The iliohypogastric nerve, measuring 2.2 mm in diameter, enters the abdominal cavity and descends laterally between the anterior surface of the quadratus lumborum and the posterior surface of the inferior pole of the kidney to continue onto the transverse abdominis (Anloague and Huijbregts, 2009; Linder, 1989; Mahadevan, 2008; Moore and Dalley, 1999; Palastanga et al., 1998; Pratt, 1991; Sauerland, 1994; Standring, 2016; Williams, 2005). The iliohypogastric nerve pierces the surface of the posterior aspect of transverse abdominis and travels parallel to the iliac crest between the transverse abdominis and the internal abdominal oblique. The nerve then divides into two branches giving rise to the lateral cutaneous (iliac) nerve and the hypogastric (anterior) nerve (Anloague and Huijbregts, 2009; Griffin, 1891). The iliac branch pierces the internal abdominal oblique muscles and travels across the tubercle superior to the iliac crest. Immediately superior it pierces the external abdominal oblique aponeurosis and splits into two cutaneous branches with one providing sensory innervation of the skin over the tensor fasciae latae on the lateral aspect of the upper thigh, and the other cutaneous branch providing sensory information of the integument over the gluteus medius and lateral third of gluteus maximus muscles at the level of the greater trochanter. The hypogastric branch continues to travel between the transverse abdominis and internal abdominal oblique muscles, providing motor innervation to both muscles, until reaching the level of the anterior iliac spine, where it enters the internal abdominal oblique muscle. It will then run parallel to the inguinal ligament ventromedially between the internal and external abdominal oblique muscles. Along a vertical line drawn from the midpoint of the outer margin of the superficial abdominal ring, the hypogastric nerve pierces the external abdominal oblique aponeurosis, providing sensory innervation to the suprapubic integument (Griffin, 1891). The iliohypogastric nerve enters the internal abdominal oblique at 1.5–8 cm medial to the ASIS on the left and 2.3–3.6 cm medial to the anterior iliac spine on the right (Avsar et al., 2002). The iliohypogastric nerve pierced the abdominal wall 2.8 ± 1.3 cm (range, 1.1–5.5 cm) medial and 1.4 ± 1.2 cm (range, 0.6–5.1 cm) inferior to the ASIS and coursed on path to terminate 4.0 ± 1.3 cm (range, 2.0–12.6 cm) lateral to the linea alba (Klaassen et al., 2011).

Variations

The iliohypogastric nerve can exhibit variability in several ways. The iliohypogastric nerve may be absent in up to 20% of lumbar plexuses. This absence of the iliohypogastric leads to minimal sensory deficients as the sensory regions of the genitofemoral and ilioinguinal nerves largely overlap with that of the iliohypogastric nerve (Anloague and Huijbregts, 2009). The iliohypogastric nerve can also vary in its point of origin and can be classified into morphological Types I–IV. In 7%, the iliohypogastric nerve arose at T12 and was classed as Type I. Type II, noted in 14%, arose conjointly from T12 and L1. Type III, which occurred in 10%, had its origin from L1, while Type IV (6%) started from both T11 and T12 (Klaassen et al., 2011). The iliohypogastric nerve can also communicate with other nerves in the lumbar plexus including the lateral femoral cutaneous and ilioinguinal via small accessory nerve branches that run over the surface of the transversalis muscle in 5% and 55%, respectively (Bardeen, 1901; Bardeen, 1906; Hollinshead, 1956a,b; Klaassen et al., 2011; Moosman and Oelrich, 1977; Netter, 2003; Sasaoka et al., 2005; Webber, 1961). Additionally, the subcostal nerve can directly contribute to the iliohypogastric nerve (Anloague and Huijbregts, 2009; Bergman et al., 1984; Hollinshead, 1956a,b; Klaassen et al., 2011; Mandelkow and Loeweneck, 1988). Morphological variability of the nerve has been observed as well. For example, the ilioinguinal nerve can be found in place of the hypogastric branch of the iliohypogastric nerve prior to exiting the superficial inguinal ring (Anloague and Huijbregts, 2009). A common trunk between the iliohypogastric and subcostal nerves can be found in as many as 30% of cases. In these cases, the division of the nerve can have three possible locations: posterior to the kidneys, between the internal abdominal oblique muscles and the transversus abdominis, and, in a few cases, between the internal and external abdominal oblique muscles. These common trunks of the iliohypogastric and subcostal nerves can be located dorsal to the lateral arcuate ligament. The nerves separate either within the vicinity of the quadratus lumborum and transversus abdominis muscles or laterally between the internal abdominal oblique and transversus abdominis.

Landmarks

Surgeons should know the relevant landmarks of the iliohypogastric nerve while operating to avoid intraoperative injury, which commonly occurs during an appendectomy, inguinal hernia repair, hysterectomy, or cesarean section. The nerve first appears ventrally on the surface of the quadratus lumborum muscle near the lateral border of the psoas muscle at the L1-L2 vertebral level approximately 1 cm paravertebrally. On the right, the iliohypogastric nerve travels posterior to the central portion of the right kidney, appearing 2 cm superior to the inferior pole on the lateral aspect of the kidney. The left iliohypogastric nerve travels 2 cm higher than the right, at the level of the kidney in 66% of cases. The nerve then traverses the fibers of the transversus abdominis aponeurosis superior to the iliac crest, equidistant from the crest and the tip of the 12th rib. The nerve can be located up to 3 cm medial at the level of the ASIS between the layers of the transversus abdominis and internal abdominal oblique muscles. At this level, the nerve pierces the internal abdominal oblique muscle and courses 4 cm superior and parallel to the inguinal ligament, deep to the aponeurosis of the external abdominal oblique muscle, and with its terminal branches penetrating its aponeurosis 4 cm lateral to the midline. At the lateral peak of the iliac crest between the transversus abdominis and the internal abdominal oblique muscles, the lateral cutaneous branch of the iliohypogastric nerve branches off and innervates the integument superficial to the tensor fasciae latae (Pećina et al., 1997).

Pathology

Iliohypogastricus syndrome results from injury to the iliohypogastric nerve and can cause abdominal dysfunction leading to weakened flexion and rotation. There can be sensory dysfunction associated with episodic pain aggravated by walking or sitting accompanied by stabbing, burning, shooting, or pricking sensation in the lower abdominal region, upper thigh, or pelvic area (Choi et al., 1996; Soldatos et al., 2013; Vuilleumier et al., 2009; Whiteside et al., 2003). The injury may be traumatic in nature such as iatrogenically during surgical procedures or from tractional injuries. The most common surgical causes of iliohypogastric nerve injury arise from incisions within the lower abdominal wall, suture entrapment, ilium harvesting for grafting, lymph node dissection within the inguinal region, femoral catheterization, orchiectomy (Pećina et al., 1997; van Ramshorst et al., 2009), and trocar placement during laparoscopic surgery within the lower abdominal wall (Alfieri et al., 2006). Tractional or entrapment injuries can also occur because the nerve courses between muscular layers leaving it susceptible to being pulled and stretched (Papadopoulos and Katritsis, 1981; Vuilleumier et al., 2009). Injury of the iliohypogastric nerve may also be induced by compressive forces such as tumors arising in the lower kidney or lower lumbar region. These tumors can directly impinge the nerve given the close proximity the nerve has to these structures and can even arise from blunt abdominal trauma, which would lead to the development of a hematoma (Vuilleumier et al., 2009).

Surgery

As previously noted, the major cause of iliohypogastric nerve injury is a result of surgical intervention within the lower abdominal wall. One study using univariate and multivariate analysis showed that failure to identify the iliohypogastric nerve significantly correlated to the presence of chronic pain and the risk of developing inguinal pain (Stulz and Pfeiffer, 1980). This further emphasizes the need for thorough anatomical knowledge of the course of the iliohypogastric nerve to preclude such injuries. Several surgical incisions of the abdominal wall can lead to a particular pathology and can affect the iliohypogastric nerve. For example, particular care should be taken into consideration to avoid injuring the anterior branch of this nerve during an appendectomy when using a lateral incisional approach (Condon and Nyhus, 1971). Surgeons can avoid incising the area 3 cm superior and medial to the ASIS to ensure the safety of the nerve. The iliohypogastric nerve can also be compromised during inguinal hernia repair. When an oblique incision is performed, the anterior branches of the nerve can be injured as the incision is expanded medially (Loos et al., 2008a,b). Incisions of the abdominal wall endanger the iliohypogastric nerve 4 cm superior to the inguinal ligament. Finally, in an oblique lumbar incision (Pfannenstiel incision), the iliohypogastric nerve can be harmed if the dissection is too close to the lateral border of the rectus abdominis muscle. This can potentially lead to the development of a neuroma (Khedkar et al., 2015).

Imaging

Although no studies have been conducted to ascertain which imaging modality is best to visualize the iliohypogastric nerve and associated nerve pathology, several imaging techniques can be used to guide therapy and identify pathology. In preparation for various surgical procedures of the lower abdominal or suprapubic region, iliohypogastric nerve block can be performed with ultrasound guidance. Variations of the nerve were better appreciated using an ultrasound-guided nerve block technique resulting in an increased effectiveness of the anesthetics. This was characterized by a decrease in the required dose or anesthetic preoperatively and a reported decrease in postoperative pain levels (Anloague and Huijbregts, 2009; Courtney et al., 2002; Eichenberger et al., 2006; Papadopoulos and Katritsis, 1981; Pećina et al., 1997). Magnetic resonance neurography can easily reveal an entrapped or enlarged iliohypogastric nerve, although its main function is to visualize tumors along the anatomical pathway of the iliohypogastric nerve. Electrophysiological data are inaccurate for diagnostic purposes, and it may be necessary to achieve nerve block with local anesthesia to confirm this diagnosis (Whiteside et al., 2003).

Treatment

The primary presentation associated with iliohypogastric nerve injury is chronic postoperative pain. There are several approaches to treating postsurgical pain ranging from conservative management to surgical excision of the nerve, depending on the severity of the pain and the patient's preference. In one study of 5506 patients with inguinal hernias undergoing herniography, 125 patients reported severe to extremely severe pain, which remained long term in as many as 25% of patients (Hakeem and Shanmugam, 2011). Antidepressants and antiepileptics seem to be more efficacious in relieving the neuropathic groin pain associated with nerve injury than conventional analgesics such as nonsteroidal antiinflammatory drugs, opioids, and muscle relaxants. However, in most cases, patients experience recurrence because tolerance develops to analgesics (Amid and Hiatt, 2007). Ultrasound-guided nerve blockade has been used to treat the pain associated with iliohypogastric neuropathy with a high accuracy and selectivity (Courtney et al., 2002). It is recommended that surgical intervention be considered at least 6 months postoperatively to allow neuropraxia to disappear on its own or be medically treated.

Surgery is suggested when pain is refractory to the aforementioned treatment options. Neurectomy should be only used after pain relief cannot be achieved through the use of a nerve blockade (Amid and Hiatt, 2007). There is still debate as to whether only the iliohypogastric nerve should be excised in cases of iliohypogastric neuropathy associated with the groin, or if all three nerves supplying the groin region (iliohypogastric, ilioinguinal, and genitofemoral nerves) should be removed. This is because the remaining nerves can still transmit pain signals (Amid and Hiatt, 2007).

THE ILIOINGUINAL NERVE

Anatomy

The ilioinguinal nerve (Fig. 6.4) originates from the anterior rami of the L1 spinal nerve but can often receive contributions from T12, L2, and L3 (Amin et al., 2016; Klaassen et al., 2011; Rab and Dellon, 2001; Schaeffer, 1953; Thane, 1895; Vanetti et al., 2016). It has a diameter of 2.2 mm ranging from 1.3 to 3.3 mm and is inversely proportional to the

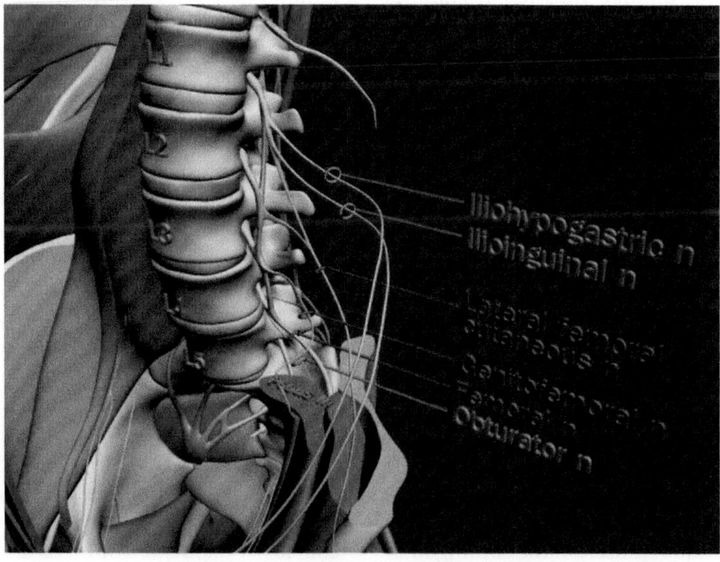

FIG. 6.4 Branches of the lumbar plexus.

iliohypogastric nerve running laterally and inferior to it (Klaassen et al., 2011; Ndiaye et al., 2007). In a minority of cases, 20% according to Klaassen et al., the ilioinguinal nerve forms a common trunk with the iliohypogastric nerve but separates shortly after exiting the intervertebral foramen (Klaassen et al., 2011; Walji and Tsui, 2016). Communicating branches with the subcostal lateral femoral cutaneous nerves (LFCNs) have been reported (Schaeffer, 1953). The ilioinguinal nerve continues laterally as it courses past the proximal and lateral border of the psoas major muscle approximately 4.4–8.6 cm cranial to the posterior superior iliac spine, and more generally passing anterior to the inferior pole of the kidney (Amin et al., 2016; Reinpold et al., 2015; Walji and Tsui, 2016). Continuing to descend inferolaterally (Schaeffer, 1953; Thane, 1895), it travels anterior to the quadratus lumborum and transversus abdominis, moving inferiorly toward the lower pole of the kidney, posterior to the ascending colon when describing the right orientation (descending colon if describing the left orientation). It then pierces the transversus abdominis cranially to the midpoint between the superior iliac spine and the iliac crests, up to 3.0 cm, and in 13% of cases, it passes slightly inferior to the midpoint of the superior iliac spines (Rab and Dellon, 2001; Reinpold et al., 2015). In the transversus abdominis plane (area between the transversus abdominis and internal abdominal oblique), the ilioinguinal nerve may communicate with the hypogastric branch of the iliohypogastric nerve through small accessory fibers (Schaeffer, 1953; Thane, 1895). After traveling for a short distance between the transversus abdominis and internal abdominal oblique muscles, it supplies the inferior fibers of the transversus abdominis with motor innervation. It will also penetrate the internal abdominal oblique and supply motor innervation to the muscle (Amin et al., 2016; Standring, 2015; Tsui, 2016; Walji and Tsui, 2016). According to Avsar et al. (2002), this penetration occurs 4.85 cm inferomedially (ranging from 3 to 6.4 cm) from the ASIS on the right, 3.37 cm inferomedially (ranging from 2 to 5 cm) on the left, 2.99 cm (ranging from 0.2 to 6.1 cm) from McBurney's point on the right, and 3.74 cm (ranging from 1.8 to 7.5 cm) on the left (Avsar et al., 2002). Whiteside et al. found a similar proximity to the ASIS (Whiteside et al., 2003), and in pediatric patients, there was an even closer proximity (Schoor et al., 2005). On a line connecting the ASIS to the umbilicus, the ilioinguinal nerve is 1.9 mm from the ASIS (range 0.61–4.01 mm) on the left and 2.0 mm (range 0.49–3.44 mm) on the right (Schoor et al., 2005). Between the external and internal abdominal oblique muscles, the ilioinguinal nerve is concealed by the fascia of the external abdominal oblique muscle until it reaches the round ligament or spermatic cord (Klaassen et al., 2011; Ndiaye et al., 2007). According to Ndiaye et al., it perforates the external abdominal oblique muscle fascia before reaching the spermatic cord or round ligament in 28.72% of cases allowing the nerve to travel on an extra-aponeurotic path. It passes over the superficial aspect of the internal abdominal oblique muscle about 1.015 cm (range 0–4 cm) from the inguinal ligament, but that distance is less than 1 cm in 66% of cases (Ndiaye et al., 2007). As it passes between the external and internal abdominal oblique muscles, it pierces the canal wall to enter the inguinal canal rather than passing through the deep inguinal ring. According to Rab et al., the ilioinguinal nerve and its sensory aspect course in the inguinal canal through one of two distinct pathways (Rab and Dellon, 2001). In type A (43.7%), the cutaneous aspect of the nerve joins the genitofemoral nerve either between the internal and external abdominal oblique muscles lateral to the deep inguinal ring, within the deep inguinal ring, or near the lateral aspect of the inguinal canal, with the genital branch of the genitofemoral nerve running ventrally on the spermatic cord or round ligament (Rab and Dellon, 2001). In types B (28.1%), C (20.3%), and D (7.8%), the genital branch of the genitofemoral nerve and the cutaneous portion of the ilioinguinal nerve enter the deep inguinal canal, and the ilioinguinal nerve courses on the ventral aspect of the round ligament or spermatic cord (Rab and Dellon, 2001). Types B, C, and D differ mainly in the course of the genital branch of the genitofemoral nerve and genitofemoral branch to the cremaster muscle compared with the round ligament or spermatic cord, but, similar to type A, the ilioinguinal nerve will pass ventral to the spermatic cord (Moosman and Oelrich, 1977; Rab and Dellon, 2001; Standring, 2015). The classification developed by Rab et al. is supported by earlier work from Moosman and Oelrich (1977). In the "aberrant" course described by Moosman and Oelrich, the sensory component of the ilioinguinal nerve was incorporated into the genital branch of the genitofemoral nerve in 35% of cases, located posteriorly within the spermatic cord (or posterior to the round ligament), and continuing inferior, deep to the cremasteric layer (Moosman and Oelrich, 1977); Wijsmuller et al., 2007). This variant path matches the type A classification from Rab et al., while types B–D mirror the "classical" course (Moosman and Oelrich, 1977; Rab and Dellon, 2001; Wijsmuller et al., 2007). However, other literature has reported fewer instances of the variant course (Al-dabbagh, 2002). As it exits the inguinal canal through the superficial inguinal ring, it lies superior to the spermatic cord or round ligament (Al-dabbagh, 2002). After emerging from the superficial inguinal ring with the spermatic cord, the cutaneous aspect of the ilioinguinal nerve supplies the proximal medial thigh, external genitalia, skin over the inguinal canal, anterior hemiscrotum, and the root of the penis in males, or the mons pubis and lateral aspect of labia majora in females (Amin et al., 2016; Moosman and Oelrich, 1977; Schaeffer, 1953; Standring, 2015; Thane, 1895; Tsui, 2016; Vanetti et al., 2016; Walji and Tsui, 2016). The distribution of the genital branch of the genitofemoral nerve overlaps with this area and also provides cutaneous innervation to the anteromedial thigh, anterior hemiscrotum, or mons pubis and labia majora (Rab and Dellon, 2001; Standring, 2015). The overlapping cutaneous distributions of these two nerves were also classified by Rab et al., type A (43.7%) having contributions only from the genital branch of the genitofemoral nerve, type B (28.1%) only from the cutaneous aspect of the ilioinguinal nerve, and the remainder from both nerves. Type C (20.3%) also has cutaneous branches of the ilioinguinal nerve to the mons pubis, inguinal crease, and root of the penis or labia majora, while the genital branch of the genitofemoral nerve innervates the inferior aspects of the inguinal and anteromedial thigh regions. In type D (7.8%), both nerves contribute to these regional distributions (Rab and Dellon, 2001). It should be noted that several studies found the ilioinguinal nerve to be absent in about 7% of inguinal dissections, often unilaterally (Al-dabbagh, 2002; Ndiaye et al., 2007; Salama et al., 1983; Wijsmuller et al., 2007). There have been reports of distal anastomotic terminal branches with the iliohypogastric nerve as well (Rab and Dellon, 2001). The pubic symphysis receives innervation from branches of the iliohypogastric, ilioinguinal, and pudendal nerves.

Pathology

Ilioinguinal nerve injury is commonly iatrogenic in origin, incurred during lower abdominal surgery or by nerve entrapment developed from scarring following surgery and pathological impingement (Amin et al., 2016; Knockaert et al., 1989; Luijendijk et al., 1997; Murinova et al., 2016). The surgeries that frequently injure the ilioinguinal nerve include herniorrhaphy (most common), laparoscopic procedures in abdomen, treatment of stress incontinence in women, and surgeries using a Pfannenstiel incision such as cesarean section births, appendectomy, prostatectomy, inguinal hernioplasty, and abdominal hysterectomy (Amin et al., 2016; Loos et al., 2008a,b; McCrory and Bell, 1999; Poobalan et al., 2003; Purves and Miller, 1986; Whiteside et al., 2003). The nerve can be directly injured during surgery if the path of the incision crosses the nerve or if the nerve is stretched while the surgical field is being manipulated, common in the Pfannenstiel incision and open hernia repairs (Dittrick et al., 2004; Gaines, 1978; Loos et al., 2008a,b; Luijendijk et al., 1997; Wijsmuller et al., 2007). A Pfannenstiel incision is made 2–3 cm superior to the pubic symphysis followed by stretching 8–15 cm, and cutting through the skin, subcutaneous fat, rectus sheath. Cuts will also be made laterally through the fasciae of the transversus abdominis, internal abdominal oblique muscles, and external abdominal oblique muscles. The anterior fascia and linear alba are separated from the rectus and pyramidalis muscles to gain access to the peritoneum causing a midline separation (Loos et al., 2008a,b; Luijendijk et al., 1997; Murinova et al., 2016). This incision and surgical field passes through the area occupied by the ilioinguinal nerve, which can lead to direct injured or injury due to scarring. Open hernia repair can cause ilioinguinal neuralgia as a result of stretching of the abdominal wall, accidental incising of the nerve, or using a mesh that may allow a neuroma to form (Gaines, 1978; Hahn, 2011; Ndiaye et al., 2007; Vernadakis et al., 2003). Direct iatrogenic injury to the nerve is most likely when splitting the internal abdominal oblique aponeurosis, manipulating the spermatic cord or manipulating the surgical field because the ilioinguinal nerve runs parallel to the inguinal canal (Ndiaye et al., 2007; Stark et al., 1999). Surgeons should be cautious when approaching or operating in the triangle of doom, between the vas deferens and the spermatic vessels, and the triangle of pain, the space created by the overlapping courses of the femoral, genitofemoral, and LFCNs. These areas often contribute to the high probability of ilioinguinal nerve injury (Demirer et al., 2006; Reinpold et al., 2015; Rosenberger et al., 2000). Ilioinguinal nerve entrapment can arise from fibrosis and postoperative scar tissue formation. The nerve can also become entrapped from the sutures, stapes, prosthetic materials or mesh from the surgery (Amid, 2004; Amin et al., 2016; Demirer et al., 2006; Loos et al., 2008a,b; Miller et al., 2008; Vernadakis et al., 2003), which can cause the development of a neuroma (Amin et al., 2016; Gaines, 1978; Knockaert et al., 1989; Murinova et al., 2016; Rosenberger et al., 2000). The nerve can also become injured or entrapped as a result of nonsurgical trauma to the lower quadrants of abdominal wall or inguinal region, and stretching of the abdominal walls following pregnancy, endometriosis, or tumors (Hahn, 2011; McCrory and Bell, 1999; Poobalan et al., 2003). Muscle entrapment of the ilioinguinal nerve commonly occurs at the iliac crest, the paravertebral area and the rectus border, classified specifically as an abdominal cutaneous nerve entrapment (Amin et al., 2016; Kopell et al., 1962; Murinova et al., 2016). "Spontaneous entrapment," resulting from trauma to the abdominal wall, usually involves the transverse abdominis and internal abdominal oblique muscles as the nerve courses in a "zigzag fashion" through them (Amin et al., 2016; Knockaert et al., 1989; Kopell et al., 1962). The symptoms of ilioinguinal nerve injury, from entrapment or incision, generally present as sensory changes throughout the nerve distribution (Amin et al., 2016; McCrory and Bell, 1999; Miller et al., 2008; Rab and Dellon, 2001; Vanetti et al., 2016). The clinical triad of symptoms to confirm ilioinguinal nerve injury has some variations, but most often reports of (1) hyperesthesia and/or dysesthesia of the medial aspect of the superior thigh and scrotum or labia majora, (2) pain exacerbated by hip extension and pressure applied to or medially to the ASIS, lateral rectus muscle or the likely area of entrapment, and (3) pain relieved by injections of the ilioinguinal nerve (Amin et al., 2016; Hahn, 2011; Knockaert et al., 1989; Rab and Dellon, 2001; Starling and Harms, 1989; Stulz and Pfeiffer, 1982). Other symptoms include motor weakness; alterations in the cremasteric reflex; chronic "difficult to pin down" pelvic, abdominal, or suprapubic pain; burning pain from the incision to the nerve distribution; a bulge of the abdomen; or a "stabbing pain" during walking due to the extension of the hip joint (Acar et al., 2013; Amin et al., 2016; McCrory and Bell, 1999; Stulz and Pfeiffer, 1982). The ilioinguinal pain or discomfort is diminished by hip flexion and lateral recumbent positioning (Amin et al., 2016; Vanetti et al., 2016). The different locations of entrapment can be detected through palpation, which elicits tenderness for the afflicted nerve. Rectus border entrapment is detected with palpation of the rectus border inferior to the umbilicus (Amin et al., 2016). To detect entrapment around the iliac crest, palpate the free edge of the external abdominal oblique muscle near the iliac crest, and to diagnose paravertebral entrapment, palpate the paravertebral space of L1 (Amin et al., 2016).

The symptoms of ilioinguinal nerve neuralgia are frequently confused with those of appendicitis, tendonitis of the abdominal muscles, lumbar radiculopathy, endometriosis, myofascial pain, upper lumbar facet pathology, interstitial cystitis, rectus sheath neuromas, and irritable bowels (Amin et al., 2016). Clinicians can eliminate these possibilities after identifying the clinical triad, and identifying abdominal or pelvic surgeries in the patient's history (Amin et al., 2016). The overlap of the nerve distribution from the genitofemoral, ilioinguinal, and iliohypogastric nerves complicates the diagnosis because it is possible to have injury to more than one of these nerves (Amin et al., 2016; McCrory and Bell, 1999; Rab and Dellon, 2001).

Surgery

The main operations involving the ilioinguinal nerve are performed either to prevent ilioinguinal neuralgia from presenting postoperatively or to resolve it. During repairs of inguinal hernias through a Lichtenstein herniorrhaphy or laparoscopic approach, the ilioinguinal nerve can be excised in order to avoid postoperative neuralgia, but the long-term effects of this method show some doubt (Alfieri et al., 2011; Barazanchi et al., 2016; Dittrick et al., 2004; Kingman et al., 2016; Khoshmohabat et al., 2012; Malekpour et al., 2008; Moosman, 1977; Mui et al., 2006; Picchio et al., 2004). For laparoscopic surgeries, Kingman et al. suggest excision of the ilioinguinal nerve as it traverses over the quadratus lumborum muscle, with clips secured proximal and distal to the site of excision. This potentially prevents neuroma formation and may provide a radiographic landmark if a nerve block procedure is required postoperatively (Kingman et al., 2016). For open hernia repair, Malekour et al. and Khoshmohabat et al. recommend neurectomy 1–2 cm lateral to the deep inguinal ring, with 3–4 cm of nerve excised. Mui et al. recommend excising the ilioinguinal nerve from its entrance to the rectus abdominis muscle to "as lateral of the deep ring as possible." However, it should be noted that there is no standardized method for ilioinguinal neurectomy due to the lack of evidence (Alfieri et al., 2011; Barazanchi et al., 2016; Picchio et al., 2004; Wijsmuller). Alternatively, nerve blocks and resections are the most common methods for relieving ilioinguinal neuralgia resulting from pelvic or abdominal surgery. Ilioinguinal nerve blocks can either be performed blind using landmarks and fascial clicks, but are more commonly performed with ultrasound guidance. When landmarks alone are used, the ASIS is identified and the needle is inserted one-fourth to one-third lateral from the ASIS on a path towards the umbilicus (Bugada and Peng, 2015; Tsui, 2016). However, van Schoor et al. suggested that 2.5 mm from the ASIS would be a more accurate injection site in a pediatric patient (Schoor et al., 2005; Tsui, 2016). The needle, inserted either at a 45° angle or perpendicularly, produces a "click" after piercing the internal abdominal oblique muscle (Tsui, 2016). The first sound may be heard when the external abdominal oblique muscle is initially pierced, but in this location it could be an aponeurosis from the muscle. Levobupivacaine or bupivacaine is injected once the fascial "click" of the internal abdominal oblique muscle is heard, and the injection is in position as the nerve courses between the transversus abdominis and internal abdominal oblique muscles (Bugada and Peng, 2015; Tsui, 2016). For the injection, the angle of the needle can be placed in the direction of the groin or umbilicus with the needle angle maintained while applying the anesthetic. After injecting anesthetic superficial to the internal abdominal oblique, the needle can slowly be withdrawn as the anesthetic is applied back out of the external abdominal oblique muscle (Tsui, 2016). The complications of the procedure lie with improper needle placement, usually associated with difficulty identifying the fascial planes, leading to colonic puncture, femoral nerve block, or injection into the peritoneum (Bugada and Peng, 2015).

To increase the accuracy of ilioinguinal nerve blocks, ultrasound is frequently used to ensure the correct placement of the needle. For an ultrasound-guided nerve block, a high-frequency linear probe, 6–15 MHz, is used with the patient lying supine (Hong et al., 2010; Tsui, 2016). For obese patients, a medium frequency and a curved probe is used, and recent literature demonstrates that a lateral decubitus position has proven to be beneficial (Mathers et al., 2015; Tsui, 2016). The ASIS is identified and the probe is used to trace the trajectory to the umbilicus (Amin et al., 2016; Hong et al., 2010; Thomassen et al., 2013; Tsui, 2016). The abdominal wall layers must be identified along with the iliohypogastric and ilioinguinal nerves that lie between the internal abdominal oblique muscle and either the external abdominal oblique or the transversus abdominis muscle (Thomassen et al., 2013; Tsui, 2016). This visualization is more evident in pediatric patients, but fluid may be required for contrast in adults (Tsui, 2016). However, if visualization is unsuccessful, anesthetic can be placed in the planes superficial and deep to the internal abdominal oblique muscle (Tsui, 2016). The needle can be inserted either "in-plane," medial, or lateral at a shallow angle towards the anterior superior iliac. The needle can be placed "out-of-plane" at a 45° angle, but with the probe positioned obliquely (Tsui, 2016). In both approaches, the location of the needle, ultrasound is used to confirm correct position. The anesthetic that surrounds the nerves will appear hypoechoic (Gofeld and Christakis, 2006; Tsui, 2016). Fluoroscopy can also be used for a nerve block, which mirrors the procedures of a nerve root block or transforaminal epidural rather than that of the ultrasound-guided technique (Amin et al., 2016). A peripheral nerve stimulator is used to identify the pathology. When approaching for paravertebral injections, fluoroscopy is used on a patient lying prone to identify the foramen, and a peripheral nerve stimulator is used to distinguish the ilioinguinal nerve from a selective nerve root technique (Amin et al., 2016). The other main solution to ilioinguinal neuralgia is neurectomy. There are many approaches to the ilioinguinal nerve, but all of them start with a nerve block using the procedures previously highlighted (Aasvang and Kehlet, 2005; Hahn, 2011). Kline et al. describe a method using vital blue dye along with the anesthetic during the nerve block in order to stain the relevant areas. The incision is made above the injection site and through the external abdominal oblique aponeurosis, which is where the dye should be found (Kline et al., 2013). The stained tissue is resected with the accompanying nerve portion, including the external abdominal oblique fascia, subcutaneous fat, and potentially the internal abdominal oblique muscle (Kline et al., 2013). If opening the scar tissue superior to the external abdominal oblique aponeurosis is not an option, Campanelli et al. suggest approaching anteriorly with a transverse incision over the inguinal canal. This approach implicates identifying the surgical equipment responsible, such as sutures or mesh from previous abdominal or pelvic surgery, removing the ilioinguinal nerve from its entrapment, and then excising the nerve. Using a similar incision, the ilioinguinal nerve can be accessed for resection as it crosses over the ASIS or the quadratus lumborum muscle, cranial to the psoas major (Campanelli et al., 2013). Hahn suggests a 6–8 cm oblique incision from the anterior iliac spine, which allows the external abdominal oblique fascia to be accessed and incised. The ilioinguinal nerve, medial and deep to the iliac spine, can be identified, cauterized, and then transected (Hahn, 2011).

THE LATERAL FEMORAL CUTANEOUS NERVE

Anatomy and Function

The LFCN is formed by contributions from the ventral rami of the L2 and L3 spinal nerves (Fig. 6.4). It is a cutaneous nerve providing innervation to the lateral aspect of the thigh. Along its highly variable course, it initially emerges from beneath the lateral border of the psoas muscle and traverses the pelvis by running obliquely past the iliacus muscle. It then approaches the ASIS parallel to the iliac crest where it will proceed to exit the pelvis. At this point, the LFCN distributes sensory innervation to the parietal peritoneum of the iliac fossa. On the left side, it passes behind the lower segment of the descending colon, and on the right side, it courses posterolaterally past the cecum. It exits the pelvis and enters the thigh region by piercing through the fascia lata beneath the inguinal ligament (Apaydin, 2015; Mirjalili, 2015). As it travels through the thigh and beneath the inguinal ligament, the LFCN courses subcutaneously laterally and distally. Along its descent through the thigh, it divides into anterior and posterior branches. 10 cm distal to the ASIS, its anterior branch becomes superficial providing sensory innervation from the skin of the anterolateral thigh down to the knee. The anterior branch also connects with cutaneous branches of the anterior femoral nerve and the infrapatellar branch of the saphenous nerve to form the peripatellar plexus. The posterior branch pierces through the fascia lata superior to the anterior branch and further divides to provide innervation from the lateral skin of the greater trochanter to halfway down the thigh. This nerve can also be responsible for supplying the gluteal skin (Apaydin, 2015; Mirjalili, 2015). An analysis of the LFCN by Ray et al. revealed that this nerve is usually flattened at the inguinal ligament, where it is engulfed by a concentrically arranged thick perineurium (Ray et al., 2010). Its mean cross-sectional area at this point was recorded as 1.921 ± 0.414 mm^2. The LFCN was also found to contain three to six fascicles at this location, with a mean of 4.5 fascicles per nerve and a mean fascicular area of 0.647 ± 0.176 mm^2. The cadaveric study by Ray et al. also reported that the mean distance from the ASIS to the point at which the LFCN passes the inguinal ligament is 1.87 ± 0.48 cm, and the average distance from the ASIS to the point at which it crosses the lateral border of the sartorius muscle is 6.15 ± 1.79 cm (Ray et al., 2010).

Variations

As mentioned earlier, the exact path taken by the LFCN during its descent through the pelvis and anterolateral thigh has a great deal of variation. De Ridder et al. found some degree of anatomical variation in the LFCN in at least 25% of the patient population (De Ridder et al., 1999). This variability may contribute to the occurrence of iatrogenic injury to the nerve during surgical procedures as a result of the inability to predict the nerve's exact course (Carai et al., 2009; Dibenedetto et al., 1996; Williams and Trzil, 1991). The first source of variability lies in the nerves that contribute to the formation of the LFCN. Normally, it arises from the posterior divisions of L2 and L3, but evidence has proven the LFCN can also arise from L1 and L2 ("high form"), and from L3 and L4 ("low form"). It may also emerge from the femoral nerve or as a distinct branch of the lumbar plexus (Apaydin, 2015). Sim and Web found that the LFCN arose from the first two lumbar nerves in 22 of 60 subjects, solely from the L2 ventral ramus in one subject, and from the femoral nerve in six subjects, with almost half showing some degree of variation in the nerves from which the LFCN was derived (Sim and Webb, 2004). Webber identified at least eight distinct patterns of neural origin and derivatives of the LFCN (Bergman et al., 1988). Carai et al. (2009) found that the LFCN was absent in almost 9% of patients who required operative intervention for meralgia paresthetica (Carai et al., 2009). Some specimens have shown an absence of the nerve on either side, but with anterior femoral cutaneous nerve acting in its place (Bergman et al., 1988). Another significant area of variability is the point at which the LFCN exits the pelvis and enters the thigh region. Normally, it exits medial to the ASIS, while it runs underneath the inguinal ligament (Tomaszewski et al., 2016). Aszmann et al. distinguished five categories of anatomical variation in the LFCN's exit from the pelvis and entry to the thigh during their cadaveric studies, which have been corroborated by other studies (Aszmann et al., 1997; Majkrzak et al., 2010; Ropars et al., 2009; Surucu et al., 1997). Aszmann et al. defined type A with the LFCN running posterior to the ASIS and across the iliac crest; type B as anterior to the ASIS and superficial to the sartorius muscle, but within the inguinal ligament; type C as medial to the ASIS, and enclosed fully within the tendinous origin of the sartorius muscle; type D as medial to the sartorius muscle, and deep to the inguinal ligament, while running between the tendon of the sartorius and the thick fascia of the iliopsoas muscle; and type E as the most medial, deep to the inguinal ligament, and embedded within a sheet of loose connective tissue. It was also noted that type E contributed to the femoral branch of the genitofemoral nerve (Aszmann et al., 1997; Cheatham et al., 2013). Finally, there are reports of a variety of branching patterns with bifurcations within the pelvis, in the thigh, and near the point where the nerve will exit the pelvis. Grothaus et al. found that the LFCN bifurcates into additional branches before traveling underneath the inguinal ligament in 27.6% of 29 cadavers studied (Grothaus et al., 2005). Rudin et al. recently proposed a classification system for the various branching patterns seen when the LFCN travels past the ASIS. In the sartorius-type pattern, a dominant anterior branch travels along the lateral border of the sartorius muscle with only a very thin posterior branch. The posterior-type has a posterior branch at least as thick as the anterior branch. This posterior branch leaves laterally and travels across the medial border of the tensor fascia latae muscle, which lies distal to the ASIS. Finally, the fan-type pattern displays many branches of similar thickness that fan out across the anterolateral thigh, traveling across the lateral border of the sartorius and the tensor fasciae latae muscles (Rudin et al., 2016). Trifurcation and quadrification have also been reported in a few studies (Surucu et al., 1997; Tomaszewski et al., 2016).

Pathology and Surgery

Given the unpredictable course of the LFCN and the number of anatomical variations reported in the literature, the nerve is extremely vulnerable to iatrogenic or accidental injury. This risk is greatest along the anterior or anterolateral proximal thigh, when it courses alongside the inguinal ligament. Mechanisms of iatrogenic injury include accidental damage to the nerve during incision, suture ligation, and transection of the nerve. This occurs most often during procedures involving the abdomen, pelvis, or hip. Surgeries that can injure the LFCN include inguinal hernia repair, inguinal lymph node biopsy, femoral artery catheterization, and any procedure involving an anterior or anterolateral approach to the hip or an ilioinguinal approach to the acetabulum. Noniatrogenic injury can occur secondary to use of belts and braces, or as a result of trauma (Mirjalili, 2015). Irritation of the LFCN produces a syndrome referred to as meralgia paresthetica (Bernhard-Roth syndrome), which occurs secondary to entrapment of the LFCN as it exits in the pelvis and passes deep to or through the inguinal ligament (Ray et al., 2010). Meralgia paresthetica produces a symptomology of pain, paresthesias, and loss of sensory functionality within the distribution of the LFCN along the anterolateral thigh (Cheatham et al., 2013). The syndrome was first described by Hager and further defined by Roth, who also named the nerve (Hager, 1885; Roth, 1895). Its incidence may be higher in diabetic patients and those with a long-term history of strenuous activities (Cheatham et al., 2013; Parisi et al., 2011; Ulkar et al., 2003). Other associated factors include obesity, constricting garments, postural alterations, and activities or physical states such as pregnancy that place a greater demand on the abdominopelvic region. The LFCN is most susceptible to compression and iatrogenic injury at its emergence from the pelvis, and the high variability in that region contributes to the development of meralgia paresthetica following surgical procedures within close proximity (Sunderland, 1970).

Meralgia paresthetica commonly occurs in patients with hip replacement procedures and spine surgeries (Cheatham et al., 2013). Analyses of patients undergoing hip surgery have revealed a high incidence of postoperative LFCN neuropraxia. Goulding et al. found that complications arose in 91% of patients who underwent anterior approach hip resurfacing and 67% of those who underwent anterior approach total hip arthroplasty (Goulding et al., 2010). Rudin et al. concluded that iatrogenic injury to the LFCN during anterior hip procedures could be avoided depending on the type of branching pattern it follows as it passes the ASIS. For a sartorius-type branching pattern, a more lateral incision further from the lateral border of the sartorius muscle is recommended. The posterior-type and fan-type branching patterns are more susceptible to incisions, and those made more laterally may not prevent injury. Rudin et al. recommend restricting skin incisions to superficial levels of the subcutaneous tissue. They also posit that injury to the posterior branch could be prevented by blunt dissection techniques and proximal mobilization of the branch with its accompanying vessels (Rudin et al., 2016). Gupta et al. found that 12% of their patients who underwent posterior lumbar spine surgery had postoperative neuropraxia within the region innervated by the LFCN (Gupta et al., 2004). They hypothesized that because patients are placed in a prone position for prolonged periods during this procedure, the resultant compression of the anterior hip leads to development of meralgia paresthetica (Cheatham et al., 2013; Gupta et al., 2004). Others have reported a similar incidence of LFCN neuropraxia following spinal procedures where patients were placed in a prone position (Cho and Lee, 2008; Yang et al., 2005).

THE GENITOFEMORAL NERVE

Anatomy

The genitofemoral nerve (historically known as the genitocrural nerve) arises from the lumbar plexus (Fig. 6.3). It is formed by the union of spinal nerve branches from L1 and L2 ventral rami within the psoas major muscle. The second lumbar nerve provides the majority of the contributions to this nerve, although it is also partly derived from the first lumbar nerve and the connective fibers between the first and second lumbar nerves (Schaeffer, 1953; Schafer and Thane, 1895; Standring, 2016). Although the anatomy of this nerve is well described, a wide range of variety exists among its anatomical path, and many variations have been identified (Rab and Dellon, 2001). The nerve innervates components of both the external genital organs and parts of the thigh (Cesmebasi et al., 2015; Maldonado et al., 2014; Schafer and Thane, 1895). Awareness of these variations is important, especially for surgeons who operate in the lower abdominal, pelvic, and upper leg areas. This understanding helps to avoid iatrogenic injury to fibers of the genitofemoral nerve (Cesmebasi et al., 2015; Tagliafico et al., 2015).

Anatomy and Variations

The genitofemoral nerve is formed within the psoas major muscle and is derived from both the first and second lumbar nerves. When comparing these contributions, the vast majority arise from the second lumbar nerve although the genitofemoral nerve does receive some input from the first lumbar nerve as well as communicating fibers between L1 and L2 (Schafer and Thane, 1895; Standring, 2016). Once formed within the psoas muscle, the genitofemoral nerve courses in the muscle and emerges from the medial border of the psoas muscle at the L3-L4 vertebral level traveling obliquely and inferiorly. At this point, the genitofemoral nerve lies on fascia that covers the anterior surface of the psoas muscle (Brown et al., 2000; Schafer and Thane, 1895), which will then divide into an internal or genital branch, and an external or femoral (crural) branch. This point of division can occur at variable heights but is most often proximal to the inguinal ligament shortly after crossing the ureter posteriorly (Schaeffer, 1953; Schafer and Thane, 1895; Standring, 2016). In some cases, it divides closer to its origin of the plexus, where the two separate branches will travel through the psoas muscle along a variety of trajectories (Rab and Dellon, 2001; Schafer and Thane, 1895; Standring, 2016). The genital branch of the genitofemoral nerve (also termed as the external spermatic nerve in males) is found proximal to the external iliac artery where it crosses the inferior portion of the artery. It continues into the deep inguinal ring after perforating the transversalis fascia and courses through spermatic cord in males or the round ligament in females. The genital branch goes on to provide motor innervation to the cremaster muscle in males and cutaneous innervation to the external genitalia in both males and females (Schaeffer, 1953; Schafer and Thane, 1895; Standring, 2016). The femoral branch (crural branch) descends inferiorly along the psoas muscle and lateral to the external iliac artery. It then traverses over the deep circumflex iliac artery and continues behind the inguinal ligament on its descent to enter the femoral sheath, which lies lateral to the femoral artery (Cesmebasi et al., 2015; Rab and Dellon, 2001; Schaeffer, 1953; Schafer and Thane, 1895; Standring, 2016). Evidence has shown the femoral branch communicating with the middle cutaneous branch of the anterior femoral nerve, and some supporting filaments may attach it to the femoral artery (Schafer and Thane, 1895). It is important to be aware of the anatomical variations that can exist at the origin, course, and point of division because of its vulnerability to iatrogenic injury during particular procedures, especially abdominal incisions (Brown et al., 2000). Variations may exist in the division of this nerve because the genital and femoral branches may arise independently from the lumbar plexus in certain individuals. Occasionally, the genital branch will come from the last thoracic and first lumbar nerves (Schafer and Thane, 1895). Another variation observed is the absence of one division completely, or the nerve entirely. In these cases, the fibers that normally contribute to the genitofemoral nerve will join another nerve instead. The fibers that typically form the genital branch may be associated with the ilioinguinal nerve, and the fibers that normally contribute to the femoral nerve may be interlocked with the external cutaneous or anterior femoral nerves (Schafer and Thane, 1895; Standring, 2016). The genitofemoral nerve may also penetrate the psoas muscle across varying distances and locations. An analysis by Rab and colleagues demonstrated that in roughly two-thirds of sampled specimens, the nerve is observed with a single nerve trunk penetrating the psoas muscle between 4 and 12 cm from the sacral prominence. After traveling an average of 7 cm (±3.5 cm), it divides into its two branches. In the remaining one-third of specimens, the branches penetrated the psoas muscle independently of each other and descended as separate nerve fibers. In these cases, the distance between the site of penetration and the sacral prominence ranged from 1.5 to 13 cm for the femoral branch, and from 4 to 13 cm for the genital branch (Rab and Dellon, 2001). Surgeons should consider variations in the course of the genitofemoral nerve as it courses through the lower abdominal and pelvic regions. Three varying trajectories of the genitofemoral nerve have been distinguished on the basis of the nerve's course along the psoas muscle (Geh et al., 2015). In the first, the genitofemoral nerve emerges from the psoas muscle as a single trunk and bifurcates into the genital and femoral branches. In the second category, it emerges from the psoas muscle as a single trunk but continues inferiorly as a single trunk toward the inguinal ligament. In the third category, the genital and femoral branches emerge separately from the psoas muscle. Studies found that the first category was most common, seen in about 50% of cases. The second category was observed in 30% and identified the third category in 20% of specimens (Geh et al., 2015). There are clinical applications and surgical significance at the vertebral level at which the genitofemoral nerve emerges from the psoas muscle. Using the transverse process of L2 and the iliac crest as landmarks, studies show that the nerve can emerge superior to the L2 transverse process, between the L2 transverse process and the iliac spine, or inferior to the iliac crest. A recent analysis found that the nerve emerges from between the L2 transverse process and the iliac spine in 70% of specimens, inferior to the iliac crest in 20% of cases, and superior to the L2 transverse process in 10% (Geh et al., 2015). Understanding the possible anatomical variations will help surgeons avoid unintended iatrogenic injury.

Innervation and Functional Variations

The genitofemoral branch carries both sensory and motor fibers. The genital branch provides motor innervation to the cremaster muscle and sensory innervation to the anterior third of the scrotum in males, but in females, supplies the mons pubis and labium majora. The femoral branch is responsible for cutaneous innervation to the anteromedial thigh (Cesmebasi et al., 2015; Rab and Dellon, 2001; Schaeffer, 1953; Standring, 2016). Although the innervation and function of the genitofemoral branch have been well established, variations do exist in the innervation patterns observed across individuals, and four different cutaneous branching patterns have been observed in the inguinal region. Adding further complexity, a recent analysis by Rab et al. showed that only 40.6% of cases studied displayed bilateral symmetry (Rab and Dellon, 2001). The first pattern of innervation was identified in 43.7% of cases, and described as having a dominant genitofemoral nerve, with no sensory contributions from the ilioinguinal nerve. The skin of the pubis, ventral scrotum/labia, and ventromedial thigh was innervated by the genital branch of the genitofemoral nerve, which entered the inguinal canal through the deep inguinal ring and coursed along the ventral surface of the spermatic cord. The nerve was also responsible for supplying motor innervation to the cremaster muscle in the male specimens. The cutaneous division of the genital branch coursed along the dorsal aspect of the spermatic cord/round ligament as it exited through the superficial inguinal ring (Rab and Dellon, 2001). The second pattern of innervation was observed in 28.1% of specimens and was described as having a dominant ilioinguinal nerve. In this pattern, the genitofemoral nerve shared a branch with the ilioinguinal nerve, and supplied motor innervation to the cremaster muscle, but gave no sensory contributions to the groin area. The skin of the pubis, ventral scrotum/labia, and ventromedial thigh was innervated by the cutaneous component of the ilioinguinal nerve. The genital branch of the genitofemoral nerve entered the inguinal canal through the deep inguinal ring and coursed along the ventral side of the spermatic cord, supplying motor innervation to the cremaster muscle. In male cadavers, it shared several branches with the cutaneous division of the ilioinguinal nerve within the inguinal canal and became integrated into the ilioinguinal nerve in the female cadavers with no cutaneous branches from the nerve in males or females (Rab and Dellon, 2001). The third pattern of innervation was observed in 20.3% of specimens and contained a dominant genitofemoral branch. The ilioinguinal nerve supplied sensory fibers to the mons pubis and inguinal crease together with an interproximal part of the root of the penis or labia majora. The cutaneous division of the genital branch of the genitofemoral nerve supplied the remaining lower parts of the inguinal and ventromedial thigh areas. The genital branch and the ilioinguinal nerve both entered the inguinal canal similar to the second pattern of innervation. The genital branch contained both motor fibers for the cremaster muscle and cutaneous fibers. The cutaneous division of the ilioinguinal nerve and motor supply to the cremaster muscle from the genitofemoral nerve both coursed ventrally to the spermatic cord, whereas the cutaneous division of the genital branch of the genitofemoral nerve coursed dorsally. In females, it ran along the dorsal side of the round ligament (Rab and Dellon, 2001).

The fourth pattern of innervation was observed in 7.7% of specimens, and had the cutaneous branches emerging from both the genitofemoral and ilioinguinal nerves. In these individuals, the ilioinguinal nerve supplied the mons pubis and inguinal crease together with the anteroproximal part of the root of the penis and labia majora. The pattern of entrance into the inguinal canal, and the relationship of the motor and cutaneous divisions of both the genitofemoral and ilioinguinal nerves to the spermatic cord/round ligament showed similarities to the third pattern of innervation previously described. However, in the fourth category, the ilioinguinal nerve contributed cutaneous innervations to the pubis, inguinal, and ventromedial thigh regions (Rab and Dellon, 2001).

Clinical Significance and Injury

The genitofemoral nerve is susceptible to injury during abdominal procedures, particularly those involving the left and/or right lower quadrants, or the psoas muscle (Cesmebasi et al., 2015; Rab and Dellon, 2001; Schaeffer, 1953; Schafer and Thane, 1895; Standring, 2016). The resulting condition is termed genitofemoral neuralgia and characterized by a pattern of chronic neuropathic pain that can become debilitating (Cesmebasi et al., 2015). The condition results in constant or intermittent pain in the regions innervated by the genitofemoral nerve and its terminal branches. This pain and discomfort usually increases when walking, standing, stooping, or performing hip extension, but relieved by recumbency. The clinical symptoms present are groin pain, paresthesias, and a burning sensation extending from lower abdomen to the medial aspect of the thigh (Cesmebasi et al., 2015; Verstraelen et al., 2015). Most commonly, this neuropathy results from iatrogenic injury to the genitofemoral nerve during surgical procedures such as femoral or inguinal herniorrhaphy. As a result of the overlap among the cutaneous distribution of the genitofemoral nerve, the other inguinal nerves, and the variability in cutaneous innervations described previously, selective nerve blocking is often a necessary diagnostic tool. Genitofemoral neuralgia can be treated with both invasive and noninvasive procedures ranging from TCAs, combination of analgesic and anesthetic injections to radiofrequency ablation, cryoablation, nerve blocking techniques, and neurectomy (Acar et al., 2013; Cesmebasi et al., 2015; Shanthanna, 2014). Some cases may have difficulties when trying to identify a single nerve as the cause of neuropathy, and a paravertebral block of the L1 and L2 nerve plexus, or a triple neurectomy will be necessary to relieve pain (Cesmebasi et al., 2015; Brown et al., 2000).

The genitofemoral nerve is also thought to play a role in the inguinoscrotal phase of testicular descent (Hutson et al., 2013; Standring, 2016). Animal models have highlighted the important role this nerve may play in successful descent of the testes (Cousinery et al., 2016; Su et al., 2012). Hutson and colleagues detailed the different stages of testicular descent and extrapolated data from murine to human males. They noted that calcitonin gene-related peptide (CGRP) is critical for testicular descent. CGRP, which is released by the genitofemoral nerve, induces rhythmic contractility in the developing cremaster muscle of the gubernaculum and provides a chemotactic gradient that stimulates gubernacular migration toward the scrotum. It was also proposed that exposure of the genitofemoral nerve to androgens is essential for its masculinization and for preprogramming the gubernacular proliferative response to CGRP (Cousinery et al., 2016; Hutson et al., 2013; Su et al., 2012).

THE FEMORAL NERVE

The femoral nerve (Figs. 6.3-6.5), which is the largest branch of the lumbar plexus, runs laterally and caudally through the psoas major muscle and anterior to the iliacus muscle (the latter of which it supplies) at a mean sagittal angle of approximately 27.78 degrees (Anloague and Huijbregts, 2009; Cho Sims et al., 2016; Choy et al., 2013; Pećina et al., 1997; Van Beek, 1998). It originates from the posterior divisions of the ventral rami of the second, third, and fourth lumbar spinal nerves within the psoas major muscle (approximately 9 cm from the skin surface) and runs between the LFCN and the obturator nerve (Farny et al., 1994; Gustafson et al., 2009; Moore and Stringer, 2011). The femoral nerve emerges from the lateral border of the psoas major muscle 4 cm superior to the inguinal ligament and beneath the fascia of the iliacus muscle (Gustafson et al., 2009). After entering the retroperitoneal space and tracing the ilium, it follows the external iliac vessels, exits the pelvis via the femoral canal, and enters the thigh traveling along the iliacus muscle while passing under the inguinal ligament through the lateral space of the lacuna muscularis, which is approximately half the medial-lateral distance between the ASIS and the pubic symphysis (Gustafson et al., 2009; Pećina et al., 1997; Van Beek, 1998). It enters the thigh lateral to the femoral artery, which lies outside the femoral sheath (Choy et al., 2013; Gustafson et al., 2009). The femoral nerve emerges from beneath the inguinal ligament about midway between the ASIS and the pubic tubercle. The femoral neurovascular bundle is contained within the femoral triangle at the level of the inguinal crease and covered by layers of skin, fat, and fascia lata (Vloka et al., 1999). The femoral triangle is formed laterally by the sartorius muscle, medially by the adductor longus muscles, and superiorly by the inguinal ligament (Vloka et al., 1999). Approximately, 1.50 ± 0.47 cm distal to the inguinal ligament (others have reported a distance of 3–5 cm), before the femoral crease, the femoral nerve splits into numerous posterior and anterior branches. These branches have been observed in 80% of cases to be divided by the lateral circumflex femoral artery (Gustafson et al., 2009; Lonchena et al., 2006; Moore and Stringer, 2011; Orebaugh, 2006; Pećina et al., 1997). One anatomical study showed that most cadavers (83.3%) possessed a

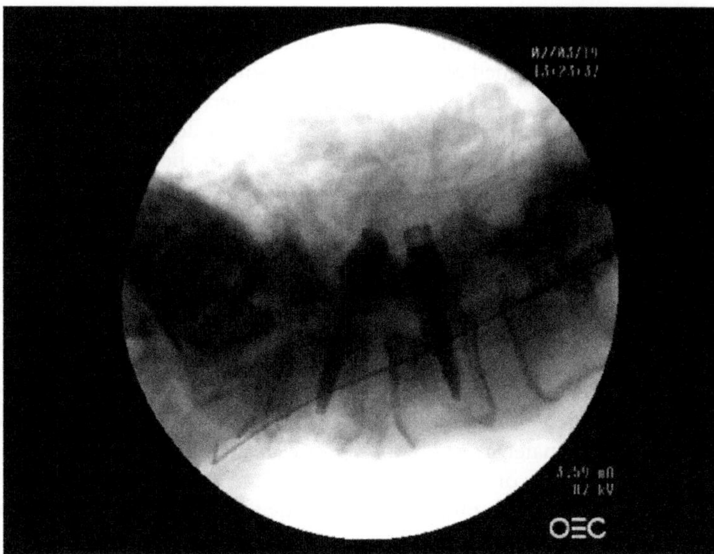

FIG. 6.5 Lateral fluoroscopy of the relationship of the lumbosacral spine and femoral nerve with a metal wire laid along its course.

femoral nerve located anterior to the deep femoral artery, whereas the femoral nerves in the remainder were posterior to this structure (16.7%) (Choy et al., 2013). The nerve receives its blood supply from the iliolumbar artery when traveling through the pelvis, the deep circumflex iliac artery when traversing the inguinal region, and the lateral circumflex femoral artery upon entering the thigh (Moore and Stringer, 2011). Some have discovered that the deep circumflex iliac artery on the left side gives fewer branches than its equivalent on the right, potentially rendering the femoral nerve on left side more susceptible to ischemic injury (Moore and Stringer, 2011). Three different lymphatic routes have been known to drain the femoral nerve. In the iliac fossa, one or two routes may drain the femoral nerve, which then moves to lymph nodes near the external iliac artery (Sunderland, 1978). The third lymphatic route drains to the lymph nodes near the femoral canal after leaving the nerve where the femoral nerve passes under the inguinal ligament (Sunderland, 1978). The femoral nerve displays a variation in its structure and relationship with other structures as it descends into the leg. It is nearly 50% wider and significantly closer to the fascia lata (6.8 vs. 26.4 mm) at its location in the inguinal crease rather than at the inguinal ligament (Vloka et al., 1999). It is partially covered by the femoral artery at the level of the inguinal crease in approximately 70% of cases, but 11.7% of cases in the inguinal ligament region (Vloka et al., 1999). The spatial arrangement within the femoral neurovascular bundle seems more consistent at the level of the inguinal crease (where the nerve is also more superficial) than at the level of the inguinal ligament (Vloka et al., 1999). Ultrasound imaging has shown that as the nerve travels distally it becomes flatter, wider, and less compact (Lonchena et al., 2016). Below the inguinal ligament, the branch-free length of the nerve is approximately 1.0–1.5 cm (Gustafson et al., 2009). Cross sections of the compound femoral nerve (the portion of the nerve between the inguinal ligament and the first branch formed in the thigh) are oval, with average major and minor diameters of approximately 10.5 and 2.3 mm, respectively (Gustafson et al., 2009). Closer to the lumbar plexus, before the flattening of the nerve, the thickness is between approximately 4.52 and 4.85 mm (Cho Sims et al., 2016). The medial cutaneous branches and nerves of the vastus medialis, vastus intermedius, vastus lateralis, and rectus femoris were dissected and found to be organized from medial toward the lateral (Gustafson et al., 2009). Within the femoral nerve, the anterior division is made up of a muscular branch to the sartorius muscle and two sensory branches (the intermediate and medial cutaneous branches of the thigh), while the posterior division comprises the motor nerves to the quadriceps femoris and articularis genus, and the saphenous nerve (Moore and Stringer, 2011). In the thigh, the most medial branch is running to the pectineus muscle, although some authors contending that this is the most anterior portion of the nerve. Others have suggested that the branch to the sartorius muscle holds this distinction (Gustafson et al., 2009). Another contention is that while some claim the medial cutaneous nerve and adductor longus branch of the femoral nerve are the first to branch away in the thigh, others claim that the medial cutaneous nerve branches more distal to the pectineus and sartorius innervating branches (Gustafson et al., 2009). Some variations in these structures may be due to the capacity of the obturator nerve to give rise to several of these muscle-bound branches (Gustafson et al., 2009). One study showed the femoral nerve was found to be made up of three-layered intrinsic divisions organized from superficial to deep (Aizawa, 1992). The first division was an intrinsic structure in the femoral nerve. The middle layer, or second division, was predominately connected to the sartorius muscle. The deepest layer or third division included the saphenous nerve and muscular branches to the quadriceps femoris. The most superficial layer contained the cutaneous branches crossing over the proximal part of the sartorius muscle. These often communicated with the femoral lateral cutaneous nerve with some fibers moving out toward the lateral aspect of the thigh instead of the main trunk of the femoral lateral cutaneous nerve. These branches were always derived from the most superficial layer of the femoral nerve before its division beneath inguinal ligament. These cutaneous branches usually divided containing both cutaneous branches and muscular branches. The cutaneous branches penetrated the sartorius muscle, and the muscular branches that supplied the sartorius muscle were in the middle layer of the femoral nerve. The most superficial layer also contained muscular branches approaching the pectineus muscle and cutaneous branches moving toward the medial aspect of the thigh. These cutaneous branches showed a close correlation with the femoral lateral cutaneous nerve (Aizawa, 1992). One key facet about the fascicular anatomy of the femoral nerve is that branches with individual fascicles or groups of fascicles within the compound femoral nerve can be traced back to their branching points and into the subsequently formed nerves (Gustafson et al., 2009). These traceable fascicles include those to the sartorius, pectineus, vastus medialis, vastus intermedius, vastus lateralis, and rectus femoris muscles, as well as, the medial cutaneous and saphenous nerves (Gustafson et al., 2009). Fascicles that formed the branches to the vastus medialis, vastus intermedius, and vastus lateralis distally were consistently observed to be in the center and dorsally within the proximal femoral nerve (Gustafson et al., 2009). Fascicles for the sensory nerves, such as the saphenous, medial cutaneous, and the nerve innervating the rectus femoris, were consistently located on the periphery (Gustafson et al., 2009). The fascicles making up the sartorius nerve generally branch away ventrally, and they are often located in the lateral, medial, or central portions of the nerve (Gustafson et al., 2009). Fascicles that formed the pectineus nerve are often located in a ventral position (Gustafson et al., 2009). Few fascicular anastomoses are seen between the distal nerve branches and the proximal compound femoral nerve with no interfascicular plexus formed (Gustafson et al., 2009).

The muscles that the femoral nerve innervates are primarily responsible for leg extension at the knee joint and flexion of the thigh, ultimately making this nerve a key component in standing (for which the three vasti muscles are primarily designed) and stepping (Gustafson et al., 2009). Other muscles innervated by this nerve include the rectus femoris and sartorius, which are also involved in standing (Gustafson et al., 2009). This nerve also has several sensory branches carrying sensation from the anteromedial thigh (medial cutaneous nerve) and sensation in the medial side of the leg and foot (saphenous nerve) (Anloague and Huijbregts, 2009; Gustafson et al., 2009; Moore and Stringer, 2011). With increasing knowledge about the fascicular anatomy of the femoral nerve, new therapies involving functional electrical stimulation to spinal cord injuries have been attempted and studied (Gustafson et al., 2009). As primary muscles in necessary motion, the vastus lateralis and vastus intermedius are most commonly targeted by neural prostheses in the hopes of achieving ambulation following spinal cord injury (Gustafson et al., 2009). Neural prostheses currently target muscles rather than nerves (Gustafson et al., 2009). Epimysial electrodes attached to the muscle at the point of nerve entry, or intramuscular electrodes near the innervating neural structure, are surgically implanted and have shown promise in improving hand grip in patients with mid-cervical tetraplegia (Gustafson et al., 2009). A nerve cuff electrode can be placed after mapping the specific branch fascicles within the compound femoral nerve (Gustafson et al., 2009). One of the most clinically relevant applications of the anatomy of the femoral nerve is femoral nerve block. Despite many scenarios that call for a femoral nerve block, the procedure remains relatively underutilized (Vloka et al., 1999). Some have speculated that this could be due to inconsistency in the literature concerning where the needle should be placed for the block (Vloka et al., 1999). One study established that there was no evidence of a femoral nerve sheath substantial enough to communicate methylene blue to the lumbar plexus or the obturator nerve, which suggests that the three-in-one blockade is limited generally to the LFCN and femoral nerve, but not the lumbar plexus or obturator nerve (Ritter, 1995). Knowledge of the anatomy of the femoral nerve is essential for this procedure, and improper placement can lead to various sequelae, such as needle penetration of the nerve or creation of a hematoma or pseudoaneurysm, which could compress the nerve over time (Mirjalili, 2015). Traditionally, the femoral artery has been used as a reference for needle insertion, so that the needle is inserted immediately lateral to this structure (Orebaugh, 2006). With such topography, it should come as no surprise that vascular puncture (often that of the lateral circumflex femoral artery) is sometimes associated with the procedure (approximately 6% of the time according to some reports) (Orebaugh, 2006). Any injury to the nerve itself can lead to permanent motor and/or sensory deficits in these patients (Moore and Stringer, 2011). It may also disrupt sensation to the anteromedial thigh and medial leg, impeding the ability to extend the knee, and lead to atrophy of the quadriceps muscle (Moore and Stringer, 2011). However, the variant anatomy is not the primary cause of such injury (Moore and Stringer, 2011). This iatrogenic injury is considered rare because it is often self-limiting, and many have speculated that its incidence is underreported (Moore and Stringer, 2011). Several studies have been performed in an attempt to decrease the incidence of sequelae from this particular procedure. One study found that the generally accepted insertion point of the needle (at the level of the inguinal crease, and next to the lateral border of the femoral artery) caused the greatest frequency of contact with the femoral nerve (71%) of all methods attempted (Vloka et al., 1999). This may be due to various previously discussed anatomical characteristics of the nerve at this location, such as its greater width (Vloka et al., 1999). Other methods include insertion of the needle at the level of the inguinal ligament, but detractors claim that this location has more anatomical variation (Vloka et al., 1999). Many trials have shown that instead of inserting the needle on the lateral border of the femoral artery, inserting it at the level of the inguinal crease but 20 mm lateral to the femoral artery (which proved to be lateral to the femoral nerve) caused no needle-femoral nerve contact (Vloka et al., 1999). This was consistent with another study, which found that the lateral circumflex femoral artery and its equivalent vein were within 1 cm of the inguinal crease in 50% of cases (Orebaugh, 2006). Others have documented the use of ultrasound scanning at the femoral crease before inserting the needle and have found that some patients have branching vessels lateral to the main femoral artery, indicating the benefits of imaging before inserting the needle (Muhly and Orebaugh, 2011). Similar injuries can be induced by drawing blood from the femoral artery or during angiography (Mirjalili, 2015). Optimal visualization of the femoral nerve calls for a specific method of imaging. Ultrasound cannot consistently follow the branching of the femoral nerve at the femoral crease and generates more inconsistent measurements than gross anatomy (Lonchena et al., 2016). On full volume maximum intensity projection image MRI, the lumbosacral plexus and its branches are more effectively visualized at 3.0 T than at 1.5 T (Mürtz et al., 2015). The branches of the lumbosacral plexus could be traced significantly further at 3.0 T, and the sharpness of the nerves was increased by 97%–169% (Mürtz et al., 2015). Several pathological states, like metabolic syndrome, can injure the femoral nerve (Rodrigues de Souza et al., 2015). Rats with elevated plasma glucose, mild hypertension, and polyneuropathy consistent with metabolic syndrome have a decreased axonal cross-sectional area, myelin thickness, and myelin fiber count in the femoral nerve (Rodrigues de Souza et al., 2015). These rats also have granules of lipofuscin in their unmyelinated fiber axons and a higher rate of injury in large myelinated fibers than controls (Rodrigues de Souza et al., 2015). It was determined that rats with metabolic syndrome express changes in their peripheral nerves consistent with early onset aging of the structure (Rodrigues de Souza et al., 2015). Another pathology involving the femoral nerve is compression due to impingement by surrounding muscle. Slippage of the iliacus muscle has even been implicated in splitting of the femoral nerve (Vázquez et al., 2007). The slippage of this muscle was as high as 7.9% in one cadaveric study and has been correlated with nerve entrapment because it is relatively close to the nerve (Vázquez et al., 2007). This muscle-related splitting caused the nerve to enter the thigh as several branches instead of a single unit (Vázquez et al., 2007). Another study found that in 68 cadavers, 4 (5.9%) had slippages of the iliacus and psoas major muscles (Spratt et al., 1996). In three cadavers, the femoral nerve was actually pierced by the slippage (Spratt et al., 1996). There was an anomaly found to cause tension on the nerve from an accessory slip of the iliacus muscle due to an iliolumbar ligament passing inferiorly and anterior to it and traversing the nerve, with its tendon splitting and attaching proximally to the lesser trochanter (Spratt et al., 1996). Iliacus tunnel syndrome can also present with femoral nerve compression (Pećina et al., 1997). The cause could range from arteriovenous malformation and vascular aneurysm to iatrogenic problems such as femoral vessel catheterization (Pećina et al., 1997). The location of the lesion (high vs. low) can be estimated on the basis of the patient's presenting symptoms (Pećina et al., 1997). For example, patients with high lesions will present with difficulty standing up when seated (Pećina et al., 1997). Those with a lower injury of the nerve will be unable to extend their knee without difficulty and will experience atrophy of the anterior thigh (Pećina et al., 1997). Losses in sensation can also accompany iliacus tunnel syndrome, and result in a loss in patellar reflex strength (Pećina et al., 1997). Difficulty in ambulating also develops in any pathology that causes compression of the nerve (Mirjalili, 2015). If sweating is retained, a complete lesion of the nerve can be ruled out (Mirjalili, 2015). Injury to the nerve can cause a series of events leading to fibrosis within the nerve itself (Azuelos et al., 2005). Any injury that causes compression of the nerve is accompanied by some element of ischemia (Azuelos et al., 2005). A progressive or repetitive force causes the nerve to become "ribbonlike" and the increase in intraneural pressure, which can retard venous flow, resulting in edema and increased pressure (Azuelos et al., 2005). This in turn can cause fibroblasts to respond and increase epineural and perineural fibrosis (Azuelos et al., 2005). Blood flow can then be impinged and ischemic injury can result, reducing the nerve's ability to repair and regenerate axons (Azuelos et al., 2005). Treatment is indicated under the following conditions: (1) the symptoms are bothersome to the patient and do not resolve within a "reasonable period" under postural treatment and antiinflammatory medications or (2) the symptoms include severe motor/sensation deficits or pain (Azuelos et al., 2005). Surgery is often the course of action for impingement or pressure on the nerve, and fortunately it tends to have a good prognosis in cases with iatrogenic causes, with about a 12-month recovery in "pure" entrapment cases (Azuelos et al., 2005). However, many are opposed to surgical intervention as the risks are considered too high, and conservative therapy, like physical therapy and reversal of coagulopathies, should be pursued instead if possible (Pećina et al., 1997). Surgeries close to the femoral nerve have sometimes caused iatrogenic injury to it. A recent study suggested that the transpsoas lateral surgical approach, which had been proposed as an alternative for the anterior approach to the L4-L5 disc space, can cause postoperative thigh pain, paresthesia, and/or weakness secondary to femoral nerve injury (Davis et al., 2011). It has been speculated that the debilitating cause during surgery is retractor dilation due to self-retaining ring retractors (Davis et al., 2011; Mirjalili, 2015). Surgery in the pelvis in general has also been implicated in femoral nerve injury and is the most common cause of femoral nerve compression (Pećina et al., 1997). Other surgeries that can damage the nerve are those involving the abdomen and hip, including appendectomies, inguinal hernia repairs, biopsies or removal of lymph nodes for malignancies in the inguinal region, and hip arthroplasties (Mirjalili, 2015; Sunderland, 1978). Compression of the nerve or the vessels supplying the nerve, and direct injury from instruments such as trocars, has been implicated in very thin or obese patients (Mirjalili, 2015). Pfannenstiel incisions have also been correlated with femoral nerve injuries (Mirjalili, 2015). Certain positionings of the body can also exert stress on the nerve, such as the lithotomy position, extreme flexion, extreme abduction, and extreme external rotation at the hip joint (Mirjalili, 2015). In the lithotomy position, the femoral nerve can be damaged by the inguinal ligament (Mirjalili, 2015). To protect against nerve injury, it is recommended to palpate the femoral arteries before and after positioning the patient to detect significant change in the pulse indicating pressure on the femoral arteries, which would result in pressure on the femoral nerves (Sunderland, 1978). Injury has also been sustained in anticoagulated patients undergoing surgery leading to compression of the nerve from a hematoma in one of the surrounding muscles (Mirjalili, 2015). Hematomas near the femoral triangle can result in flaccid paralysis of the quadriceps, loss of knee jerk, and loss of sensation from the anterior and medial aspects of the thigh to the medial side of the leg, foot, and toe (Sunderland, 1978). In hip surgery, lateral and anterolateral approaches to the joint call for caution with respect to the femoral nerve (Mirjalili, 2015). Iatrogenic injury to the saphenous nerve is most closely associated with total stripping of the great saphenous vein, resulting from its proximity to the vessel below the level of the knee (Mirjalili, 2015). Injury to the saphenous nerve can also be a result of improper placement of braces or stirrups during operations for positioning of the patient (Sunderland, 1978). Femoral nerve injury following surgery can present as the patient falling when attempting to stand postoperatively (Mirjalili, 2015). Patients experiencing falls with a loss in sensation over pertinent regions of the leg following surgery, near the femoral nerve, should be monitored and have femoral nerve injury ruled out (Mirjalili, 2015). Traumatic injuries, including acute stretching of the femoral nerve during forced extension of the lower limb and fractures of the pubis, can damage or even lead to transection of the femoral nerve. Other injuries to the femoral nerve in the absence of trauma include spreading inflammatory reactions from benign or malignant masses and effects of radiation to the pelvis in patients with ovarian or uterine malignancies (Sunderland, 1978). If a patient exhibits symptoms of femoral nerve injury, the surgeon must use motor and sensory deficits to determine where the injury may be located, how to approach the nerve, and whether a graft is necessary (Van Beek, 1998). If a femoral nerve is injured proximally, a midline abdominal incision is preferred, allowing control and access to the vasculature with a clear view of the entire femoral plexus and the obturator nerve (Van Beek, 1998). This consists of palpating the artery; marking the ASIS, the pubic symphysis, and the femoral artery; and drawing a line to connect the first two structures listed (Pirela-Cruz, 1998). A line should also be drawn to indicate the location of the femoral artery so that it intersects the previously drawn line (Pirela-Cruz, 1998). Based on the patient's body habitus, the incision should roughly follow the lines drawn and should commence halfway between the vertical line and the ASIS, which is just distal to the oblique line (Pirela-Cruz, 1998). This cut should be continued in a medial direction until it is approximately 2.0 cm lateral to the vertical line, whereupon it should be curved in a caudal direction (Pirela-Cruz, 1998). The ilioinguinal nerve requires special attention when opening (Davis et al., 2011). Medially, the incision should continue to the external abdominal oblique muscle and to the inguinal ligament on the anterior thigh (Pirela-Cruz, 1998). Retraction of the peritoneum in a cranial and central direction should expose the fascia of the iliacus muscle (Pirela-Cruz, 1998). Once the fascia over the psoas muscle is opened, the femoral nerve can be identified on the lateral border of the muscle; use of a nerve stimulator can help in the identifying the location of its motor branches (Pirela-Cruz, 1998). If the nerve injury is more distal, a direct approach is sometimes preferred as this allows the injury to be visualized optimally, but if the injury is close to the inguinal ligament, the literature suggests using a "step cut" technique (Van Beek, 1998). A nerve graft is often needed during femoral nerve surgery if there is a gap of more than 4 cm (Van Beek, 1998). If the hip was flexed during surgical repair of the nerve, then flexion should be maintained in a cast for approximately 3 weeks during convalescence, to avoid nerve injury (Van Beek, 1998). Generally speaking, femoral nerve grafting yields good results if the cause is iatrogenic (Van Beek, 1998). Like any other structure in the body, the femoral nerve and the lumbosacral plexus exhibit considerable variation in the general population (Anloague and Huijbregts, 2009). Five out of 18 specimens in one study did not exhibit a standard femoral nerve with contributions from L2 to L4 and forming at the level of L4-L5 (Davis et al., 2011). One study investigating iatrogenic injury to the nerve found that the most clinically relevant variation was an altered position of the nerve at its entrance into the thigh. The nerve was between the femoral artery and vein, instead of lying lateral to the femoral artery (Moore and Stringer, 2011). However, many other variations of the nerve have been documented (Anloague and Huijbregts, 2009). A study exclusively investigating variations of the femoral nerve revealed instances in which the nerve branched into two or three slips around the psoas major muscle fibers (these slips rejoined after bypassing the muscle and before passing under the inguinal ligament) or gave off only one anterior femoral cutaneous nerve instead two (Anloague and Huijbregts, 2009). In this study, a surprising 88% of patients showed some kind of variation within the lumbosacral plexus, while 35.29% had a variation specifically in the femoral nerve (Anloague and Huijbregts, 2009). As mentioned earlier, a slip in the psoas major muscle is not uncommon, and one study reported its incidence as high as 2.2% (Anloague and Huijbregts, 2009).

THE OBTURATOR NERVE

Anatomy

The obturator nerve is derived from the second to fourth ventral rami, sharing its roots with the femoral nerve (Fig. 6.6). Its largest and smallest contributors are typically from L2 and L3, respectively (Schaeffer, 1953; Standring, 2016; Sunderland, 1978; Thane, 1895; Tubbs et al., 2015). Its primary function is to supply motor function to the major adductor muscles of the lower limb (obturator externus, adductor brevis, adductor longus, adductor magnus, gracilis, and, at times, pectineus), and sensation to the medial thigh. Through communicating fibers, it can also contribute to articular innervation of the knee and sensation of a small area of the medial leg. The obturator nerve travels through a complex pathway deep within the pelvis. It descends medially along the posterior wall, just lateral to the lumbar vertebral column, anterior to the quadratus lumborum and iliacus muscles, and posterior to the psoas muscle. It passes the sacroiliac joint, posterior to the common iliac artery, and lateral to the internal iliac vessels. At the pelvic inlet, it moves anteriorly and slightly inferiorly, adjacent to the medial side of the pelvic wall, following the arcuate line, which is just superior to the obturator internus muscle. Throughout this

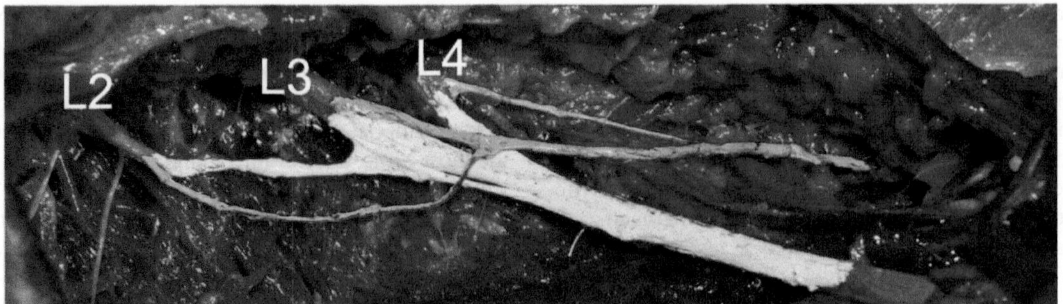

FIG. 6.6 Cadaveric dissection of the origin of the right femoral (yellow) and obturator nerves (green).

course, the nerve is enveloped in the subperitoneal cellular tissue of the region, flattening and enlarging the nerve (Cruveilhier, 1844). On this trajectory, it reaches the obturator canal, a small opening within the superior aspect of the larger obturator foramen (Fig. 6.7). The obturator foramen is covered by the obturator membrane, aside from the opening of the canal, which is located 2.7 cm lateral and 1.7 cm inferior to the pubic tubercle (Jo et al., 2016). The canal is bordered by the obturator sulcus of the pubic bone superiorly, the internal and external obturator muscles inferiorly, with the obturator membrane forming the floor of the tunnel (Pećina et al., 1997). Branching off from the internal iliac vessels, the obturator artery and vein travel just inferior to the nerve along the pelvic wall and through the obturator canal to exit the pelvis (Cruveilhier, 1844). As the nerve exits the obturator canal, it splits immediately into an anterior and posterior branch. Leaving the obturator canal, the anterior branch supplies the hip joint via the articular branch and branches a "twig" to the accessory obturator nerve (AON), if that nerve is present (Schaeffer, 1953). The anterior division descends within a flat plane on the anterior surface of the obturator externus and adductor brevis muscles, deep to the pectineus and adductor longus muscles (Martinoli et al., 2013; Schaeffer, 1953). Within this pathway, it supplies the adductor longus, gracilis and may supply the adductor brevis and pectineus muscles

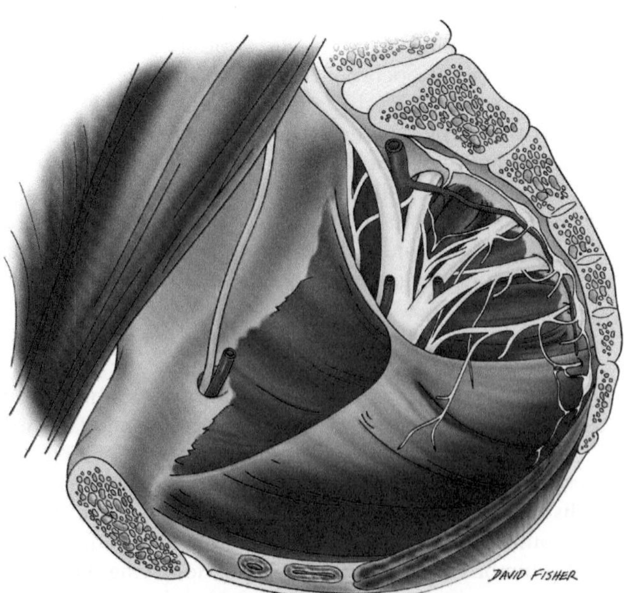

FIG. 6.7 Medial view of the distal course of the obturator nerve in the pelvis.

(Sunderland, 1978; Tubbs et al., 2015). As it travels to the inferior border of the adductor longus, an arterial branch supplies the femoral artery, and a cutaneous branch communicates with the medial cutaneous nerve of the thigh and the saphenous nerve, forming the subsartorial nerve plexus. This plexus is responsible for providing cutaneous sensation to the medial thigh (Standring, 2016; Sunderland, 1978; Tubbs et al., 2015). Occasionally, this "subsartorial" cutaneous branch can provide sensation to the medial leg (Schaeffer, 1953; Thane, 1895). The posterior branch of the obturator nerve pierces the anterior surface of the obturator externus muscle and then descends posterior to the adductor brevis muscle and anterior to the adductor magnus muscle. Within this pathway, the nerve divides into branches to supply the obturator externus, adductor magnus, and adductor brevis muscles. Articular filaments are also sent to the knee joint, either by entering the adductor magnus distally, or by passing via the adductor hiatus to the posterior knee, with the femoral artery. Within the popliteal fossa, the nerve descends with the popliteal artery and pierces the oblique posterior ligament, which will provide sensory innervation to the cruciate ligaments and synovial membrane (Schaeffer, 1953; Standring, 2016; Sunderland, 1978; Tipton, 2008).

Variations in Topography

Many variations exist as the obturator nerve distinguishes itself from its lumbar roots. The obturator nerve may have additional roots from the first or fifth lumbar nerve. More specifically, the obturator nerve can arise in a "high" or "prefixed" form from L1 to L4 or less commonly from L1 to L3. It can also arise in a "low" or "postfixed" form from L2 to L5. Typically, the branch arising from the third lumbar nerve is the largest while the branch arising from the second is often very small and may not contribute in some variations (Standring, 2016; Sunderland, 1978; Tubbs et al., 2015). Among these variations, differences in route may be found. The branch from the main nerve trunk to the obturator externus muscle can pass to the lateral instead of the usual medial side (Tubbs et al., 2015). The articular branch to the hip has been identified leaving the main branch and running independently of the hip joint before passing the obturator foramen; its origin has also been recognized as the posterior, rather than the anterior branch (Schaeffer, 1953; Sunderland, 1978). The distribution of the obturator nerve branches has degrees of variation. The nerve sometimes gives a branch to the pectineus or obturator internus (Sunderland, 1978). The anterior cutaneous branch can be absent, in which case the cutaneous sensation of the medial thigh is innervated by the femoral nerve (Tubbs et al., 2015). Similarly, when the anterior branch is missing, the posterior branch will innervate the adductor brevis and obturator externus (Standring, 2016). Multiple branches have been reported to the following structures: obturator internus, obturator artery, pectineus, and periosteum of pubis pelvic surface (Sunderland, 1978). When the communicating cutaneous nerve from the obturator is large, it can travel from the subsartorial plexus, pierce the deep fascia lata at the knee, and communicate with the saphenous nerve to provide cutaneous sensation for the medial leg (Standring, 2016; Sunderland, 1978; Thane, 1895). In this variation, the medial cutaneous nerve of the thigh is typically small and ends within the subsartorial plexus after providing a few cutaneous filaments (Standring, 2016). Another reported variation includes the presence of an AON. Its prevalence has been documented to be approximately 8%–9% (Pećina et al., 1997; Sunderland, 1978); however, numbers as high as 17% and 30% have also been reported (Henry, 1973; Sunderland, 1978). It is usually small and arises from the ventral rami of the third and fourth lumbar nerve roots, although combinations of single to triple nerve roots ranging between L2 and L5 have been identified (Sunderland, 1978; Tubbs et al., 2015). After leaving the nerve roots, it typically descends just anterior (often adherent) to the main obturator trunk, medial to the psoas major muscle, and traverses the superior pubic ramus (Henry, 1973; Schaeffer, 1953). The nerve then descends within the psoas sheath, under the Poupart's ligament, and runs posterior to the pectineus (Henry, 1973; Schaeffer, 1953; Sunderland, 1978). In this path, it provides branches that may innervate one or more of the following: deep pectineus, hip joint, anterior branch of obturator, and adductor longus (Henry, 1973; Schaeffer, 1953; Standring, 2016). If only one branch is present, it typically innervates the deep pectineus and the hip joint, in lieu of the femoral branch (Tubbs et al., 2015).

Intraneural Topography

The intraneural topography of the obturator has been documented by examining the cross-sectional composition of the nerve in sections proximal to, at, and distal to the obturator foramen. Proximal to the foramen, the nerve divides into superior, intermediate, and inferior groups, based on cross-sectional areas. The superior group comprises bundles from the gracilis, cutaneous fibers, adductor longus, and adductor brevis muscles. The intermediate group consists of bundles from the obturator externus muscle and hip-joint fibers. The inferior group is made of bundles from the adductor magnus, obturator externus, and obturator vessels. In the proximal half of the pelvic section, toward the sacroiliac joint, the superior and inferior groups are intermingled in plexus formations. The nerve travels toward the distal half of the pelvis, and the superior bundle is rarely engaged in plexus formation with the inferior group. At the obturator foramen, the fibers for the gracilis, adductor longus, and adductor brevis lie toward the anteromedial portion of the bundle, while the fibers to obturator externus and adductor magnus are in a posterolateral position. Distal to the foramen, the obturator nerve courses through most of its muscles as bundles ranging from 1 to 8 funiculi. Moving distally from the nerve roots, the aforementioned "superior group" of the obturator nerve largely corresponds to fibers that run along the anteromedial portion of the nerve when it reaches the foramen and becomes the anterior branch when distal to the foramen. On the other hand, the "intermediate" and "inferior group" within the pelvis largely corresponds to fibers that run along the posterolateral portion of the nerve when it reaches the foramen and becomes the posterior branch when distal to the foramen. The average percentage cross-sectional area of the obturator nerve occupied within the funiculi has been measured at the foramen, midway along the lateral pelvic wall, and at the level of the sacroiliac joint and found to be 41%, 49%, and 52%, respectively (Sunderland, 1978).

Pathology

The most common cause of obturator pathology is compression, as a result of its deep anatomy. Some common sites of compression include within the obturator canal near the vascular bundle of obturator vessels; in the fibromuscular canal anterior to the obturator membrane but posterior to the obturator externus; in the muscular tunnel where the posterior division separates the obturator externus; within the fascia located deep to the pectineus and adductor brevis muscles, but superficial to the obturator externus; and the proximal third of the adductor magnus (Kumka, 2010). The female reproductive anatomy can predispose women to obturator pathologies. In parturition, the fetal head can compress the obturator nerve against the pelvic wall, causing "obstetrical palsy" (Pećina et al., 1997). Similarly, pelvic masses such as obturator hernias and ovarian tumors may produce the same signs and symptoms (Sunderland, 1978). Other compressive etiologies include bone osteophytes, obturator artery aneurysms, and retroperitoneal lesions (Pećina et al., 1997; Standring, 2016). Due to the proximity of surrounding pelvic structures, disease processes can affect the nerve. For example, as the obturator runs toward the obturator canal, it runs under or near the sigmoid colon. Cases of carcinoma of the large intestine and other pathologic growths in the pelvis must be kept in mind as differentials. Infection in the pelvis has been seen to follow the posterior branch into the thigh. Furthermore, the articular branch to the hip and filaments sent to the sacroiliac joint can be involved in joint pathology (Schaeffer, 1953). Isolated mononeuropathy of the obturator nerve is rare. For example, in pathologies secondary to direct trauma, patients are more likely to present with complex comorbidities, as a pelvic fracture severe enough to lesion the obturator nerve will likely also injure other structures such as spinal nerves, the lumbosacral plexus, and other peripheral leg nerves (Stewart, 2000). Labral tears of the hip can lead to acetabular labral cysts that not only impinge on the obturator nerve, but also injure other nerves near the hip joint, such as the femoral and posterior sciatic nerves (Kim et al., 2014; Yukata et al., 2005). There are reports of idiopathic obturator neuropathy, but no significant evidence for true entrapment in anatomical variations such as a narrow obturator foramen. While obturator palsy has been reported in newborns, this is thought not to be congenital, but secondary to a prolonged abnormal leg position in utero that overstretches the obturator nerve, which usually has a recovery within 2 weeks (Stewart, 2000; Sunderland, 1978). In cases of idiopathic meralgia paresthetica, mechanical friction has been proposed as a cause of pseudoganglia swellings caused by irritation of the nerve, thickening the epineurium as it crosses over the linea terminalis (Tubbs et al., 2003). The "Howship-Romberg sign" describes patients with compression of the obturator nerve, often from an obturator hernia, causing pain referred to the hip, medial thigh, and knee (Standring, 2016). This sign should not be confused with the "Obturator sign," which is used to describe irritation of the obturator internus muscle, typically caused by appendicitis. Isolated lesions of the obturator nerve are extremely rare but may occasionally occur as a result of direct trauma (sometimes during parturition) or anterior dislocations of the hip. A more distal nerve entrapment syndrome causing chronic medial thigh pain has been described in athletes with large adductor muscles.

There are several iatrogenic etiologies behind obturator neuropathy including hip arthroplasty, abdominal surgery, plastic surgery, forceps delivery, compression from retractor or surgical cement placement, and hematoma secondary to femoral venipuncture while anticoagulated (Yukata et al., 2005). Following hip arthroplasty, nerves close to the obturator foramen can be injured if methyl methacrylate escapes inferiorly from the acetabulum and exerts pressure on the obturator nerve near the superior ramus of the pubis (Sunderland, 1978). Obturator paralysis has also been seen postoperatively in patients positioned on operating tables with the thighs acutely flexed, i.e., lithotomy position, to such an extent that the nerve leaves the bony obturator foramen (Sunderland, 1978). However, iatrogenic injury more commonly involves the sciatic and femoral nerves (Stewart, 2000). Iatrogenic complications, when they occur, need not be limited to obturator neuropathy. For instance, the tension-free vaginal tape technique has been implicated in significant vascular and bowel injuries, accompanied by neuropathy (Kumka, 2010). Musculoskeletal variations have also been shown to cause obturator nerve disturbances. Athletes with large adductor muscles can develop chronic medial thigh pain secondary to distal entrapment of the nerve (Standring, 2016). They can also develop chronic groin pain due to chronic denervation of the adductor muscles (Tipton, 2008). Conversely, atrophied or weak adductors may lead to snapping hip syndrome (Oh et al., 2014).

Imaging and Diagnostics

Ultrasound can be useful for exploring the nerve segments of the lower limb. The obturator nerve is best visualized when the patient is positioned with the leg straight and in a slight external rotation. However, the deep anatomical course underlying this region and the requisite patient positioning limit the usefulness of this imaging modality because there are only six nerves that can be imaged in the hip (the lateral femoral cutaneous, femoral, sciatic, obturator, superior and inferior gluteal, and pudendal nerves) (Soong et al., 2007). The best-established confirmation of obturator nerve lesions is identifying electromyography (EMG) abnormalities in the hip adductors. In such cases, the EMG of the adductor brevis, adductor longus, and gracilis muscles shows high amplitude, long duration, complex motor unit potentials, and longer fibrillation potentials, corresponding to denervation and atrophy of these muscles (Tipton, 2008). These EMG findings can help differentiate obturator nerve deficits from similar pathologies such as lumbar and diabetic (Jo et al., 2016). Alternatively, on T2-weighted MRI, an increased signal intensity in the medial thigh indicates that the muscles are undergoing denervation or atrophy with fatty infiltration. Specifically, the imaging signals that correspond to obturator neuropathy are more focal, more proximal, and spare the obturator externus (Yukata et al., 2005).

Surgical Interventions

There are several treatments for patients with obturator neuropathy. Most cases will use a combination of conservative management, physical therapy, and NSAIDs for analgesia. For many patients, a return to regular activity is expected within 6 weeks (Tipton, 2008). Surgical intervention may be required in cases with identifiable pelvic pathology, or when pain and weakness prove to be resistant to conservative management (Tipton, 2008). Percutaneous radiofrequency lesioning is a form of treatment used to alleviate refractory pain; however, it does have several complications including neuritis, neuroma formation, sensory loss, loss of motor function, and transient hematoma formation if the patient is on anticoagulation medications (Chaiban et al., 2013). Cryoanalgesia is another useful analgesic treatment modality but it carries the risk of deafferentation pain (Rigaud et al., 2008). Alternatively, percutaneous thermocoagulation is a procedure used to denature proteins in the peripheral nerves, which will provide pain relief. This method provides a longer duration of analgesia and entails a greater risk of inducing loss of motor function, neuroma formation, neuritis, and postprocedural nerve inflammation (Yavuz et al., 2013). Regional anesthetic blockade is a key intervention for various neuropathies. Appropriate use of obturator nerve blocks have been associated with reduced consumption of NSAIDs and sustained pain relief for up to several months. For patients undergoing transurethral bladder tumor resection, there is a greater than 50% incidence of adductor muscle spasm postsurgery (Tekgul et al., 2014). Obturator nerve blockade can be of great help to these patients by providing analgesia and managing spasticity for the pelvis and thigh (Jo et al., 2016). Obturator nerve blocks can be modified for various applications. In patients with refractory, progressive hip displacement that reach the maximum dose of botulinum toxin treatment, obturator nerve blocks using ethyl alcohol have proven to be an alternate remedy (Park et al., 2014). In patients requiring general anesthesia, obturator nerve blockade with spinal analgesia may be used (Khorrami et al., 2012). Despite the utility of nerve blockades, some risks are involved. Incomplete nerve blocks can lead to bladder wall perforation or dissemination of a tumor secondary to thigh adductor muscle contractions (Soong et al., 2007). The obturator nerve also has the highest failure rate of blockade among the triad of nerves involved in a three-in-one nerve block (Soong et al., 2007). However, as techniques advance, the risks and difficulties involved with this procedure will undoubtedly decrease. In an anatomical study, a vertical obturator blocking technique landmarking only by palpation of a single anatomical structure has been shown to have a high degree of accuracy (93.75%) (Fiegl et al., 2013). In certain presentations, surgery may be unavoidable. A patient presenting with neuropathy secondary to arthroplasty might have a nerve encased in cement. Such patients should be observed carefully, with surgical exploration to follow if the symptoms fail to resolve. In cases of neuropathy resulting from pelvic trauma or intraoperative laceration, the patient could require nerve repair and grafting. For cases of progressive symptoms with unidentified causes, surgical exploration of the obturator canal should be conducted in search of a hernia or other tissue, e.g., endometriosis (Stewart, 2000).

Denervation or phenol injections are two other alternatives to treat adductor contractures, particularly when nerve blockage is unfeasible (Sunderland, 1978). Denervation has been used constructively to avoid adductor contractures in paraplegic patients and avoid intraoperative complications during transurethral resection due to obturator nerve irritation (Kendir et al., 2008). Furthermore, studies suggest that the obturator nerve can serve as a potential nerve donor or graft site for various procedures. Surgical applications of the obturator nerve in facial reanimation procedures have been shown to be feasible (Rozen et al., 2013). In femoral nerve neurotization, the obturator nerve has been successfully used as a distal donor nerve. Autografting of motor nerves from the obturator to pudendal has also been done (Houdek et al., 2014). One technique particularly useful for high-level nerve lesions is to transfer the anterior branch of the obturator nerve which has been shown to successfully return power to at least part of the quadriceps femoris muscle (Tung et al., 2012). However, this procedure involves neurorrhaphy within the pelvis, which complicates the procedure, and attempts near the muscle have been performed in hopes of decreasing recovery time (Goubier et al., 2012).

The Furcal Nerve

The lumbosacral plexus receives less attention than the brachial plexus most likely due to decreased reports of injuries on the plexus. The lumbar plexus is often formed by a contribution from the 12th thoracic (subcostal) nerve, the first three lumbar ventral rami and the greater part of the fourth lumbar ventral ramus. The lumbosacral plexus is formed by the remaining small part of the fourth lumbar nerve and the fifth lumbar nerve (lumbosacral trunk) (Gray, 1918) and the upper sacral nerves (Harshavardhana and Dabke, 2014). Various types of lumbosacral nerve root anomalies have been described in the literature. The existing classifications of nerve root abnormalities take into consideration convergence, intradural or extradural anastomosis, and division (Chotigavanich and Sawangnatra, 1992; Haijiao et al., 2001). The furcal nerve has been variably defined, but many identify it as the nerve that enters into the formation of both the lumbar and sacral plexuses (Fig. 6.8). This is because the nerve divides between the two plexuses

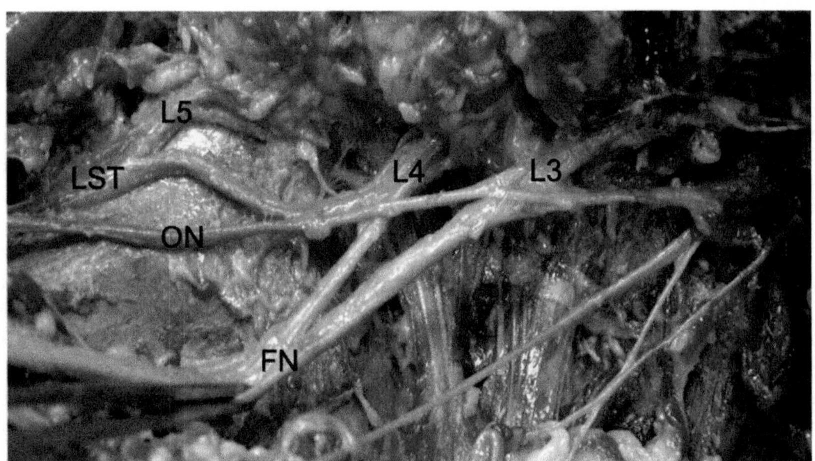

FIG. 6.8 Left-sided cadaveric dissection noting the lower lumbar ventral rami. L4 or the furcal nerve is seen giving branches to the obturator (ON), femoral (FN), and lumbosacral trunk nerves (LST).

(Clemente, 1985; Hollinshead, 1964; Schaeffer, 1946; Standring, 2005) serving as a link between them. For example, a part of the L4 ventral ramus joins with L5 ventral ramus to form the lumbosacral trunk. Some, however, have described the furcal nerve as a separate nerve traveling alongside the L4 nerve root in the intervertebral foramen, having separate anterior and posterior root fibers, its own dorsal root ganglion and thus indicating that it is its own independent nerve root. It also has fibers contributing to neighboring nerves, 26% to the femoral nerve, 18% to the obturator nerve, and 16% to the lumbosacral trunk (Kikuchi et al., 1986). Schaeffer described the furcal nerve as "when the fourth nerve enters into the formation of both lumbar and sacral plexuses, it may be called the furcal nerve, but this name is also applied to any of the nerves that enter into the formation of both plexuses, so there may be one or more furcal nerves" (Schaeffer, 1946). Others have defined the furcal nerve simply as the entire ventral ramus of the L4 spinal nerve.

Variations of the Furcal Nerve

The variability is a result of a deviation from the normal fetal development during the first 4 weeks of life. Kikuchi et al. performed cadaveric dissections including coronal and sagittal sectioning of the lumbosacral region in order to better delineate the anatomy of the furcal nerve. The furcal nerve was found in up to 93% of their dissections and mainly as L4. The furcal nerve has been referred to as the boundary root (Kikuchi et al., 1986). However, although most furcal nerves arise at the L4 level, they can occur at any level from L1 to S1 (Haijiao et al., 2001; Hollinshead, 1964; Romanes, 1981; Schaeffer, 1946; Standring, 2005). When the furcal nerve arises cranial to L4, the lumbar plexus is termed prefixed, while a more caudal emergence is identified as postfixed (Clemente, 1985; Hollinshead, 1964; Romanes, 1981; Schaeffer, 1946; Standring, 2005). In Bardeen and Elting's findings, 42.3% were found to be normal, 36% prefixed, and 21.5% postfixed (Bardeen, 1901). Several other variations of the furcal nerve have also been described. The furcal nerve may consist of L3 and L4 in some cases and other times, L4 and L5. These "doubled" furcal nerves have an incidence of 0.8% (L3 and L4 more common than L4 and L5) (Harshavardhana and Dabke, 2014; Bergman et al., 1988). At times, the L4 branch to the lumbosacral plexus is missing, leaving L5 as the sole furcal nerve or boundary root. In rhesus monkeys, as a rule, there are seven lumbar vertebrae, and the L5 ventral ramus is usually the furcal nerve (Paterson, 1894). Kikuchi et al. further classified the anatomical variations of the furcal nerve into six types (A through F) on the basis of the level at which they arose. In A, two furcal nerves were at the L3 and L4 root levels; in B, one furcal nerve was at the cephalad side of the L4 root; in C, one furcal nerve root was at the L4 level, following the same course as the proper L4; in D, two furcal nerves at the cephalad side of the L4 root; in E, two furcal nerves arose at L4 and L5 roots, respectively; and in F, a furcal nerve was at the cephalad side of the L5 nerve root (Kikuchi et al., 1986). Earlier reports suggested the prevalence of extra connections to be as high as 20%, although this was reported in patients with radicular symptoms, and not in cadavers (D'Avella and Mingrino, 1979; Haijiao et al., 2001; Maiuri and Gambardella, 1986).

Clinical Significance

These variations described above create several controversies including the atypical sciatica presentation and discrepancy between clinical presentation and imaging. Interestingly, there are few reports regarding the detailed anatomy of the furcal nerve with respect to its involvement in different clinical conditions such as lumbosacral radicular symptoms (D'Avella and Mingrino, 1979; Kikuchi et al., 1984; Parke and Watanabe, 1987). For patients with radiculopathy, a selective spinal nerve root blockade approach is used, and the root chosen for the blockade is usually determined as a result of clinical presentation and imaging identification of nerve root compression. L5 or S1 radiculopathy usually presents as pain below the knee up to the foot, whereas, L2-L4 radiculopathy is perceived as pain projecting to the knee, thigh or groin. However, in a subset of patients, the clinical picture is confusing and there are a number of reasons for this, including variable furcal nerve contribution (Bartynski et al., 2010; Kikuchi et al., 1986). In a study by Bartynski, L4 injection provoked typical gluteal, hip, or posterior thigh pain (sciatica) in 5 out of 32 patients, consistent with a prominent furcal nerve contribution to the sacral plexus and reported three patients complaining of pain projecting to the ankle or foot (Bartynski et al., 2010). Clinical suspicion and a thorough MRI examination can be useful in identifying this subset of patients (Harshavardhana and Dabke, 2014). With an increased prevalence of posterolateral approaches to the spine, surgeons must pay attention to the various presentations of a furcal nerve to avoid nerve injury. It is also important to be able to recognize patients with atypical sciatica because those patients may have a furcal nerve with a conjoined nerve root. A thorough understanding of anatomical variations and insight into the anomalies of the lumbosacral plexus reduce the incidence of failed back surgery and enhances surgical success.

THE ACCESSORY OBTURATOR NERVE

The AON (Fig. 6.9) was first reported in 1672 by Isbrand van Diemerbroeck, who stated that it was identified in about one in three people and originated from the third and fourth lumbar nerves (Swanson, 2015). It was not described in depth until Schmidt had done so in 1794. Once discovered, the nerve was termed the anterior internal crural nerve, accessory nerve of the internal crural nerve, and the nerve of the coxofemoral articulation (Cruveilhier, 1844). Some have proposed that the AON should be named the accessory femoral nerve owing to its typical derivation from the posterior part of the anterior division of L3 and L4, its function, and its anatomical course over the pubic ramus (McMinn, 2003).

Origin

When present, the AON arises from L3 or more commonly L3 and L4 between the roots of the femoral and obturator nerves. It can also arise from variable combinations of L2, L3, and L4, or from the obturator nerve directly (Bergman et al., 1984; Bergman et al., 1988). Katritsis et al. found it was formed by roots from the anterior primary divisions of L3 and L4 in 63.6% of specimens, L2, L3, and L4 in 10.6% of specimens, L2 and L3 in 7.6% of specimens, L3 in 6.1% of specimens, or from the trunk of the obturator nerve in 12.1% of specimens (Katritsis et al., 1980). Ellis reported one case in which the AON arose from the trunk of the obturator nerve (Ellis, 1887). Quain described the obturator nerve as originating in association with the anterior crural nerve in two cases (Quain et al., 1867).

Anatomy

The prevalence of the AON has consistently been reported as ranging from 10% to 30% (Hollinshead, 1956a,b; Lennon and Horlocker, 2006; Woodburne, 1956). Population samples in individual studies have been too small for reliable estimates of the overall prevalence of the AON. Most studies have failed to record sex or unilateral bias. Studies have reported a greater prevalence in females and of left-sided AON, but these results could be misleading owing to the low sample size (Akkaya et al., 2008; Sim and Webb, 2004). The

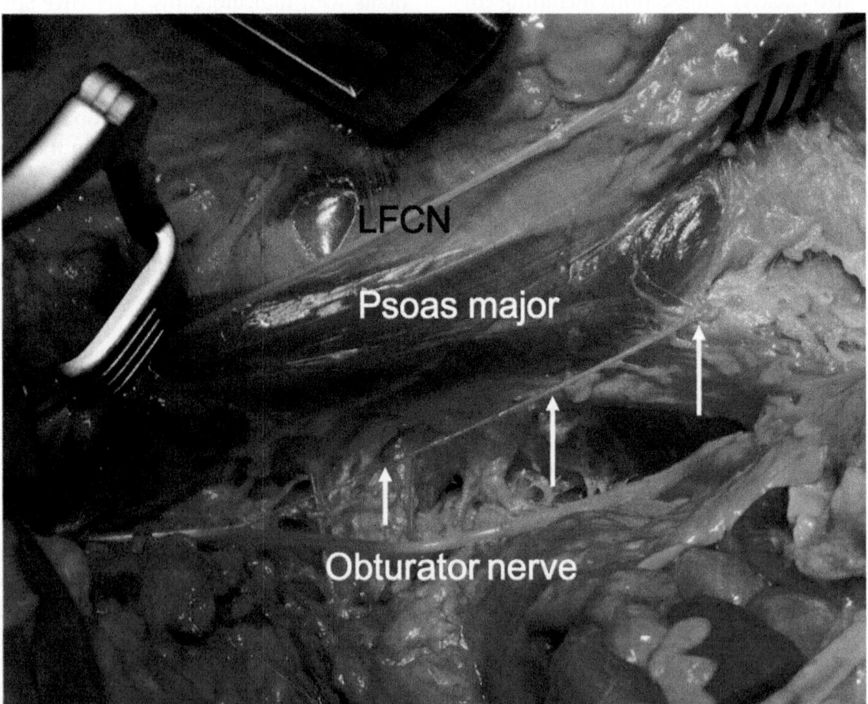

FIG. 6.9 Left-sided cadaveric dissection noting the lateral femoral cutaneous nerve (LFCN), which in this case, pierced the anterior surface of the psoas major. Medial to the psoas major, the obturator nerve is seen giving off the smaller accessory obturator nerve (arrows), which here, is ending on the periosteum of the pubis.

largest study by Katritsis et al., which examined 1000 plexuses, revealed no sex difference in the prevalence of an AON in the lumbar plexus but showed left-sided dominance in unilateral cases (Katritsis et al., 1980). This suggests a lack of association between side dominance and sex. The AON, which often branches from the trunk of the obturator nerve (12.1%) (Katritsis et al., 1980), has also been suggested to be termed the accessory femoral nerve. Misidentification of the AON can lead to surgical complications such as those in a case reported by Jirsch, which demonstrated the importance of these variations in surgical practice (Jirsch and Chalk, 2007). In this case, the AON was mistaken as obturator nerve, which led to the obturator nerve being injured during elective laparoscopic tubal occlusion.

In 100% of the plexuses examined that had an AON, Katritsis et al. found that it passed 2–3 cm anterolateral to the obturator nerve and medial to the psoas major toward the obturator foramen, but instead of passing through the canal it passed over the superior pubic ramus, lying medial to the psoas muscle (Katritsis et al., 1980). Woodburne (1956) described the AON as passing directly over the pubic ramus, under the femoral vein. After crossing the pubic ramus, the nerve descends dorsally to the pectineus muscle, where it typically divides into three branches: one entering the anterior hip joint, another entering the dorsomedial aspect of the pectineus muscle, and the third moving medially to anastomose with the anterior branch of the obturator nerve (Standring, 2008; Woodburne, 1956). In a rare case reported by Rohini et al., the AON emerged on the medial side of the psoas major, entered the femoral triangle, divided into its three typical terminal branches, and passed superficial to the pectineus muscle, instead of deep to it (Rohini et al., 2012).

Variations

Katritsis et al. (1980) studied 1000 plexuses (132 with AON) and found that 36.4% of AONs had variant origins. Although most of these variations were not drastically different, the AON has shown to derive from the trunk of the obturator, or the anterior crural nerve (Quain et al., 1867). Multiple variations of the three terminal divisions have been reported. Katritsis et al. found that after supplying the pectineus, the AON branched off behind the pectineus muscle, and supplied the anterior branch (14.3%), posterior branch (4.65%), trunk of the obturator nerve (6.1%), or the femoral nerve (2.3%) (Katritsis et al., 1980). Woodburne (1959) also reported that a single branch supplying the adductor longus is not uncommon, along with other additional branches. A very common variation of the AON makes it the sole innervation of the pectineus muscle rather than the typical dual innervation with the femoral nerve (Woodburne, 1956). Quain et al. (1867) described a small cutaneous branch that supplies the inner thigh and proximal inner leg. Shakespeare reported a similar finding of the AON anastomosing with the obturator nerve and supplying cutaneous innervation to the inner thigh. In one case reported by Tubbs et al., a pseudoganglion was found in association with an AON (Allen and Shakespeare, 1883; Tubbs et al., 2003).

Landmarks

Akkaya et al. (2008) reported that the AON had an average distance of 1.6 cm from the femoral nerve and was 2.0 cm superior and 2.0 cm anterior to the upper wall of the external opening of the obturator canal, 4.0 cm from the pubic tubercle, and 4.6 cm from the median plane (Akkaya et al., 2008). Although no measurements of the AON have been reported, it has been described as "smaller than the usual obturator nerve" (Gray, 1867; Quain et al., 1867; Woodburne, 1956). Because of the close proximity of the LFCN to the AON in the pelvis, it is important to be able to distinguish them from each other. The LFCN is usually formed from the posterior division of L2 and L3 (Anloague and Huijbregts, 2009). It passes laterally to the psoas muscle instead of medially as the AON does.

Embryology

There are conflicting accounts of the embryological origin of the AON. According to the original hypothesis of its derivation, the AON arises from a splitting of the obturator nerve caused by the developing obturator foramen (Beziehungenzwischen, 1894; Woodburne, 1956). The fact that the pubis develops around the obturator nerve, enclosing it in the obturator foramen, brought doubt on this proposal (Howell, 1936; Woodburne, 1956). Howell also asserted that when the pubis develops around the obturator nerve, it separates itself from the AON (Howell, 1936). Yasar reported an AON in 4 of 20 lumbar plexuses in 10 fetuses between gestational ages 24 and 28 weeks (Yasar et al., 2014). Woodburne (1956) described the pectineus as a "border muscle" in embryological development. This is because it is located between the muscles typically innervated by the obturator and femoral nerves. It is located in the anterior thigh, but its function is similar to that of an adductor medial thigh muscle. The development of this muscle and its innervation questions whether the AON and its innervation of this border muscle represents the femoral or the obturator nerve.

The AON innervates the pectineus on its dorsomedial aspect, while the femoral branch that arises distally to the inguinal ligament turns medially, travels dorsal to the femoral vessels, and finally innervates the muscle on the ventrolateral aspect (Woodburne, 1956). As a result, there have been disputes naming the AON "the accessory femoral nerve." Woodburne (1956) proposed that the innervation might differ because the dorsomedial obturator portion of the pectineus muscle was phylogenetically separate from the ventrolateral femoral portion. This questions whether the phylogenetic separation of the pectineus muscle may lead to embryological development of the AON. Leche (1900) suggested that in some mammals there is an obturator intermedius muscle in addition to the obturator externus during development. He proposed that this obturator intermedius becomes associated with the pectineus muscle, leading to dual innervation by both the femoral nerve and the AON. Grafenberg described a 6-week-old human embryo in which the muscles of the anterior and medial thigh developed from a single primordial muscle (Grafenberg, 1904; Woodburne, 1956), which was innervated by both the femoral and obturator nerves. Uneven splitting of this muscle could account for the changes in innervation leading to the development of the AON. Visual evidence for this was suggested in a study by Bardeen, who believed that a mass associated with the embryonic external obturator and pectineus muscles was the area where the obturator nerve would innervate (Bardeen, 1906). Further support is provided by its course and location on the dorsal aspect of the pectineus muscle after crossing the linea terminalis, before splitting into its terminal branches. The proposal that the AON first formed because of a phylogenic separation is supported by its atypical path over the pubic ramus (which is the known path for innervation of the anterior thigh muscles) instead of through the obturator canal.

Clinical Implications

Akkaya et al. (2008) reported that an AON could negatively affect the clinical efficacy of an obturator nerve block. He stated that if the patient had an AON, it might also need to be blocked. AON blockage can be recommended for thigh surgeries, treatment of pain, and diagnosis of hip joint pain (Rohini et al., 2012). Akkaya et al. showed that in 12 cadavers the AON was located a mean distance of 4 cm lateral to the pubic tubercle, which should be used as a reference for AON block (Akkaya et al., 2008). Positioning for such a block should be 2 cm lateral and caudal to the pubic tubercle. The needle should then be rotated 30° lateral and inserted toward the superior edge of the superior pubic ramus (Akkaya et al., 2008).

REFERENCES

Aasvang, E., Kehlet, H., 2005. Surgical management of chronic pain after inguinal hernia repair. Br. J. Surg. 92, 795–801.

Acar, F., Ozdemir, M., Bayrakli, F., Cirak, B., Coskun, E., Burchiel, K., 2013. Management of medically intractable genitofemoral and ilioinguinal neuralgia. Turk. Neurosurg. 23 (6), 753–757.

Aizawa, Y., 1992. On the organization of the plexus lumbalis. On the recognition of the three-layered divisions and the systematic description of the branches of the human femoral nerve. Okajimas Folia Anat. Jpn. 69 (1), 35–74.

Akkaya, T., Comert, A., Kendir, S., 2008. Detailed anatomy of accessory obturator nerve blockade. Minerva Anestiol. 74, 119–122.

Al-dabbagh, A., 2002. Anatomical variations of the inguinal nerves and risks of injury in 110 hernia repairs. Surg. Radiol. Anat. 24, 102–107.

Alfieri, S., Rotondi, F., Di Giorgio, A., Fumagalli, U., Salzano, A., Di Miceli, D., Ridolfini, M.P., Sgagari, A., Dogletto, G., 2006. Influence of preservation versus division of ilioinguinal, iliohypogastric, and genital nerves during open mesh herniorrhaphy. Ann. Surg. 243 (4), 553–558.

Alfieri, S., Amid, P., Campanelli, G., Izard, G., Kehlet, H., Wijsmuller, A.R., Di Miceli, D., Doglietto, G.B., 2011. International guidelines for prevention and management of post-operative chronic pain following inguinal hernia surgery. Hernia 15, 239–249.

Allen, H., Shakespeare, E.O., 1883. A System of Human Anatomy: Bones and Joints, 2 ed. H. C. Lea's Son & Company, p. 566.

Amid, P., 2004. Causes, prevention, and surgical treatment of postherniorrhaphy neuropathic inguinodynia: triple neurectomy with proximal end implantation. Hernia 8, 343–349.

Amid, P.K., Hiatt, J.R., 2007. New understanding of the causes and surgical treatment of post herniorrhaphy inguinodynia and orchalgia. J. Am. Coll. Surg. 205 (2), 381–385.

Amin, N., Krashin, D., Trescot, A.M., 2016. Ilioinguinal and Iliohypogastric Nerve Entrapment: Abdominal. Peripheral Nerve Entrapments. Springer, pp. 413–424.

Anloague, P.A., Huijbregts, P., 2009. Anatomical variations of the lumbar plexus: a descriptive anatomy study with proposed clinical implications. J. Man. Manip. Ther. 17 (4), 107–114.

Apaydin, N., 2015. Variations of the lumbar and sacral plexuses and their branches. In: Tubbs, R.S., Rizk, E., Shoja, M.M., Loukas, M., Barbaro, N., Spinner, R.J. (Eds.), Nerves and Nerve Injuries, vol. 1. Elsevier, San Diego, pp. 614–617, 2010.

Aszmann, O.C., Dellon, E.S., Dellon, A.L., 1997. Anatomical course of the lateral femoral cutaneous nerve and its susceptibility to compression and injury. Plast. Reconstr. Surg. 100, 600–604.

Avsar, F.M., Sahin, M., Arikan, B.U., Avsar, A.F., Demirci, S., Ethan, A., 2002. The possibility of nervus ilioingionalis and nervus Iliohypogastricus injury in lower abdominal incisions and effects on hernia formation. J. Surg. Res. 107 (2), 179–185.

Azuelos, A., Corò, L., Alexandre, A., 2005. Femoral nerve entrapment. Acta Neurochir. Suppl. 92, 61–62.

Barazanchi, A.W.H., Fagan, P.V.B., Smith, B.B., Hill, A.G., 2016. Routine neurectomy of inguinal nerves during open onlay mesh hernia repair: a meta-analysis of randomized trials. Ann. Surg. 264, 64–72.

Bardeen, C.R., 1901. A statistical study of the abdominal and border nerves in man. Am. J. Anat. 1, 203–228.

Bardeen, C.R., 1906. Development and variation of the nerves and the musculature of the inferior extremity and of the neighboring regions of the trunk in man. Am. J. Anat. 6, 259–390.

Bartynski, W.S., Kang, M.D., Rothfus, W.E., 2010. Adjacent double–nerve root contributions in unilateral lumbar radiculopathy. AJNR Am. J. Neuroradiol. 31, 327–333.

Bergman, R.A., Thompson, S.A., Afifi, A.K., 1984. Catalogue of Human Variations. Urban & Schwarzenberg, Baltimore, pp. 158–161.

Bergman, R.A., Thompson, S.A., Afifi, A.K., Saadeh, F., 1988. Compendium of Human Anatomic Variation. Urban and Schwarzenberg, Baltimore, pp. 143–148.

Beziehungenzwischen, B., 1894. Skelett, Muskulatur nervender extremitaten. MowhJb 21, 241–277.

Brown, J.S., Butrick, C.W., Carter, J.E., Doleys, D.M., El-Minawi, A.M., Howard, F.M., Kinback, K.M., Lowery, D.C., Perry, C.P., 2000. Pelvic Pain Diagnosis and Management. Lipincott Williams and Wilkins, Philadelphia.

Bugada, D., Peng, P.W., 2015. Ilioinguinal, iliohypogastric, and genitofemoral nerve blocks. In: Regional Nerve Blocks in Anesthesia and Pain Therapy. Springer, pp. 707–715.

Cahill, K.S., Martinez, J.L., Wang, M.Y., Vanni, S., Levi, A.D., 2012. Motor nerve injuries following the minimally invasive lateral transpsoas approach. J. Neurosurg. Spine 17 (3), 227–231.

Campanelli, G., Bertocchi, V., Cavalli, M., Bombini, G., Biondi, A., Tentorio, T., et al., 2013. Surgical treatment of chronic pain after inguinal hernia repair. Hernia 17, 347–353.

Carai, A., Fenu, G., Sechi, E., Crotti, F.M., Montella, A., 2009. Anatomical variability of the lateral femoral cutaneous nerve: findings from a surgical series. Clin. Anat. 22, 365–370.

Cesmebasi, A., Yadav, A., Gielecki, J., Tubbs, R.S., Loukas, M., 2015. Genitofemoral neuralgia: a review. Clin. Anat. 28 (1), 128-13.

Chaiban, G., Paradis, T., Atallah, J., 2013. Use of ultrasound and fluoroscopy guidance in percutaneous radiofrequency lesioning of the sensory branches of the femoral and obturator nerves. Pain Pract. 14 (4), 343–345.

Cheatham, S.W., Kolber, M.J., Salamh, P.A., 2013. Meralgiaparesthetica: a review of the literature. Int. J. Sports Phys. Ther. 8, 883–893.

Cho, K.T., Lee, H.J., 2008. Prone position-related meralgiaparesthetica after lumbar spinal surgery: a case report and review of the literature. J. Korean Neurosurg. Soc. 44, 392–395.

Cho Sims, G., Boothe, E., Joodi, R., Chhabra, A., 2016. 3D MR Neurography of the lumbosacral plexus: obtaining optimal images for selective longitudinal nerve depiction. AJNR Am. J. Neuroradiol. 37, 2158–2162.

Choi, P.D., Nath, R., Mackinnon, S.E., 1996. Iatrogenic injury to the ilioinguinal and iliohypogastric nerves in the groin: a case report, diagnosis, and management. Ann. Plast. Surg. 37 (1), 60–65.

Chotigavanich, C., Sawangnatra, S., 1992. Anomalies of the lumbosacral nerve roots-An anatomic investigation. Clin. Orthop. Relat. Res. 278, 47–50.

Chou, D., Storm, P.B., Campbell, J.N., 2004. Vulnerability of the subcostal nerve to injury during bone graft harvesting from the iliac crest. J. Neurosurg. Spine 1 (1), 87–89.

Choy, K.W., Kogilavani, S., Norshalizah, M., Rani, S., Aspalilah, A., Hamzi, H., Farihah, H.S., Das, S., 2013. Topographical anatomy of the profunda femoris artery and the femoral nerve: normal and abnormal relationships. Clin. Ter. 164 (1), 17–19.

Clemente, C.D., 1985. Gray's Anatomy, 30th American ed. Lea and Febiger, Philadelphia, pp. 1225–1235.

Condon, R.E., Nyhus, L.M., 1971. Complications of groin hernia and of hernial repair. Surg. Clin. N. Am. 51 (6), 1325–1336.

Courtney, C.A., Duffy, K., Serpell, M.G., O'Dwyer, P.J., 2002. Outcome of patients with severe chronic pain following repair of groin hernia. Br. J. Surg. 89 (10), 1310–1314.

Cousinery, M.C., Li, R., Vannitamby, A., Vikraman, J., Southwell, B.R., Hutson, J.M., 2016. Neurotrophin signaling in a genitofemoral nerve target organ during testicular descent in mice. J. Pediatr. Surg. 51 (8), 1321–1326.

Cranfield, K.A., Buist, R.J., Nandi, P.R., Baranowski, A.P., 1997. The twelfth rib syndrome. J. Pain Symptom Manag. 13 (3), 172–175.

Cruveilhier, J., 1844. The Anatomy of the Human Body, 1 ed. Harper & Brothers, New York.

Dakwar, E., Vale, F.L., Uribe, J.S., 2011. Trajectory of the main sensory and motor branches of the lumbar plexus outside the psoas muscle related to the lateral retroperitoneal transpsoas approach. J. Neurosurg. Spine 14 (2), 290–295.

Davis, T.T., Bae, H.W., Mok, J.M., Rasouli, A., Delamarter, R.B., 2011. Lumbar plexus anatomy within the psoas muscle: implications for the transpsoas lateral approach to the L4–L5 disc. J. Bone Joint Surg. Am. 93 (16), 1482–1487.

De Ridder, V.A., de Lange, S., Popta, J.V., 1999. Anatomical variations of the lateral femoral cutaneous nerve and the consequences for surgery. J. Orthop. Trauma 13, 207–211.

Demirer, S., Kepenekci, I., Evirgen, O., Birsen, O., Tuzuner, A., Karahuseyinoglu, S., Ozban, M., Kutedam, E., 2006. The effect of polypropylene mesh on ilioinguinal nerve in open mesh repair of groin hernia. J. Surg. Res. 131, 175–181.

Dibenedetto, L.M., Lei, Q., Gilroy, A.M., Hermey, D.C., Marks Jr., S.J., Page, D.W., 1996. Variations in the inferior pelvic pathway of the lateral femoral cutaneous nerve: implications for laparoscopic hernia repair. Clin. Anat. 9, 232–236.

Dittrick, G.W., Ridl, K., Kuhn, J.A., McCarty, T.M., 2004. Routine ilioinguinal nerve excision in inguinal hernia repairs. Am. J. Surg. 188, 736–740.

D'Avella, D., Mingrino, S., 1979. Microsurgical anatomy of lumbosacral spinal roots. J. Neurosurg. 51, 819–823.

D'Souza, L., Jagannathan, S., McManus, F., 1994. Subcostal nerve: anatomical awareness in Salter's innominate osteotomy. J. Pediatr. Orthop. 14 (5), 660–661.

Eichenberger, U., Greher, M., Kirchmair, L., Curatolo, M., Moriggl, B., 2006. Ultrasound-guided blocks of the ilioinguinal and iliohypogastric nerve: accuracy of a selective new technique confirmed by anatomical dissection. Br. J. Anaesth. 97 (2), 238–243.

Ellis, G., 1887. Demonstrations of Anatomy, vol. 11, pp. 543–631.

Fahim, D.K., Kim, S.D., Cho, D., Lee, S., Kim, D.H., 2011. Avoiding abdominal flank bulge after anterolateral approaches to the thoracolumbar spine: cadaveric study and electrophysiological investigation. J. Neurosurg. Spine 15 (5), 532–540.

Farny, J., Drolet, P., Girard, M., 1994. Anatomy of the posterior approach to the lumbar plexus block. Can. J. Anaesth. 41 (6), 480–485.

Feigl, G.C., Ulz, H., Pixner, T., Dolcet, C., Likar, R., Sander-Kiesling, A., 2013. Anatomical investigation of a new vertical obturator nerve block technique. Ann. Anat. 195 (1), 82–87.

Gaines, R.D., 1978. Complications of groin hernia repair: their prevention and management. J. Natl. Med. Assoc. 70, 195.

Geh, N., Schultz, M., Yang, L., Zeller, J., 2015. Retroperitoneal course of iliohypogastric, ilioinguinal, and genitofemoral nerves: a study to improve identification and excision during triple neurectomy. Clin. Anat. 28 (7), 903–909.

Gofeld, M., Christakis, M., 2006. Sonographically guided ilioinguinal nerve block. J. Ultrasound Med. 25, 1571–1575.

Goubier, J., Teboul, F., Yeo, S., 2012. Transfer of two motor branches of the anterior obturator nerve to the motor portion of the femoral nerve: an anatomical feasibility study. Microsurgery 32 (6), 463–465.

Goulding, K., Beaule, P.E., Kim, P.R., Fazekas, A., 2010. Incidence of lateral femoral cutaneous nerve neuropraxia after anterior approach hip arthroplasty. Clin. Orthop. Relat. Res. 468, 2397–2404.

Grafenberg, E., 1904. Die entwickelung der MenschlichenBeckenmuskulatur. Anat. Hefte 259–390. Mowh. Jb, 21: 241-277. 23: 431-493.

Gray, H., 1867. Anatomy, Descriptive and Surgical, first ed., p. 582

Gray, H., 1918. Anatomy of the Human Body. URL: http://www.bartleby.com/107/212.html.

Griffin, M., 1891. Some varieties of the last dorsal and first lumbar nerves. J. Anat. Physiol. 26, 48–55.

Grothaus, M.C., Holt, M., Mekhail, A.O., Ebraheim, N.A., Yeasting, R.A., 2005. Lateral femoral cutaneous nerve: an anatomic study. Clin. Orthop. Relat. Res. 437, 164–168.

Gupta, A., Muzumdar, D., Ramani, P.S., 2004. Meralgiaparesthetica following lumbar spine surgery: a study in 110 consecutive surgically treated cases. Neurol. India 52, 64–66.

Gustafson, K.J., Pinault, G.C., Neville, J.J., Syed, I., Davis Jr., J.A., Jean-Claude, J., Triolo, R.J., 2009. Fasucular anatomy of human femoral nerve: implications for neural prostheses using nerve cuff electrodes. J. Rehabil. Res. Dev. 46 (7), 973–984.

Hager, W., 1885. Neuralgia femoris: resection des nerv, cutan, femoris anterior externus. Dtsch. Med. Wochenschr. 11, 218.

Hahn, L., 2011. Treatment of ilioinguinal nerve entrapment—a randomized controlled trial. Acta Obstet. Gynecol. Scand. 90, 955–960.

Haijiao, W., Koti, M., Smith, F., Wardlaw, D., 2001. Diagnosis of lumbosacral nerve root anomalies by magnetic resonance imaging. J. Spinal Disord. 14, 143–149.

Hakeem, A., Shanmugam, V., 2011. Current trends in the diagnosis and management of post-herniorraphy chronic groin pain. World J. Gastrointest. Surg. 3 (6), 73–81.

Harman, N.B., 1898. The caudal limit of the lumbar visceral efferent nerves in man. J. Anat. Physiol. 32 (3), 403–421.

Harshavardhana, N.S., Dabke, V.H., 2014. The furcal nerve revisited. Orthop. Rev. 6 (3), 5428, 2014.

Henry, A.K., 1973. Extensile Exposure, second ed. Churchill Livingstone, London.

Hollinshead, W.H., 1956a. Anatomy for Surgeons. In: The Thorax, Abdomen and Pelvis, vol. 2. Hoeber-Harper, New York, pp. 850–870.

Hollinshead, W.H., 1956b. Anatomy for Surgeons. In: The Thorax, Abdomen and Pelvis, vol. 2. Cassell & Co, London, pp. 636–638.

Hollinshead, W.H., 1964. Anatomy for Surgeons, vol. 3. Harper and Row, New York, pp. 597–605.

Hong, J.Y., Kim, W., Koo, B., Kim, Y., Jo, Y., Kil, H., 2010. The relative position of ilioinguinal and iliohypogastric nerves in different age groups of pediatric patients. Acta Anaesthesiol. Scand. 54, 566–570.

Houdek, M.T., Wagner, E.R., Wyles, C.C., Moran, S.L., 2014. Anatomical feasibility of the anterior obturator nerve transfer to restore bowel and bladder function. Microsurgery 34 (6), 459–463.

Howell, A.B., 1936. The phylogenetic arrangement of the muscular system. Anat. Rec. 66, 295–316.

Hutson, J.M., Southwell, B.R., Li, R., Lie, G., Ismail, K., Harisis, G., Chen, N., 2013. The regulation of testicular descent and the effects of cryptorchidism. Endcor. Rev. 34 (5), 725–752.

Izci, Y., Gurkanlar, D., Ozan, H., Gonul, E., 2005. The morphological aspects of lumbar plexus and roots: an anatomical study. Turk Neurosurg. 15, 87–92.

Jirsch, J.D., Chalk, C.H., 2007. Obturator neuropathy complicating elective laparoscopic tubal occlusion. Muscle Nerve 36, 104–106.

Jo, S.Y., Chang, J.C., Bae, H.G., Oh, J., Heo, J., Hwang, J.C., 2016. A Morphometric study of the obturator nerve around the obturator foramen. J. Korean Neurosurg. Soc. 59 (3), 282–286.

Katritsis, E., Anagnostopoulou, S., Papadopoulos, N., 1980. Anatomical observations on the accessory obturator nerve (based on 1000 specimens). Anat. Anzeiger 148, 440–445.

Kendir, S., Akkaya, T., Comert, A., et al., 2008. The location of the obturator nerve: a three-dimensional description of the obturator canal. Surg. Radiol. Anat. 30 (6), 495–501.

Khedkar, S.M., Bhalerao, P.M., Yemul-Golhar, S.R., Kelkar, K.V., 2015. Ultrasound-guided ilioinguinal and iliohypogastric nerve block, a comparison with the conventional technique: an observational study. Saudi J. Anaesth. 9 (3), 293–297.

Khorrami, M., Hadi, M., Javid, A., et al., 2012. A comparison between blind and nerve stimulation guided obturator nerve block in transurethral resection of bladder tumor. J. Endourol. 26 (10), 1391-1322.

Khoshmohabat, H., Panahi, F., Alvandi, A.A., Mehrvarz, S., Mohebi, H.A., Koushki, E.S., 2012. Effect of ilioinguinal neurectomy on chronic pain following herniorrhaphy. Trauma Mon. 17, 323.

Kikuchi, S., Hasue, M., Nishiyama, K., Ito, T., 1984. Anatomical and clinical studies of radicular symptoms. Spine 9, 23–29.

Kikuchi, S., Hasue, M., Nishiyama, M., Ito, T., 1986. Anatomic features of the furcal nerve and its clinical significance. Spine 11, 1002–1007.

Kim, S., Seok, H., Lee, S.Y., Park, S.W., 2014. Acetabular paralabral cyst as a rare cause of obturator neuropathy: a case report. Ann. Rehabil. Med. 38 (3), 427–432.

Kim, K.S., Ji, S.R., Hong, M.K., Kwon, Y.J., Hwang, J.H., Lee, S.Y., 2015. Intercostal nerve schwannoma encountered during a rib-latissimus dorsi osteomyocutaneous flap operation. Arch. Plast. Surg. 42 (6), 800–802.

Kingman, S.A., Amid, P.K., Chen, D.C., 2016. Laparoscopic triple neurectomy. In: The Sages Manual of Groin Pain. Springer, pp. 333–342.

Klaassen, Z., Marshall, E., Tubbs, R.S., Louis Jr., R.G., Wartmann, C.T., Loukas, M., 2011. Anatomy of the ilioinguinal and iliohypogastric nerves with observations of their spinal nerve contributions. Clin. Anat. 24, 454–461.

Kline, C.M., Lucas, C.E., Ledgerwood, A.M., 2013. Directed neurectomy for treatment of chronic postsurgical neuropathic pain. Am. J. Surg. 205, 246–249.

Knockaert, D., Heygere, F., Bobbaers, H., 1989. Ilioinguinal nerve entrapment: a little-known cause of iliac fossa pain. Postgrad. Med. J. 65, 632–635.

Kopell, H.P., Thompson, W.A., Postel, A.H., 1962. Entrapment neuropathy of the ilioinguinal nerve. N. Engl. J. Med. 266, 16–19.

Kumka, M., 2010. Critical Sites of entrapment of the posterior division of the obturator nerve: anatomical considerations. J. Can. Chiropr. Assoc. 54 (1), 33–42.

Leche, W., 1900. Muskulatur. Saugethiere: Mammalia. In: Bronn's Klassen und Ordnungen des Thierreichs, vol. 6, pp. 649–919.

Linder, H.H., 1989. Clinical Anatomy. Appleton & Lange, East Norwalk, CT.

Lennon, R.L., Horlocker, T.T., 2006. Mayo Clinic Analgesic Pathway: Peripheral Nerve Blockade for Major Orthopedic Surgery and Procedural Training Manual. CRC Press, p. 6.

Lonchena, T.K., McFadden, K., Orebaugh, S.L., 2016. Correlation of ultrasound appearance, gross anatomy, and histology of the femoral nerve at the femoral triangle. Surg. Radiol. Anat. 38 (1), 115–122.

Loos, M.J.A., Scheltinga, M.R.M., Roumen, R.M.H., 2008a. Surgical management of inguinal neuralgia after a low transverse Pfannenstiel incision. Ann. Surg. 248 (5), 880–885.

Loos, M.J., Scheltinga, M.R., Mulders, L.G., Roumen, R.M., 2008b. The Pfannenstiel incision as a source of chronic pain. Obstet. Gynecol. 111, 839–846.

Lovering, R., Anderson, L., 2008. Architecture and fiber type of the pyramidalis muscle. Anat. Sci. Int. 83 (4), 294–297.

Luijendijk, R.W., Jeekel, J., Storm, R.K., Schutte, P.J., Hop, W., Drogendijk, A.C., et al., 1997. The low transverse Pfannenstiel incision and the prevalence of incisional hernia and nerve entrapment. Ann. Surg. 225, 365.

Lykissas, M.G., Kostas-Agnantis, I.P., Korompilias, A.V., Vekris, M.D., Beris, A.E., 2013. Use of intercostal nerves for different target neurotization in brachial plexus reconstruction. World J. Orthop. 4 (3), 107–111.

Machin, D.G., Shennan, J.M., 1983. Twelfth rib syndrome: a differential diagnosis of loin pain. Br. Med. J. 287 (6392), 586.

Mahadevan, V., 2008. Pelvic girdle and lower limb. In: Standring, S. (Ed.), Gray's Anatomy: The Anatomical Basis of Clinical Practice, 40th ed. Elsevier, New York, pp. 1327–1429.

Maigne, J.Y., Maigne, R., Guerin-Surville, H., 1986. Anatomic study of the lateral cutaneous rami of the subcostal and iliohypogastric nerves. Surg. Radiol. Anat. 8 (4), 251–256.

Maiuri, F., Gambardella, A., 1986. Anomalies of the lumbosacral nerve roots. Neurol. Res. 11, 130–135.

Majkrzak, A., Johnston, J., Kacey, D., Zeller, J., 2010. Variability of the lateral femoral cutaneous nerve: an anatomic basis for planning safe surgical approaches. Clin. Anat. 23, 304–311.

Maldonado, P.A., Slocum, P.D., Chin, K., Corton, M.M., 2014. Anatomic relationships of psoas muscle: clinical applications to psoas hitch ureteral reimplantation. Am. J. Obstet. Gynecol. 211 (5), 563.

Malekpour, F., Mirhashemi, S.H., Hajinasrolah, E., Salehi, N., Khoshkar, A., Kolahi, A.A., 2008. Ilioinguinal nerve excision in open mesh repair of inguinal hernia—results of a randomized clinical trial: simple solution for a difficult problem? Am. J. Surg. 195, 735–740.

Mandelkow, H., Loeweneck, H., 1988. The iliohypogastric and ilioinguinal nerves. Distribution in the abdominal wall, danger areas in surgical incisions in the inguinal and pubic regions and reflected visceral pain in their dermatomes. Surg. Radiol. Anat. 10 (2), 145–149.

Martinoli, C., Miguel-Perez, M., Gandolfo, N., Zicca, A., Tagliafico, A., 2013. Imaging of neuropathies about the hip. Eur. J. Radiol. 82 (1), 17–26.

Mathers, J., Haley, C., Gofeld, M., 2015. Ilioinguinal nerve block in obese patients: description of new technique. J. Med. Ultrasound 23, 185–188.

McCrory, P., Bell, S., 1999. Nerve entrapment syndromes as a cause of pain in the hip, groin and buttock. Sport. Med. 27, 261–274.

McMinn, R.M.H., 2003. Last's Anatomy: Regional and Applied, ninth ed. Elsevier, Australia, p. 397.

Miller, J.P., Acar, F., Kaimaktchiev, V., Gultekin, S., Burchiel, K., 2008. Pathology of ilioinguinal neuropathy produced by mesh entrapment: case report and literature review. Hernia 12, 213–216.

Mirjalili, S.A., 2015. Anatomy of the lumbar plexus. In: Tubbs, R.S., Rizk, E., Shoja, M.M., Loukas, M., Barbaro, N., Spinner, R.J. (Eds.), Nerves and Nerve Injuries, vol. 1. Elsevier, San Diego, pp. 614–617, 2015.

Moosman, D.A., Oelrich, T.M., 1977. Prevention of accidental trauma to the ilioinguinal nerve during inguinal herniorrhaphy. Am. J. Surg. 133, 146–148.

Moore, K.L., Dalley, A.F., 1999. Clinically Oriented Anatomy, fourth ed. Lippincott, Williams & Wilkins, Baltimore, MD.

Moore, A.E., Stringer, M.D., 2011. Iatrogenic femoral nerve injury: a systemic review. Surg. Radiol. Anat. 33 (8), 649–658.

Moore, K.L., Daly, A.F., Agur, A.M.R., 2010. Clinically Oriented Anatomy, sixth ed. Lippincott Williams & Wilkins, Philadelphia.

Muhly, W.T., Orebaugh, S.L., 2011. Ultrasound evaluation of the anatomy of the vessels in relation to the femoral nerve at the femoral crease. Surg. Radiol. Anat. 33 (6), 491–494.

Mui, W.L., Ng, C.S., Fung, T.M., Cheung, F.K., Wong, C.M., Ma, T.H., Bn, M.Y., Ng, E.K., 2006. Prophylactic ilioinguinal neurectomy in open inguinal hernia repair: a double-blind randomized controlled trial. Ann. Surg. 244, 27–33.

Murinova, N., Krashin, D., Trescot, A.M., 2016. Ilioinguinal nerve entrapment: pelvic. In: Peripheral Nerve Entrapments. Springer, pp. 467–477.

Mürtz, P., Kaschner, M., Lakghomi, A., Gieseke, J., Willinek, W.A., Schild, H.H., Thomas, D., 2015. Diffusion-weighted MR neurography of the brachial and lumbosacral plexus: 3.0 T versus 1.5 T imaging. Eur. J. Radiol. 84 (4), 696–702.

Nasseh, H., Pourreza, F., Saberi, A., Kazemnejad, E., Kalantari, B.B., Falahatkar, S., 2013. Focal Neuropathies following percutaneous nephrolithotomy (PCNL) – preliminary study. Ger. Med. Sci. 11 (7).

Ndiaye, A., Diop, M., Ndoye, J., Konaté, I., Mané, L., Nazarian, S., Dia, A., 2007. Anatomical basis of neuropathies and damage to the ilioinguinal nerve during repairs of groin hernias. (about 100 dissections). Surg. Radiol. Anat. 29, 675–681.

Netter, F.H., 2003. Abdomen. Atlas of Human Anatomy, third ed. Icon Learning Systems, Teterboro, NJ, p. 259.

Oh, J., Kang, M., Park, J., Lee, J.I., 2014. A possible cause of snapping hip: intrapartum obturator neuropathy. Am. J. Phys. Med. Rehabil. 93 (6), 551.

Ombregt, L., 2013. Disorders of the thoracic spine: pathology and treatment. In: A System of Orthopaedic Medicine, third ed. Churchill Livingstone, pp. 169–184.

Orebaugh, S.L., 2006. The femoral nerve and its relationship to the lateral circumflex femoral artery. Anesth. Analg. 102 (6), 1859–1862.

Palastanga, N., Field, D., Soames, R., 1998. Anatomy & Human Movement: Structure & Function, 3rded. Butterworth Heinemann, Boston, MA, p. 11.

Papadopoulos, N.J., Katritsis, E.D., 1981. Some observations on the course and relations of the iliohypogastric and ilioinguinal nerves (based on 348 specimens). Anat. Anzeiger 149, 357–364.

Parisi, T.J., Mandrekar, J., Dyck, P.J., Klein, C.J., 2011. Meralgia-paresthetica: relation to obesity, advanced age, and diabetes mellitus. Neurology.

Park, E.S., Rha, D., Lee, W.C., Sim, E.G., 2014. The effect of obturator nerve block on hip lateralization in low functioning children with spastic cerebral palsy. Yonsei Med. J. 55 (1), 191–196.

Parke, W., Watanabe, R., 1987. Lumbosacral intersegmental epispinal axons and ectopic ventral nerve rootlets. J. Neurosurg. 67, 269–277.

Paterson, A.M., 1894. The origin and distribution of the nerves to the lower limb. J Anat Physiol 28 (Pt 2), 169–193.

Pećina, M.M., Nemanić, J.K., Markieitz, A.D., 1997. Tunnel Syndromes: Peripheral Nerve Compression Syndromes, second ed. CRC Press, Boca Raton, pp. 173–175.

Picchio, M., Palimento, D., Attanasio, U., Matarazzo, P.F., Bambini, C., Caliendo, A., 2004. Randomized controlled trial of preservation or elective division of ilioinguinal nerve on open inguinal hernia repair with polypropylene mesh. Arch. Surg. 139, 755–758.

Pirela-Cruz, M.A., 1998. Surgical exposures of the peripheral nerves in the extremities. In: Omer, G.E., Spinner, M., Van Beek, A.L. (Eds.), Management of Peripheral Nerve Problems, second ed. W.B. Saunders Company, Philadelphia, pp. 197–198.

Poobalan, A.S., Bruce, J., Smith, W.C.S., King, P.M., Krukowski, Z.H., Chambers, W.A., 2003. A review of chronic pain after inguinal herniorrhaphy. Clin. J. Pain 19, 48–54.

Pratt, N.E., 1991. Clinical Musculoskeletal Anatomy. Lippincott, New York, NY.

Purves, J., Miller, J., 1986. Inguinal neuralgia: a review of 50 patients. Can. J. Surg. 29, 43–45.

Quain, J., Sharpey, W., Thomson, A., Cleland, J.G., 1867. Quain's Elements of Anatomy, 7 ed. The University of California, James Walton, pp. 663–664.

Rab, M., Dellon, A., 2001. Anatomic variability of the ilioinguinal and genitofemoral nerve: implications for the treatment of groin pain. Plast. Reconstr. Surg. 108, 1618–1623.

Ray, B., D'Souza, A.S., Kumar, B., Marx, C., Ghosh, B., Gupta, N.K., Marx, A., 2010. Variations in the course and microanatomical study of the lateral femoral cutaneous nerve and its clinical importance. Clin. Anat. 23, 978–984.

Reinpold, W., Schroeder, A., Schroeder, M., Berger, C., Rohr, M., Wehrenberg, U., 2015. Retroperitoneal anatomy of the iliohypogastric, ilioinguinal, genitofemoral, and lateral femoral cutaneous nerve: consequences for prevention and treatment of chronic inguinodynia. Hernia 19, 539–548.

Rigaud, J., Labat, J., Riant, T., Hamel, O., Bouchot, O., Robert, R., 2008. Treatment of obturator neuralgia with laparoscopic neurolysis. J. Urol. 179 (2), 590–595.

Ritter, J.W., 1995. Femoral nerve "sheath" for inguinal paravascular lumbar plexus block is not found in human cadavers. J. Clin. Anesth. 7 (6), 470–473.

Rodrigues de Souza, R., Gama, E.F., El-RaziNeto, S., Maldonado, D., 2015. Effects of metabolic syndrome on the ultrastructure of the femoral nerve in aging rats. Histol. Histopathol. 30 (10), 1185–1192.

Rohini, M., Yogesh, A.S., Banerjee, C., Goyal, M., 2012. Variant accessory obturator nerve? A case report and embryological review. J Med Health Sci 1, 7–9.

Romanes, G.J., 1981. Cunningham's Textbook of Anatomy, twelfth ed. Oxford University Press, Oxford.

Ropars, M., Morandi, X., Huten, D., Thomazeau, H., Berton, E., Darnault, P., 2009. Anatomical study of the lateral femoral cutaneous nerve with special reference to minimally invasive anterior approach for total hip replacement. Surg. Radiol. Anat. 31, 199–204.

Rosenberger, R., Loeweneck, H., Meyer, G., 2000. The cutaneous nerves encountered during laparoscopic repair of inguinal hernia. Surg. Endosc. 14, 731–735.

Roth, V.K., 1895. Meralgiaparesthetica. Med ObozrMozk 43, 678.

Rozen, S., Rodriguez-Lorenzo, A., Audolfsson, T., Wong, C., Cheng, A., 2013. Obturator nerve anatomy and the relevance to one-stage facial reanimation: limitations of a retroperitoneal approach. Plast. Reconstr. Surg. 131 (5), 1057–1064.

Rudin, D., Manestar, M., Ullrich, O., Erhardt, J., Grob, K., 2016. The anatomical course of the lateral femoral cutaneous nerve with special attention to the anterior approach to the hip joint. J Bone Joint Surg Am 98, 561–567.

Salama, J., Sarfati, E., Chevrel, J., 1983. The anatomical bases of nerve lesions arising during the reduction of inguinal hernia. Anat. Clin. 5, 75–81.

Sasaoka, N., Kawaguchi, M., Yoshitani, K., Kato, H., Suzuki, A., Furuya, H., 2005. Evaluation of genitofemoral nerve block, in addition to ilioinguinal and iliohypogastric nerve block, during inguinal hernia repair in children. Br. J. Anaesth. 94, 243–246.

Sauerland, E.K., 1994. Grant's Dissector, 11thed. Williams & Wilkins, Baltimore, MD.

Schaeffer, J.P., 1946. Morris' Human Anatomy: A Complete Systemic Treatise. The Blakiston Company, Philadelphia.

Schaeffer, J.P., 1953. Morris' Human Anatomy: A Complete Systematic Treatise, eleventh ed. McGraw-Hill Book Company, Inc., New York.

Schafer, E.A., Thane, G.D., 1895. Quain's Elements of Anatomy Vol III-Part II: The Nerves, tenth ed. Longmans, Green, and Co, London.

Schoor, A., Boon, J., Bosenberg, A., Abrahams, P.H., Meiring, J., 2005. Anatomical considerations of the pediatric ilioinguinal/iliohypogastric nerve block. Paediatr. Anaesth. 15, 371–377.

Shanthanna, H., 2014. Successful treatment of genitofemoral neuralgia using ultrasound guided injection: a case report and short review of literature. Case Rep. Anesthesiol. https://doi.org/10.1155/2014/371703.

Sim, I.W., Webb, T., 2004. Anatomy and anaesthesia of the lumbar somatic plexus. Anaesth. Intensive Care 32, 178–187.

Soldatos, T., Andreisek, G., Thawait, G.K., Guggenberger, R., Williams, E.H., Carrino, J.A., Chhabra, A., 2013. High-Resolution 3-T MR neurography of the lumbosacral plexus. RadioGraphics 33 (4), 967–987.

Soong, J., Schafhalter-Zoppoth, I., Gray, A.T., 2007. Sonographic imaging of the obturator nerve for regional block. Reg. Anesth. Pain Med. 32 (2), 146–151.

Spratt, J.D., Logan, B.M., Abrahams, P.H., 1996. Variant slips of psoas and iliacus muscles, with splitting of the femoral nerve. Clin. Anat. 9 (6), 401–404.

Standring, S., 2005. Gray's Anatomy, 39th ed. Elsevier, Philadelphia.

Standring, S., 2008. Gray's Anatomy, 40th Ed. Churchill Livingstone, London, pp. 1069–1081.

Standring, S., 2015. Gray's Anatomy: The Anatomical Basis of Clinical Practice, 41st ed. Elsevier Health Sciences, New York.

Standring, S., 2016. Gray's Anatomy: The Anatomical Basis of Clinical Practice, 41st ed. Elsevier, London.

Stark, E., Oestreich, K., Wendl, K., Rumstadt, B., Hagmüller, E., 1999. Nerve irritation after laparoscopic hernia repair. Surg. Endosc. 13, 878–881.

Starling, J.R., Harms, B.A., 1989. Diagnosis and treatment of genitofemoral and ilioinguinal neuralgia. World J. Surg. 13, 586–591.

Stewart, J.D., 2000. Focal Peripheral Neuropathies, third ed. LWW, Philadelphia, PA.

Stulz, P., Pfeiffer, K.M., 1980. Postoperative nerve irritation syndromes of peripheral nerves after routine interventions in the lower abdomen and the inguinal region. Chirurg 51 (10), 664–667.

Stulz, P., Pfeiffer, K.M., 1982. Peripheral nerve injuries resulting from common surgical procedures in the lower portion of the abdomen. Arch. Surg. 117, 324–327.

Su, S., Farmer, P.J., Li, R., Sourial, M., Buraundi, S., Bodemer, D., Southwell, B.R., Hutson, J.M., 2012. Regression of the mammary branch of the genitofemoral nerve may be necessary for testicular descent in rats. J. Urol. 188, 1443–1448.

Sunderland, S., 1970. Anatomical features of nerve trunks in relation to nerve injury and nerve repair. Clin. Neurosurg. 17, 38–62.

Sunderland, S.S., 1978. Nerves and Nerve Injuries, second ed. Churchill Livingston, Edinburgh London and New York, pp. 999–1009.

Surucu, H.S., Tanyeli, E., Sargon, M.F., Karahan, S.T., 1997. An anatomic study of the lateral femoral cutaneous nerve. Surg. Radiol. Anat. 19, 307–310.

Swanson, L.W., 2015. Neuroanatomical Terminology: A Lexicon of Classical Origins and Historical Foundations. Oxford University Press, New York, p. 29.

Tagliafico, A., Bignotti, B., Cadoni, A., Perez, M.M., Martinoli, C., 2015. Anatomical study of the iliohypogastric, ilioinguinal, and genitofemoral nerves using high-resolution ultrasound. Muscle Nerve 51 (1), 42–48.

Tekgul, Z.T., Divrik, R.T., Turan, M., Konyalioglu, E., Simsek, E., Gonullu, M., 2014. Impact of obturator nerve block on the short-term recurrence of superficial bladder tumors on the lateral wall. Urol. J. 11 (1), 1248–1252.

Thane, G.D., 1895. Quain's Elements of Anatomy In: Part 2: The Nerves, tenth ed., vol. 3. Longmans, Green, and Co., London.

Thomassen, I., van Suijlekom, J., van de Gaag, A., Ponten, J., Nienhuijs, S., 2013. Ultrasound-guided ilioinguinal/iliohypogastric nerve blocks for chronic pain after inguinal hernia repair. Hernia 17, 329–332.

Tipton, J.S., 2008. Obturator neuropathy. Curr. Rev. Musculoskeletal Med. 1 (3–4), 234–237.

Tokita, K., 2006. Anatomical significance of the nerve to the pyramidalis muscle: a morphological study. Anat. Sci. Int. 81 (4), 210–224.

Tomaszewski, K.A., Popieluszko, P., Henry, B.M., Roy, J., Sanna, B., Kijek, M.R., Walocha, J.A., 2016. The surgical anatomy of the lateral femoral cutaneous nerve in the inguinal region: a meta- analysis. Hernia 20, 649–657.

Tran, T.M., Ivanusic, J.J., Hebbard, P., Barrington, M.J., 2009. Determination of spread of injectate after ultrasound-guided transversus abdominis plane block: a cadaveric study. Br. J. Anaesth. 102 (1), 123–127.

Tsui, B.C., 2016. Ilioinguinal and iliohypogastric nerve blocks. In: Pediatric Atlas of Ultrasound and Nerve Stimulation-Guided Regional Anesthesia. Springer, pp. 477–483.

Tubbs, R.S., Sheetz, J., Salter, G., Oakes, W.J., 2003. Accessory obturator nerves with bilateral pseudoganglia in man. Ann. Anat. 185 (6), 571–572.

Tubbs, R.S., Rizk, E., Shoja, M.M., Loukas, M., Barbaro, N., Spinner, R.J., 2015a. Nerves and Nerve Injuries. In: History, Embryology, Anatomy, Imaging, and Diagnostics, vol. 1. Academic Press, Cambridge, MA.

Tubbs, R.S., Rizk, E., Shoja, M.M., Loukas, M., Barbaro, N., Spinner, R.J., 2015b. Nerves and Nerve Injuries In: Pain, Treatment, Injury, Disease, and Future Directions, first ed., vol. 2. Elsevier.

Tung, T.H., Chao, A., Moore, A.M., 2012. Obturator nerve transfer for femoral nerve reconstruction: anatomic study and clinical application. Plast. Reconstr. Surg. 130 (5), 1066–1074.

Ulkar, B., Yildiz, Y., Kunduracioglu, B., 2003. Meralgiaparesthetica: a long-standing performance-limiting cause of anterior thigh pain in a soccer pain. Am. J. Sports Med. 31, 787–789.

Van Beek, A.L., 1998. Peripheral nerve injuries of the lower extremity. In: Omer, G.E., Spinner, M., Van Beek, A.L. (Eds.), Management of Peripheral Nerve Problems, second ed. W.B. Saunders Company, Philadelphia, pp. 58–59.

van der Graaf, T., Verhagen, P.C., Kerver, A.L., Kleinrensink, G.J., 2011. Surgical anatomy of the 10th and 11th intercostal and subcostal nerves: prevention of damage during lumbotomy. J. Urol. 186 (2), 579–583.

van Ramshorst, G.H., Kleinrensink, G.J., Hermans, J.J., Terkivatan, T., Lange, J.F., 2009. Abdominal wall paresis as a complication of laparoscopic surgery. Hernia 13 (5), 539–543.

Vanetti, T.K., Luba, A.T.R., Assis, F.D., de Oliveira, C.A., 2016. Genitofemoral nerve entrapment: pelvic. In: Peripheral Nerve Entrapments. Springer, pp. 479–489.

Vázquez, M.T., Murillo, J., Maranillo, E., Parkin, I.G., Sanudo, J., 2007. Femoral nerve entrapment: a new insight. Clin. Anat. 20 (2), 175–179.

Vernadakis, A.J., Koch, H., Mackinnon, S.E., 2003. Management of neuromas. Clin. Plast. Surg. 30, 247–268.

Verstraelen, H., De Zutter, E., De Muynck, M., 2015. Genitofemoral neuralgia: adding to the burden of chronic vulvar pain. J. Pain Res. 8, 845–849.

Vloka, J.D., Hadzić, A., Drobnik, L., Ernest, A., Reiss, W., Thys, D.M., 1999. Anatomical landmarks for femoral nerve block: a comparison of four needle insertion sites. Anesth. Analg. 89 (6), 1467–1470.

Vuilleumier, H., Hübner, M., Demartines, N., 2009. Neuropathy after herniorrhaphy: indication for surgical treatment and outcome. World J. Surg. 33 (4), 841–845.

Walji, A.H., Tsui, B.C., 2016. Clinical anatomy of the lumbar plexus. In: Pediatric Atlas of Ultrasound-And Nerve Stimulation-Guided Regional Anesthesia. Springer, pp. 165–175.

Webber, R.H., 1961. Some variations in the lumbar plexus of nerves in man. Acta Anat. 44, 336–345.

Whiteside, J.L., Barber, M.D., Walters, M.D., Falcone, T., 2003. Anatomy of ilioinguinal and iliohypogastric nerves in relation to trocar placement and low transverse incisions. Am. J. Obstet. Gynecol. 189 (6), 1574–1578.

Wijsmuller, A.R., Lange, J.F., Kleinrensink, G.J., van Geldere, D., Simons, M.P., Huygen, F.J., Jeekel, J., Lange, J.F., 2007. Nerve-identifying inguinal hernia repair: a surgical anatomical study. World J. Surg. 31, 414–420.

Williams, A., 2005. Pelvic girdle and lower limb. In: Standring, S. (Ed.), Gray's Anatomy: The Anatomical Basis of Clinical Practice, 39th ed. Elsevier, New York, pp. 1456–1499.

Williams, P.H., Trzil, K.P., 1991. Management of meralgiaparesthetica. J. Neurosurg. 74, 76–80.

Williams, E.H., Williams, C.G., Rosson, G.D., Heitmiller, R.F., Dellon, A.L., 2008. Neurectomy for treatment of intercostal neuralgia. Ann. Thorac. Surg. 85 (5), 1766–1770.

Woodburne, R.T., 1956. The accessory obturator nerve and the innervation of the pectineus muscle. Anat. Rec. 136, 367–369.

Yang, S.H., Wu, C.C., Chen, P.Q., 2005. Postoperative meralgiaparesthetica after posterior spine surgery: incidence, risk factors, and clinical outcomes. Spine 30, E547–E550.

Yasar, S., Kaya, S., Temiz, C., 2014. Morphological structure and variations of lumbar plexus in human fetuses. Clin. Anat. 27, 383–388.

Yavuz, F., Yasar, E., Taskaynatan, M.A., Goktepe, A.S., Tan, A.K., 2013. Nerve block of articular branches of the obturator and femoral nerves for the treatment of hip joint pain. J. Back Musculoskelet. Rehabil. 26 (1), 79–83.

Yukata, K., Arai, K., Yoshizumi, Y., Tamano, K., Imada, K., Nakaima, N., 2005. Obturator neuropathy caused by an acetabular labral cyst: MRI findings. Am. Journal. Rev. 184, S112–S114.

FURTHER READING

Akata, T., Murakami, J., Yoshinaga, A., 1999. Life-threatening haemorrhage following obturator artery injury during transurethral bladder surgery: a sequel of an unsuccessful obturator nerve block. Acta Anaesthesiol. Scand. 43, 784–788.

Atanassoff, P.G., Weiss, B.M., Brull, S.J., 1996. Lidocaine plasma levels following two techniques of obturator nerve block. J. Clin. Anesth. 8, 535–539.

Bardeen, C.R., Elting, A.W., 1901. A statistical study of the variations in the formation and position of the lumbosacral plexus in man. Anat. Anzeiger 19, 124–209.

Mirilas, P., Mentessidou, A., 2013. The secondary external inguinal ring and associated fascial planes: surgical anatomy, embryology, applications. Hernia 17, 379–389.

Porrett, P.M., Drebin, J., 2015. The Surgical Review: An Integrated Basic and Clinical Science Study Guide. Lippincott Williams & Wilkins.

Spaw, A.T., Ennis, B.W., Spaw, L.P., 1991. Laparoscopic hernia repair: the anatomic basis. J. Laparoendosc. Surg. 1, 269–277.

Standring, S., Anand, N., Birch, R., Collins, P., Crossman, A.R., Gleeson, M., Jawaheer, G., Smith, A., Spratt, J.D., Stringer, M.D., Tubbs, R.S., Tunstall, R., Wein, A.J., Wigley, C.B., 2016. Gray's Anatomy: The Anatomical Basis of Clinical Practice, 41st ed. Elsevier, Philadelphia.

CHAPTER 7

Lumbar Vertebrae

STEPHEN J. BORDES • R. SHANE TUBBS

EMBRYOLOGY

Spinal development is heavily influenced by the notochord and formation of somites (Kaplan et al., 2005). In the third week of embryonic life, gastrulation occurs, whereby a bilaminar disk forms a trilaminar disk. By the fourth week, epiblastic cells migrate toward the primitive streak and form a prechordal plate anteriorly and a notochordal process posteriorly (Tubbs et al., 2016). The vertebral column begins to form around this latter structure. By the end of the fifth week, 42–44 pairs of somites form from the paraxial mesoderm on either side of the notochord (Tubbs et al., 2016). These somites form in a cranial to caudal direction from clefts in the dorsal paraxial mesoderm and help to age the fetus (Kaplan et al., 2005). Each somite forms a sclerotome and a dermomyotome (Tubbs et al., 2016). The sclerotome becomes part of the vertebral column while the dermomyotome is responsible for muscle and soft-tissue development (Tubbs et al., 2016). A dorsal and ventrolateral process forms at the caudal end of each somite. The dorsal segment later becomes the neural arch while the ventrolateral part, or costal element, contributes to the development of the transverse process (Kaplan et al., 2005). Fusion of each vertebra depends on the close interaction of two sclerotomes, which are divided by developing intervertebral disks. Interaction between the chordal process and somitic mesenchyme ultimately forms the vertebral centrum (Kaplan et al., 2005). The centrum continues to expand concentrically with age as new axial mesenchyme increases in thickness and density around the notochord (Kaplan et al., 2005). Dorsal processes of the mesenchyme expand laterally to the developing dorsal root ganglion and contribute to the formation of the zygapophyseal joints. Blood vessels cross the developing vertebrae and nerves form in between. Intervertebral disks develop from axial mesenchyme opposite the lower half of cranial somitic mesenchyme (Kaplan et al., 2005). Pieces of the vertebrae, such as the spinal processes, form separately from the centrum and must fuse with it (Kaplan et al., 2005). As a result of this process, 5 lumbar vertebrae progressively develop in addition to 7 cervical, 12 thoracic, and 5 sacral vertebrae.

During the sixth week of development, the mesenchyme surrounding the notochord begins to take on a cartilaginous form (Tubbs et al., 2016). Chondrification centers form in the centrum of each vertebral body and quickly chondrify this structure. Centers then appear in each neural arch, expand dorsally, and fuse together (Kaplan et al., 2005). The spinous processes emerge at this point. Chondrification centers continue to expand laterally and ventrally, thus fusing together the rest of the vertebrae. Between the 9th and 10th weeks, ossification is simultaneously occurring with chondrification (Kaplan et al., 2005). Primary ossification centers form when blood vessels invade cartilaginous structures. By the 12th-14th weeks, each arch and body contains one of these centers (Kaplan et al., 2005). They expand radially and reach the anterior surface by week 22 and the posterior surface by week 25 (Kaplan et al., 2005). Superior and inferior aspects of the vertebral bodies are left cartilaginous as these growth plates will continue to expand with age. Even at birth, the distal aspects of vertebral joints and processes are still cartilaginous to allow for growth until puberty, at which point secondary ossification centers appear (Kaplan et al., 2005). These centers are separated from the rest of the vertebrae by thin layers of cartilage. By the 25th year of life, this cartilage ossifies and the remaining ossifications centers fuse with the rest of the vertebrae (Kaplan et al., 2005).

ANATOMY

The lumbar vertebrae consist of five vertebrae (Fig. 7.1). These vertebrae consist of an anterior part, known as the body. The vertebral body has flat superior and inferior surfaces and serves substantial weight-bearing function (Figs. 7.2 and 7.3). It is not solid, but rather a crystalline, cancellous shell containing cortical bone and spongy trabeculae (Fig. 7.4) (Bogduk, 2005). The shell

Surgical anatomy of the lateral transpsoas approach to the lumbar spine. https://doi.org/10.1016/B978-0-323-67376-1.00007-0

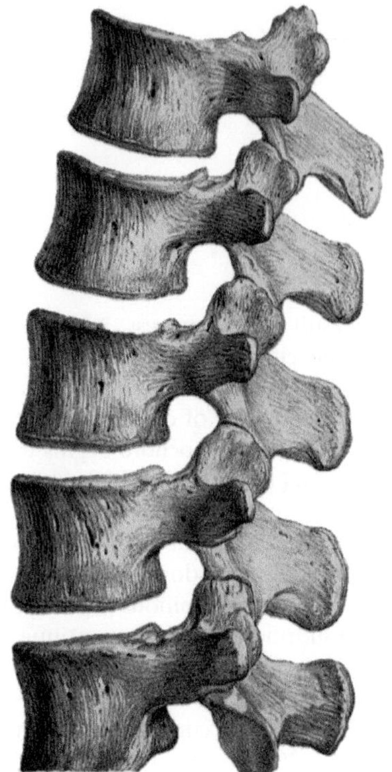
FIG. 7.1 Lateral view of the lumbar vertebrae.

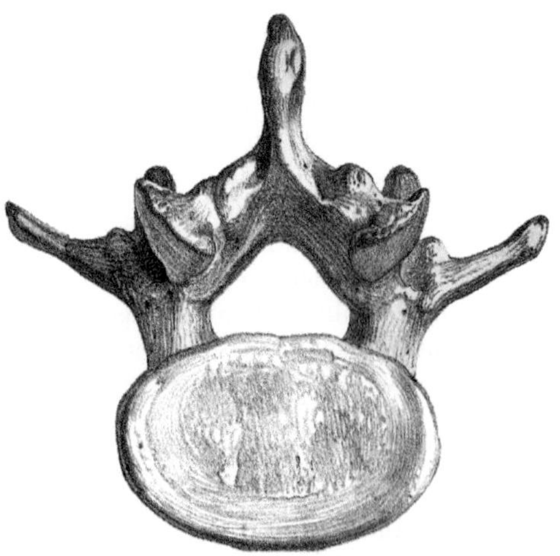
FIG. 7.2 Inferior view of a lumbar vertebra.

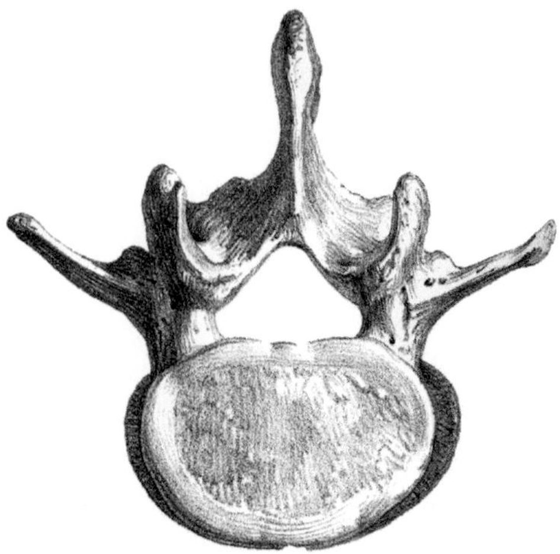
FIG. 7.3 Superior view of a lumbar vertebra.

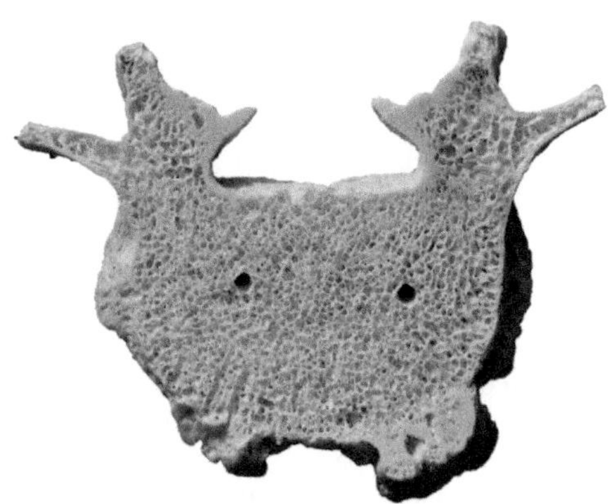
FIG. 7.4 Cross section through a lumbar vertebra noting the trabecular pattern of the body.

is supported by a meshwork of transverse and vertical trabeculae (Bogduk, 2005). Vertical trabeculae are the first to bear vertical forces; transverse trabeculae ensure that vertical trabeculae do not bend or bow with increasing longitudinal force (Bogduk, 2005). Hollow, spongy spaces, also known as the vertebral spongiosa, between the trabeculae transmit vertebral vasculature and house hematopoietic cells (Bogduk, 2005). This composition lightens the weight of each vertebra, prevents vertebral collapse, and allows the vertebrae to quickly dissipate sudden forces with a reduced risk of fracture (Bogduk, 2005). While solid bones possess great static strength, they weaken with dynamic activity. Such structure enables the vertebrae to possess great strength without sacrificing longitudinal weight-bearing integrity. As a result, articulating vertebrae can withstand immense vertical force; however, they are not designed for stability in any other directional plane (Bogduk, 2005).

Emerging from the posterior aspect of the body are two bony prominences known as the pedicles (Figs. 7.2 and 7.3). These pedicles allow for the superior and inferior orientation of the vertebra when viewed laterally (Bogduk, 2005). A lamina projects from each pedicle and fuses posteriorly at the midline (Fig. 7.3). These lamina form tentlike structures that surround and protect the neural arch (Bogduk, 2005). The laminae have sharp, jagged superolateral surfaces, smooth and round lateral surfaces, and enlarged inferolateral surfaces that become inferior articular processes (Bogduk, 2005). Four articular cartilages are present on each vertebra: two right and left, superior and inferior. Each inferior articular surface contains an articular facet on the lateral surface while each superior articular surface contains one on the medial surface (Figs. 7.2 and 7.3) (Bogduk, 2005). These facets are covered in smooth articular cartilage. Posteriorly, the superior articular process contains a smooth mammillary process (Bogduk, 2005). A spinous process emerges posteriorly from the midline junction of the two lamina and a transverse process emerges laterally from the junction of the pedicle and lamina (Bogduk, 2005). On its posterior surface, the transverse process contains an accessory process, which is a bony prominence that can vary in size and length (Bogduk, 2005). The accessory process lies inferior and lateral to the ipsilateral mammillary body (Bogduk, 2005). These two landmarks are separated by the mamillo-accessory notch (Bogduk, 2005). When viewed from above, the lumbar vertebrae contain a space between the body and neural arch, known as the vertebral foramen. This space transmits the spinal cord and associated nervous structures inside the vertebral column (Fig. 7.5).

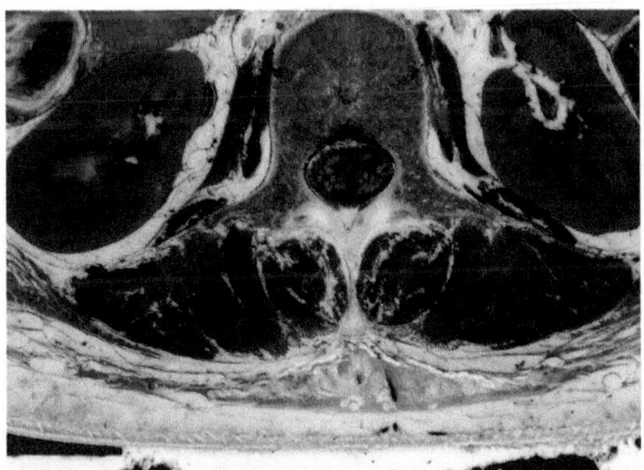

FIG. 7.5 Axial section through the lumbar spine in a cadaver. Note the relationship of the vertebra to the kidneys and deep back muscles. The cauda equina is noted within the vertebral foramen. (Image courtesy of Dr. Beom Sun Chung, Department of Anatomy, Ajou University School of Medicine, South Korea.)

When viewing the vertebrae laterally, two notches can be appreciated superior and inferior to the pedicle on either side. The superior notch is bordered anteriorly by the vertebral body, inferiorly by the pedicle, and posteriorly by the superior articular process (Bogduk, 2005). The inferior notch is much larger in size and is helpful in identifying superior and inferior borders of the vertebrae (Bogduk, 2005). It lies inferior to the pedicle and anterior to the lamina and inferior articular process (Bogduk, 2005). These notches form intervertebral foramina when they articulate with superior and inferior vertebrae.

The posterior parts of the vertebrae are able to resist many different forces that act on the column. Inferior articular processes project downward and interlock with the superior articular processes, forming synovial, zygapophyseal joints (Bogduk, 2005). This design resists the sheering and sliding forces of each body. The remaining processes, including the transverse, accessory, mammillary, and spinous, serve as sites of muscle attachment (Bogduk, 2005). Every muscle that acts of the vertebral column attaches to a posterior element (Bogduk, 2005). Psoas major and diaphragmatic crura attach to the vertebral bodies (Fig. 7.6); however, they do not act on the vertebral column (Bogduk, 2005). The laminae work to transfer forces working on various parts of the vertebral column which provides immense stability (Bogduk, 2005). Patients who have undergone laminectomy lose this support and vertebral mobility.

Vertical forces are transmitted from the laminae via to the pars interarticularis to the pedicles. The pars interarticularis is the specific part of the lamina that connects the superior and inferior articular processes (Bogduk, 2005). It comprises thicker cortical bone as this segment undergoes tremendous force by redirecting laminar forces to the horizontal plane of the pedicles and vertebral bodies (Bogduk, 2005). Weakness herein can predispose individuals to fracture.

The pedicles connect anterior and posterior elements of the vertebrae and undergo tremendous force as they function similar to a lever (Bogduk, 2005). They are made up of hollow, cylindrical cortical bone that can bend and tense in any direction which provides the qualities needed to carry out function (Bogduk, 2005). Any forces applied to the posterior vertebral elements are transferred to the vertebral bodies via the pedicles (Bogduk, 2005). These forces include those required to lock the articular processes to resist twisting and sliding in addition to the downward forces elicited by the muscles acting on the posterior elements (Bogduk, 2005).

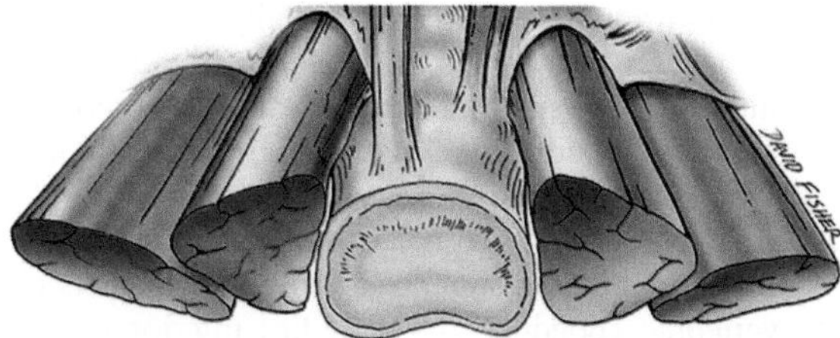

FIG. 7.6 Schematic drawing of the anterior lumbar spine noting the relationships of, from medial to lateral, the crura of the diaphragm, psoas major, and quadratus lumborum.

When two vertebrae articulate with one another, they form three intervertebral joints. The inferior articular processes of the superior vertebra form two joints via articulation with the two superior articular processes of the inferior vertebra (Bogduk, 2005). These joints are termed zygapophyseal or posterior intervertebral joints (Bogduk, 2005). The third joint is formed via articulation of the two vertebral bodies. This joint is rarely but properly referred to as the anterior intervertebral joint (Bogduk, 2005).

Zygapophyseal joints are synovial joints (Bogduk, 2005). Inferior and superior articular processes each have facets covered with articular cartilage. A synovial membrane and joint capsule span the area between these two surfaces (Bogduk, 2005). The capsule comprises dense collagenous and elastic fibers that weave around the joint's posterior, superior, and inferior borders (Bogduk, 2005). These fibers further attach to superior and inferior articular processes and form subcapsular pockets that are filled with fat (Bogduk, 2005). This fat is able to pass from the joint space to extracapsular space via small foramina at superior and inferior capsular margins (Bogduk, 2005). It functions to fill any remaining space and, as a result, is bordered externally by the capsule and internally by the synovium (Bogduk, 2005). The capsule's collagenous anterior border is replaced by the ligamentum flavum (Bogduk, 2005).

In addition to intraarticular fat, zygapophyseal joints also contain meniscoid structures (Bogduk, 2005). A small and thin connective tissue rim fills the curved margins left by articular cartilage. Adipose pads can be found at superior and inferior margins of the joint that contain fat and vasculature enclosed within a synovial fold (Bogduk, 2005). The synovial fold becomes continuous with the rest of the synovial joint as does the fat contained within it. Lastly, fibro-meniscoid structures, the longest of the meniscoid structures, extend from the joint's superior and inferior surfaces (Bogduk, 2005). These structures also contain vasculature and adipose wrapped within a layer of synovium which then become continuous with the rest of the joint (Bogduk, 2005). While the menisci may function primarily to fill, protect, and lubricate joint space, they may also help to receive and dissipate vertebral load (Bogduk, 2005).

It is important to note the orientation of the joints. Superior articular facets typically face posteromedially (Bogduk, 2005). The backward orientation of the superior joint surface prevents the superior vertebra from sliding forward as its inferior articular facet faces anteriorly (Bogduk, 2005). Furthermore, the medial orientation of the superior articular facet prevents vertebral rotation as the laterally oriented inferior articular facet locks the inferior vertebra in place (Bogduk, 2005). The degree of vertebral movement is thus limited by the orientation of the zygapophyseal joints. If a joint is oriented perpendicular to the sagittal plane, it greatly decreases forward movement but increases rotational movement (Bogduk, 2005). As a result, the orientation of the joint usually falls between 0 and 90 degrees to resist both forward and rotational movement to some degree (Bogduk, 2005).

The lumbar vertebrae have an intimate relationship with regional arteries and veins and are supplied by these neighboring structures. The abdominal aorta lies along the left anterior surface of the lumbar vertebrae and gives off lumbar arteries that supply the adjacent bone (Fig. 7.7). The inferior vena cava lies along the right anterior surface of the lumbar vertebrae and receive lumbar veins coursing over the anterior surface of the lumbar vertebral bodies. The vertebral venous plexus of Batson is related to the lumbar vertebral vertebrae at all levels (Figs. 7.8 and 7.9).

IMAGING

X-ray, CT, and MR imaging are very useful for vertebral imaging and recognition of various pathologies. Degenerative diseases are better detected with MR imaging and can be categorized according to the change (Tehranzadeh et al., 2000). In type I disease, T1-weighted images decrease in intensity while T2-weighted images increase (Tehranzadeh et al., 2000). Both indicate the presence of edema. Fatty changes, or type II changes, increase signal intensity on both T1- and T2-weighted images (Tehranzadeh et al., 2000). Finally, sclerotic, type II disease changes show a decreased intensity on both T1- and T2-weighted images (Tehranzadeh et al., 2000).

VARIATIONS

As prior research has shown, the lumbar vertebrae show the least variation when compared to the rest of the

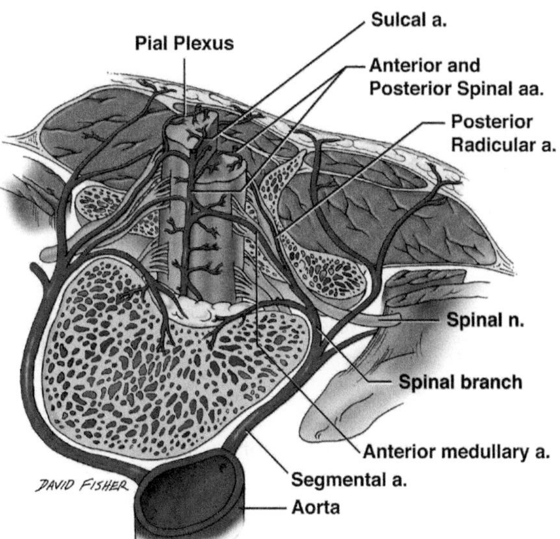

FIG. 7.7 Schematic drawing of the relationship of a lumbar vertebra and the aorta and lumbar arteries.

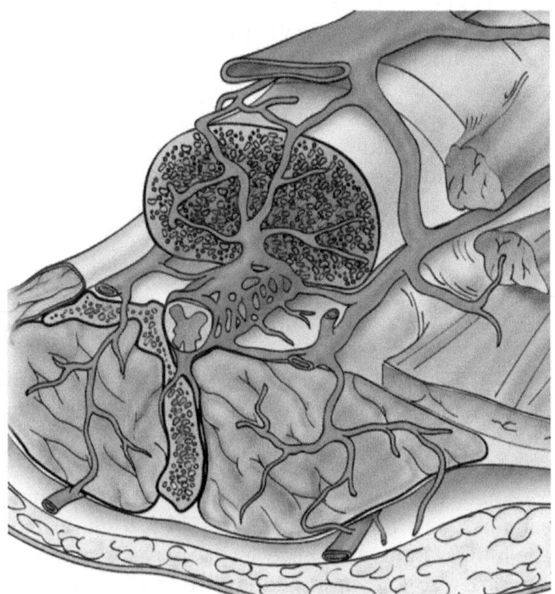

FIG. 7.8 Schematic drawing (inferior view) noting the circumferential venous relationships to the lumbar vertebra.

vertebral column (Tubbs et al., 2016). With that having been said, variants are known to exist.

The lumbosacral column is the most common vertebral site in which to find transitional vertebra. This variation typically involves L5 or S1 (Tubbs et al., 2016). In some cases, L5 can become sacralized unilaterally or bilaterally (Tubbs et al., 2016). In other cases, S1 can exhibit nonunion with the remaining four sacral vertebra and articulate directly with L5 and S2 (Tubbs et al., 2016). Such an anomaly is known as lumbarization of S1 (Tubbs et al., 2016). In these cases, intervertebral disk space tends to increase between S1 and S2 but can be small or nonexistent between L5 and S1 (Tubbs et al., 2016).

Congenital synchondrosis, also known as block vertebra, results from defective somite segmentation (Tubbs et al., 2016). Vertebral bodies adjacent to one another subsequently fuse together. In half of the cases, the apophyseal joints fuse together as well (Tubbs et al., 2016). In other cases, the adjacent vertebrae fuse entirely, forming a solid block of bone (Tubbs et al., 2016). It is not uncommon to see a remnant of the intervertebral disk in the middle of these fused vertebrae (Tubbs et al., 2016).

Fusion failure of both vertebral body halves result in sagittal cleft vertebrae (Tubbs et al., 2016). This cleft is formed from an invagination of cortical endplates (Tubbs et al., 2016). Such variation is oftentimes associated with a longitudinal extension of the notochord through the vertebral column as the cartilaginous outline begins to ossify (Tubbs et al., 2016).

Hemivertebra can form when one of the two primary ossification centers in the vertebral body fails to form (Fig. 7.10) (Fisahn et al., 2016). While disk spaces typically remain the same, the wedge-shaped lateral segment induces scoliosis when seen as an isolated deformity (Fisahn et al., 2016). Prior studies have hypothesized that lack of vasculature to a lateral vertebral half contributes to the failed development of one ossification center (Fisahn et al., 2016). Absence of the anterior vertebral body segment results in a dorsal hemivertebra (Tubbs et al., 2016). The ventral space is replaced with fibrous tissue (Tubbs et al., 2016) At the same time, a ventral hemivertebra can result from an absence of the posterior body segment (Tubbs et al., 2016). Both of these anomalies are much less common than lateral hemivertebrae (Tubbs et al., 2016).

Absence of a pedicle, while more common in the cervical spine, can occur in the lumbar spine (Tubbs et al., 2016). Failure of formation of an ossification center leads to development of a contralateral hyperplastic pedicle as well as malformed ipsilateral articular and transverse processes (Tubbs et al., 2016).

Certain endplate variations also exist. Notochordal remnants can cause a nuclear impression double hump, or Cupid's bow contour, whereas herniation of the nucleus pulposus causes a fibrotic squaring of the endplate either centrally or

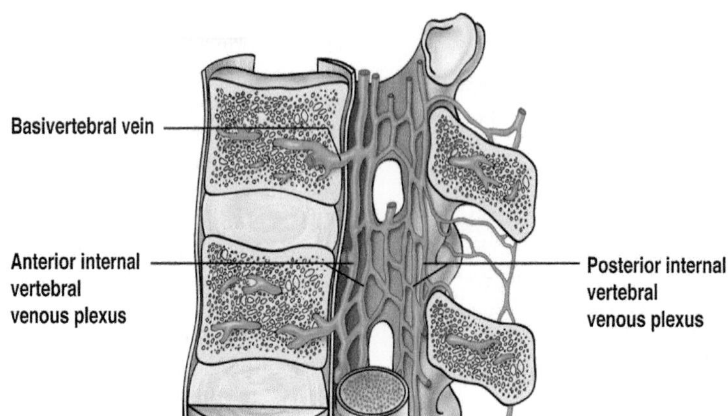

FIG. 7.9 Schematic drawing (sagittal view) noting the basivertebral vein within the body of a lumbar vertebra and its internal connections.

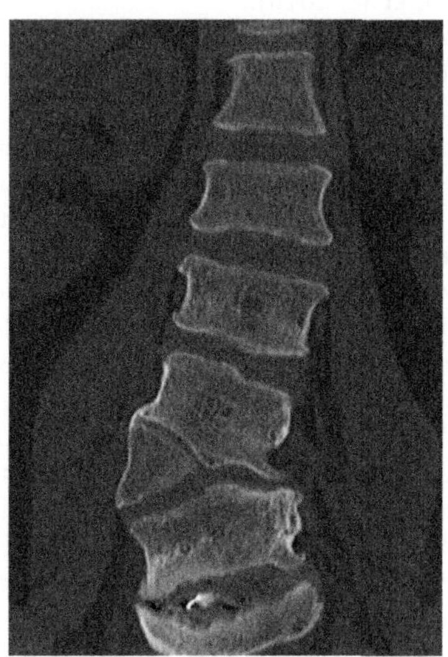

FIG. 7.10 A hemivertebra of the lumbar spine.

peripherally (Tubbs et al., 2016). The latter is known as a Schmorl's node (Tubbs et al., 2016).

Just as the notochord induces formation of the vertebral body, the neural tube influences the development of the neural arch (Tubbs et al., 2016). Failure within this signaling pathway results in vertebral arch defects (Tubbs et al., 2016). Spina bifida occulta is one of the most common variations. Failure of spinous process or lamina ossification interrupts the fusion of neural arches (Tubbs et al., 2016). The resulting defect can range in scale from a small midline malformation to a complete absence of neural arch. Spina bifida involving the S1 vertebra is known as a knife-clasp deformity as the subsequent elongation of the L5 spinous process causes extreme pain upon extension of the vertebral column (Tubbs et al., 2016). Spina bifida occulta and scoliosis have also been associated with split spinal cord malformations (Tubbs et al., 2016).

Disruption of the pars interarticularis either unilaterally or bilaterally results in spondylolysis and occurs most commonly at L5 (Tubbs et al., 2016). This causes the vertebral body to move more anterior than the body inferior to it.

Nonunion within the lumbar vertebrae is not uncommon. In this case secondary ossification centers fail to develop (Tubbs et al., 2016). This most commonly occurs at the apophyses of L1's transverse process and L3's inferior articular process (Tubbs et al., 2016).

Facet joints are also important to note. L5-S1 facet joints are oriented in the sagittal plane, whereas L1-2 and L4-5 are oriented in the coronal plane (Tubbs et al., 2016). Such can variation can exist bilaterally or unilaterally and most commonly occurs from L4-S1 (Tubbs et al., 2016).

While cervical ribs often gain more attention, lumbar ribs occur more frequently (Tubbs et al., 2016). The lumbar transverse processes can serve as rudimentary ribs, also known as gorilla ribs, in which a small rib joins the ventral aspect of a short transverse process (Tubbs et al., 2016).

REFERENCES

Bogduk, N., 2005. Clinical Anatomy of the Lumbar Spine and Sacrum, fourth ed. Elsevier.

Fisahn, C., Chapman, J.R., Oskouian, R.J., Loukas, M., Tubbs, R.S., Johal, J., 2016. Hemivertebrae: a comprehensive review of embryology, imaging, classification, and management. d 32 (11), 2105–2109. https://doi.org/10.1007/s00381-016-3195-y.

Kaplan, K.M., Spivak, J.M., Bendo, J.A., 2005. Embryology of the spine and associated congenital abnormalities. Spine J. 5, 564–576. https://doi.org/10.1016/j.spinee.2004.10.044.

Tehranzadeh, J., Andrews, C., Wong, E., 2000. Lumbar spine imaging: normal variants, imaging pitfalls, and artifacts. Radiol Clin North Am 38 (6), 1207–1253. https://doi.org/10.1016/S0033-8389(08)70004-6.

Tubbs, R.S., Shoja, M., Loukas, M., 2016. Bergman S Comprehensive Encyclopedia of Human Anatomic Variation. Wiley, Hoboken.

CHAPTER 8

Lumbar Intervertebral Discs

SKYLER JENKINS • R. SHANE TUBBS

INTRODUCTION

The intervertebral discs (Fig. 8.1) cushion the load applied on the spine as well as act to increase range of motion. The lumbar intervertebral discs are cylindrical and are approximately 4 cm in diameter by 7–10 mm in height with the anterior side being taller than the posterior (Raj, 2008). This morphological difference contributes primarily to the lordosis of the lumbar spine cranially, but caudally, the vertebral bodies are also a contributing factor (DePalma and Rothman, 1970).

EMBRYOLOGY AND DEVELOPMENT

The intervertebral disc begins its development during gastrulation and has a bimodal embryological origin. The cartilage end plates and the annulus fibrosus develop from the mesoderm, whereas the nucleus pulposus is a remnant of the notochord (Choi et al., 2008; Peacock, 1951; Walmsley, 1953; Roberts et al., 1989). In the late third week of embryogenesis, the primitive streak, three germ layers, and the notochord take their form. On both lateral sides of the notochord, three main zones develop: the paraxial, intermediate, and lateral mesoderm. The paraxial mesoderm differentiates cranio-caudally into 42–44 pairs of somites which will eventually develop into bones of the head, vertebrae, and other bony structures in the thorax and associated musculature (Kaplan et al., 2005). The development of each somite gives rise to two parts, a sclerotome and dermomyotome. Sclerotomes respond to Sonic Hedgehog (Shh) signals released by the ventral floor plate and the notochord (Ehlen et al., 2006). The cells of the sclerotome are primarily responsible for the formation of the spine.

During the fourth week of development, the cells of the sclerotome surround the notochord and the neural tube, dividing into a cranial area of loosely packed cells and a caudal area of densely packed cells, separated by a "free space" (Kaplan et al., 2005; O'Rahilly, 1996). The cells from the densely packed caudal area migrate into the "free space" beginning the formation of the annulus fibrosus (O'Rahilly, 1996). It is theorized that these regions respond to signals from Pax gene expression, mainly Pax1, Pax9, and TGFb-3 (Tomaszewski et al., 2015). The annulus is also dependent on signaling from the notochord via Noggin protein, which is synergistic with Shh to block bone morphogenetic protein signaling from the vertebral bodies (Tomaszewski et al., 2015). As the annulus fibrosus develops, the notochord retracts within the forming vertebral body to become the nucleus pulposus, composed of notochordal and large vacuolated cells (Peacock, 1951; Sivakamasundari, 2012; Aszodi et al., 1998; Pazzaglia et al., 1989). Using mouse models and lineage-tracing for Shhcre, ShhcreERT, and Noto-cre, it was determined that the notochordal cells gave rise to the nucleus pulposus (Sivakamasundari, 2012).

Approximately the third month of development, the discs can first be seen as dense cellular regions surrounding the notochord, alternating with less cellular vertebral bodies (Walmsley, 1953).

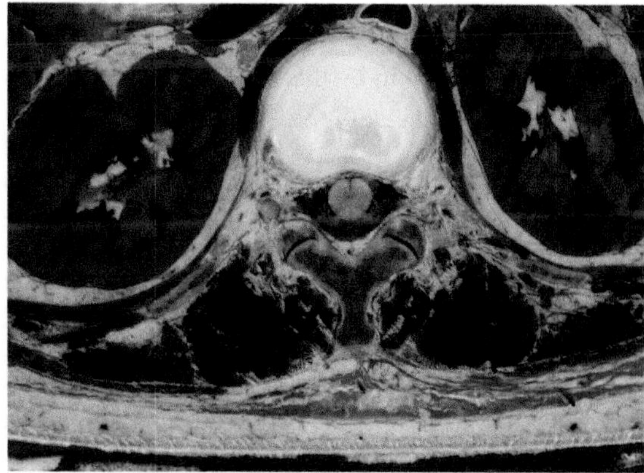

FIG. 8.1 Cadaveric axial image noting the surrounding relationships of a lumbar intervertebral disc. (Courtesy of Dr. Beom Sun Chung, Department of Anatomy, Ajou University School of Medicine, Republic of Korea.)

Surgical anatomy of the lateral transpsoas approach to the lumbar spine. https://doi.org/10.1016/B978-0-323-67376-1.00008-2

ANATOMY

The intervertebral discs (IVDs) comprise approximately 25%–33% of the spinal column length (Raj, 2008). They are wedge-shaped, found in all levels of the spine except between C1 and C2 and the coccyx and are bounded superiorly and inferiorly by cartilage endplates. Consisting of an inner gelatinous core, the nucleus pulposus, and an outer ring of fibrous cartilage, annulus fibrosus, the main function of the IVD is mechanical, transmitting physiological stresses to the entire spinal column (Raj, 2008). All regions of the disc are comprised of an extracellular collagen matrix with proteoglycans which pull water into the disc via high swelling pressure (Urban et al., 1979). Though a distinct delineation between the annulus and nucleus may be seen in early childhood, by adulthood this separation becomes more homogenous as the deep layers of the annulus merge with the outer nucleus (Bogduk, 1997). Finally, bordering the IVD on either side, the cartilaginous endplate, 1 mm thick, contains horizontally arranged collagen organized parallel to the vertebral bodies, providing tensile strength anchoring the IVD to the bone (Raj, 2008).

Structure and Composition of the Nucleus Pulposus

The nucleus pulposus comprises the central part of the IVD, approximately 40% of the disc's cross-sectional area, and exerts a swelling pressure that allows the disc to withstand axial loads (Urban et al., 1979; Bogduk, 1997). It is situated between the middle and posterior third of the disc and is comprised of a highly hydrated chondroitin and keratan-sulfate proteoglycan and aggrecan containing gel (Urban et al., 1979). Due to the high concentration of proteoglycans, 65% dry weight, water, drawn in by the anionic charge of aggrecan and osmotic gradient, is held within the nucleus (Raj, 2008; Bogduk, 1997; Yu et al., 2002). Because of the hydrostatic pressure created, the nucleus withstands the compressive forces applied to the spine and maintains the disc height (Tomaszewski et al., 2015).

The matrix of the nucleus consists of the type II collagen, aggrecan, and proteoglycan units. Type II collagen is found within the nucleus, annulus and endplates and provides a structural framework for the proteoglycans (Eyre et al., 1991). Collagen comprises 15%–20% of the dry weight of the nucleus with a majority being type II supplemented by radially placed elastin fibers and minimal amounts of noncollagenous proteins (Bogduk, 1997; Vora et al., 2010). The ratio of proteoglycans to collagen is 27:1 (Tomaszewski et al., 2015).

In a study done by Iatridis et al. (2007), it was found that the composition of proteoglycans also differed within the nucleus, providing support for theories of the relationship of disc degeneration and proteoglycan content.

Structure and Composition of the Annulus Fibrosus

Forming the outer ring of the IVD and surrounding the nucleus pulposus, the annulus fibrosus is a dense band of connective tissue organized into an outer and inner ring. The outer ring is made up of type I collagen, arranged into 15–25 concentric rings called lamellae (Fig. 8.2) (Marchand and Ahmed, 1990). The collagen fibers lay parallel within each ring and at a 65° angle with respect to the spinal axis (Raj, 2008; Hickey and Hukins, 1980). The lamellae are connected to each other by bundles of fibrillin, elastin, aggrecan, lubricin, and type IV collagen (Tomaszewski et al., 2015; Vora et al., 2010). Though the rings are concentric, there is a topographical arrangement of the lamellae. They are thicker in the central, anterior, and lateral disc, whereas they are finer, more tightly packed and thinner posteriorly (Bogduk, 1997). The inner ring is mainly comprised of type II collagen (Adams et al., 1977). These lamellae are also anchored into the cartilaginous endplate, providing support (Hickey and Hukins, 1980). Outside the collagen network in the extracellular substance, proteoglycans, glycoproteins, and elastic fibers are found.

The annulus is primarily composed of water, 60%–70% dry weight, followed by collagen and proteoglycans, primarily aggregated (Bogduk, 1997). There is also a spatial arrangement of components; a

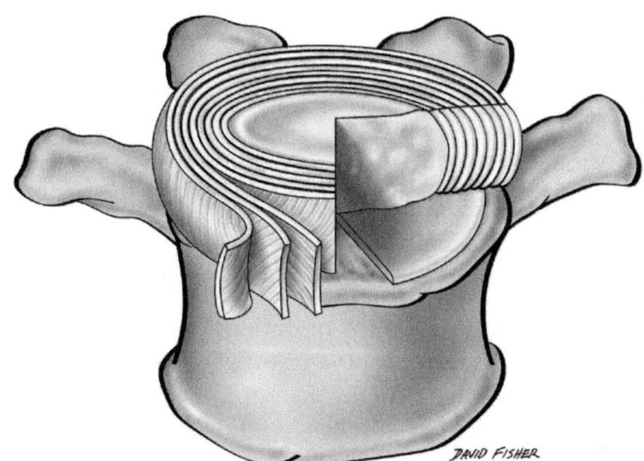

FIG. 8.2 Schematic drawing noting the layering of the annulus fibrosus.

higher concentration of water and proteoglycans are found in the anterior and superficial annulus, whereas, there is increased collagen fibril concentration in the deep annulus compared to superficial (Urban et al., 1996).

Structure and Composition of the Endplates

Bounding the superior and inferior edges of the IVD, the cartilage endplate is the interface between the IVD and vertebral body (Raj, 2008). It is a horizontal, thin layer of hyaline and fibrocartilage fibers that run parallel to the IVD, sometimes continuing into the annulus, preventing the nucleus from herniating into the adjacent vertebra, and provides a strong bond to the IVD (Roberts et al., 1989). However, the bond to the vertebral bodies is much weaker and can be severed in, for example, spinal trauma (Bogduk, 1997).

The endplate has a similar composition to the annulus and nucleus, consisting of primarily water, proteoglycans, and type II collagen fibers. However, due to its involvement in calcification, type X collagen is thought to be an essential constituent of the endplate (Tomaszewski et al., 2015). Within the endplate, collagen is found in higher concentration nearer to the bone, whereas proteoglycan concentration is greater near the nucleus (Bogduk, 1997).

INNERVATION

A variety of nerves innervate the lumbar IVDs. The sinuvertebral nerve, a meningeal branch of the spinal nerve, provides nociceptive innervation to both the posterior longitudinal ligament and the adjacent, posterior part of the outer annulus (Bogduk et al., 1981). The posterolateral aspect of the disc is supplied by both the adjacent ventral primary rami and gray rami communicantes near the junction of the two (Bogduk et al., 1981). In addition, the lateral aspects are innervated by branches of the rami communicantes.

There is also an extensive network of fine, free nerve fibers on the IVD with unmyelinated free nerve endings within the outer lamellae of the annulus; however, the inner lamellae and nucleus lack innervation (Raj, 2008; DePalma and Rothman, 1970; Yu et al., 2002; Vora et al., 2010; Bogduk et al., 1981). With progressive degenerative disc disease, however, there is a hyperinnervation of nociceptive fibers, within previous noninnervated sections. This accompanies neovascularization of the disc possibly due to the action of neurotrophins (Tomaszewski et al., 2015). The cartilaginous endplate is normally fully avascular and aneural (Raj, 2008).

BLOOD SUPPLY

In the healthy adult, the intervertebral discs are nearly avascular with their only direct blood supply from a small number of penetrating capillaries in the outermost layer of the annulus fibrosus (Weissbach et al., 2002). This supply is also contributed to by external and endplate capillary network in the surrounding soft tissue, branching off segmental arteries arising from the aorta (Grunhagen et al., 2006). Finally, "the nucleus, inner anulus, and part of the outer anulus are supplied by a capillary network arising from the vertebral arteries that penetrates the subchondral plate to terminate in loops at the bone-cartilage end-plate junction" (Grunhagen et al., 2006). Venous drainage into the subchondral venous plexus or into veins of the marrow spaces of adjacent vertebral bodies.

During embryological development through the first decade of life, blood vessels from the segmental arteries penetrate the annulus and endplate (Tomaszewski et al., 2015). However, through the course of development and early adulthood, these vascular sources are obliterated leaving the discs nearly avascular.

PATHOLOGY

According to (Raj, 2008), disc lesions can be classified as contained or herniated, in four separate grades. Grade 0: Normal, nonleaking nucleus; Grade 1: Tearing of the inner one-third of the annulus fibrosus; Grade 2: The tear has affected the entire structure of the disc; however, the outer shape of the annulus is intact and there is no bulging or protrusion of the disc; Grade 3: Tears have completely disrupted the annulus, the posterior longitudinal ligament, and have affected the posterior portion of the disc, allowing for leakage of radiocontrast fluid on discography; This classification contains a disc bulge or herniation (Raj, 2008).

IMAGING/STUDIES

Using MRI, there have been multiple morphologic grading systems for disc degeneration (Pfirrmann et al., 2002; Atlas et al., 1993; Brant-Zawadzki et al., 1995; Eyre et al., 1989). Current grading systems use the MRI signal intensity, disc structure, differentiation between the nucleus and annulus, and disc height (Pfirrmann et al., 2002).

Computerized tomography (CT) is the gold standard for the classification of annular tears and has been modified multiple times (Sachs et al., 1987). Using this classification, there are five different grades:

Grade 0: Normal disc—no contrast media leaks from the nucleus pulposus; Grade 1: Contrast material leaks only to the inner one-third of the annulus; Grade 2: Contrast material leaks to the outer two-thirds of the annulus; Grade 3: Contrast material leaked through complete thickness of the annulus, and it may cause pain; Grade 4: Contrast material spreads around the disc, encompassing greater than 30 degrees of the circumference; Grade 5: Encompasses a Grade 3 or 4 radial tear that completely ruptures the outer layer of the disc, leaking fluid into the epidural space, leading to an inflammatory process and pain (Raj, 2008).

Provocation discography with follow-up CT discogram is the gold standard for diagnosing internal disc disruption (IDD). This is done in two steps: (1) use contrast material to pressurize the disc, eliciting a painful response from the patient; (2) perform a painless discogram of the bounding discs (Raj, 2008). Because this procedure may damage discs, a gadolinium DTPA–enhanced MRI may be used (Raj, 2008).

LATERAL TRANSPSOAS APPROACH TO THE LUMBAR SPINE

In this approach, the radiographic center of the disc is identified, access to the disc space is gained through the psoas major muscle by using various dilators, and direct visualization of the disc is obtained by expansion of the blade retractor system (Park et al., 2010). This procedure has application for use in interbody fusion, far-lateral disc herniations, degenerative disc disease, spinal stenosis, degenerative scoliosis, nonunion, trauma, infection, and low-grade spondylolisthesis (Patel et al., 2012). Utilizing a minimally invasive retroperitoneal transpsoas approach to the lumbar spine, the surgeon minimizes the risk of surgical exposure and morbidity due to muscular stress, as well as increases the ease of accessibility of the upper lumbar spine by using gravity to draw the abdominal contents anteriorly (L1-L4) (Bergey et al., 2004; Madhok and Kanter, 2010; Lajer et al., 1997; Levrant et al., 1997; Regan et al., 1995; Jansen, 1997; McAfee et al., 1995). Much of the complications using this approach involved neurological injuries to the lumbar plexus (Park et al., 2010; Sofianos et al., 2012). This can be minimized by gaining access through the anterior portion of the psoas major muscle (Park et al., 2010). However, through moving access portals more anteriorly and away from the center of the disc, the left-to-right dimensions of the disc get smaller and a smaller, less-stable interbody implant is required. This also increases the risk of damaging blood vessels and the peritoneal cavity (Park et al., 2010). In addition, as the lumbosacral plexus migrates dorsal to ventral from L1 through the L5 disc spaces, these nerves have the greatest risk of being injured, by a posteriorly positioned dilator/retractor, during the transpsoas approach to the L4-5 level (Benglis et al., 2009).

REFERENCES

Adams, P., Eyre, D.R., Muir, H., 1977. Biochemical aspects of development and ageing of human lumbar intervertebral discs. Rheumatol. Rehabil. 16, 22–29.

Aszodi, A., Chan, D., Hunziker, E., Bateman, J., Fassler, R., 1998. Collagen II is essential for the removal of the notochord and the formation of intervertebral discs. J. Cell Biol. 143, 1399–1412.

Atlas, S.W., Hackney, D.B., Listerud, J., 1993. Fast spin-echo imaging of the brain and spine. Magn. Reson. Q. 9, 61–83.

Benglis, D., Vanni, S., Levi, A., 2009. An anatomical study of the lumbosacral plexus as related to the minimally invasive transpsoas approach to the lumbar spine. J. Neurosurg. Spine 10 (2), 139–144.

Bergey, D., Villavicencio, A., Goldstein, T., Regan, J., 2004. Endoscopic lateral transpsoas approach to the lumbar spine. Spine 29, 1681–1688.

Bogduk, N., 1997. Clinical Anatomy of the Lumbar Spine and Sacrum, third ed. Churchill Livingstone, New York, NY.

Bogduk, N., Tynan, W., Wilson, S., 1981. The nerve supply to the human lumbar intervertebral discs. J. Anat. 132, 39–56.

Brant-Zawadzki, M.N., Jensen, M.C., Obuchowski, N., et al., 1995. Interobserver and intraobserver variability in interpretation of lumbar disc abnormalities: a comparison of two nomenclatures. Spine 20, 1257–1263.

Choi, K., Cohn, M., Harfe, B., 2008. Identification of nucleus pulposus precursor cells and notochordal remnants in the mouse: implications for disc degeneration and chordoma formation. Dev. Dynam. 237, 3953–3958.

DePalma, A.F., Rothman, R.H., 1970. The Intervertebral Disc. W.B. Saunders Company, Philadelphia, PA.

Ehlen, H.W., Buelens, L.A., Vortkamp, A., 2006. Hedgehog signaling in skeletal development. Birth Defects Res C Embryo Today 78 (3), 267–279.

Eyre, D., Benya, P., Buckwalter, J., et al., 1989. Intervertebral disc: Part B. Basic science perspectives. In: Frymoyer, J.W., Gordon, S.L. (Eds.), New Perspectives on Low Back Pain. American Academy of Orthopaedic Surgeons, Park Ridge, IL.

Eyre, D., et al., 1991. The intervertebral disc. In: Gordon, S., Frymoyer, J. (Eds.), New Perspectives on Low Back Pain. American Academy of Orthopedic Surgeons, pp. 149–207.

Grunhagen, T., Wilde, G., Soukane, D., Shirazi-Ald, S., Urban, J., 2006. Nutrient supply and intervertebral disc metabolism. J. Bone Jt. Surg. 88 (2), 30–35.

Hickey, D., Hukins, D., 1980. X-ray diffraction studies of the arrangement of collagenous fibres in human fetal intervertebral disc. J. Anat. 131 (1), 81.

Iatridis, J., MacLean, J., O'Brien, M., Stokes, A., 2007. Measurements of proteoglycan and water content distribution in human lumbar intervertebral discs. Spine 32 (14), 1493–1497.

Jansen, R., 1997. FDA Submission. 240 BAK Laparoscopic Procedure.

Kaplan, K., Spivak, J., Bendo, J., 2005. Embryology of the spine and associated congenital abnormalities. Spine J. 5, 564–576.

Lajer, H., Widecrantz, S., Heisterberg, L., 1997. Hernias in trocar ports following abdominal laparoscopy: a review. Acta Obstet. Gynecol. Scand. 76, 389–393.

Levrant, S.G., Bieber, E.J., Barnes, R.B., 1997. Anterior abdominal wall adhesions after laparotomy or laparoscopy. J. Am. Assoc. Gynecol. Laparoscopists 4, 353–356.

Madhok, R., Kanter, A., 2010. Extreme-lateral, minimally invasive, transpsoas approach for the treatment of far-lateral lumbar disc herniation. J. Neurosurg. Spine 12, 347–350.

Marchand, F., Ahmed, A.M., 1990. Investigation of the laminate structure of lumbar disc anulus fibrosus. Spine 15, 402–410.

McAfee, P.C., Regan, J.R., Zdeblick, T., Picetti, G., Geis, W., Regan, J., Zuckerman, J., Heim, S., Fedder, I., 1995. The incidence of complications in endoscopic anterior thoracolumbar spinal reconstructive surgery: a prospective multicenter study compromising the first 100 consecutive cases. Spine 20, 1624–1632.

ORahilly, R., 1996. Human Embryology and Teratology. John Wiley & Sons, New York.

Park, D., Lee, M., Lin, E., Singh, K., An, H., Phillips, F., 2010. The relationship of intrapsoas nerves during a transpsoas approach to the lumbar spine: anatomic study. J. Spinal Disord. Tech. 23, 223–228.

Patel, V., Park, D., Herkowitz, H., 2012. Lateral transpsoas fusion: indications and outcomes. Sci. World J. 893608 (6).

Pazzaglia, U., Salisbury, J., Byers, P., 1989. Development and involution of the notochord in the human spine. J. R. Soc. Med. 82, 413–415.

Peacock, A., 1951. Observations on the prenatal development of the intervertebral disc in man. J. Anat. 85, 260–274.

Pfirrmann, C., Metzdorf, A., Zanetti, M., Hodler, J., Boos, N., 2002. Magnetic resonance classification of lumbar intervertebral disc degeneration. Spine 26, 1873–1878.

Raj, P., 2008. Intervertebral disc: anatomy-physiology-pathophysiology-treatment. Pain Pract. 8 (1), 18–44.

Regan, J.J., McAfee, P.C., Mack, M.J., 1995. Atlas of Endoscopic Spine Surgery. Quality Medical Publishing Inc, St. Louis, MO.

Roberts, S., Menage, J., Urban, J.P.G., 1989. Biochemical and structural properties of the cartilage end-plate and its relation to the intervertebral disc. Spine 14, 166–174.

Sachs, B.L., Vanharanta, H., Spivey, M.A., et al., 1987. Dallas discogram description: a new classification of CT/discography in low back disorders. Spine 12, 287–294.

Sivakamasundari, L., 2012. Bridging the gap: understanding embryonic intervertebral disc development. Cell Dev. Biol. 1 (2), 103.

Sofianos, D., Briseno, M., Abrams, J., Patel, A., 2012. Complications of the lateral transpsoas approach for lumbar interbody arthrodesis: a case series and literature review. Clin. Orthop. Relat. Res. 470, 1621–1632.

Tomaszewski, K.A., Saganiak, K., Gładysz, T., Walocha, J.A., 2015. The biology behind the human intervertebral disc and its endplates. Folia Morphol. 74 (2), 157–168.

Urban, J.P., Maroudas, A., Bayliss, M.T., Dillon, J., 1979. Swelling pressures of proteoglycans at the concentrations found in cartilaginous tissues. Biorheology 16, 447–464.

Urban, J., 1996. Disc biochemistry in relation to function. In: Wiesel, S.W., Weinstein, J.N., Herkowitz, H.N., Dvorak, J., Bell, G. (Eds.), The Lumbar Spine. Saunders, Philadelphia, pp. 271–280.

Vora, A.J., Doerr, K.D., Wolfer, L.R., 2010. Functional anatomy and pathophysiology of axial low back pain: disc, posterior elements, sacroiliac joint, and associated pain generators. Phys. Rehad. Clin. North Am. 21 (4), 679–709.

Walmsley, R., 1953. The development and growth of the intervertebral disc. Edinb. Med. J. 60, 341–364.

Weissbach, S., Rohrbach, H., Weiler, C., Spratt, K.F., Nerlich, A.G., 2002. Classification of age-related changes in lumbar intervertebral discs. Spine 27, 2631–2644.

Yu, J., Winlove, C.P., Roberts, S., Urban, J.P., 2002. Elastic fibre organization in the intervertebral discs of the bovine tail. J. Anat. 201, 465–475.

CHAPTER 9

The Ligaments of the Lumbar Spine

MARY KATHERINE CLEVELAND • R. SHANE TUBBS

INTRODUCTION

As with the other regions of the spine, the lumbar vertebrae rely on a robust collection of soft tissues to maintain their structural integrity during load bearing and movement. Of these soft tissues, the lumbar vertebral ligaments play a very important role. These highly specialized structures allow for extremes of movement while maintaining alignment of the spinal canal, intervertebral foramina, and intervertebral discs. Therefore, disruption of these structures can lead to significant neurological compromise. Spine surgeons need a detailed understanding of the anatomy of the lumbar spine ligaments.

ANTERIOR LONGITUDINAL LIGAMENT

Anatomy

The anterior longitudinal ligament (ALL) (Figs. 9.1 and 9.2) is composed of a strong band of collagenous fibers that extends along the anterior aspect of the vertebral column (Bannister et al., 1996; Bogduk, 1997; Dickman et al., 1999; Lang, 1993). The ALL is attached to the basilar occipital bone rostrally, extends to the anterior tubercle of the atlas (C1) along with the front of the body of the axis (C2), and runs caudally to the anterior of the sacrum (Bannister et al., 1996). The ALL becomes narrower and thicker over the vertebral bodies opposed to where it passes over the intervertebral (IV) discs (Bannister et al., 1996; Dickman et al., 1999). Likewise, it is also thicker and narrower in the thoracic region, as compared with its presence in the cervical and lumbar regions, and broadens as it travels caudally (Bannister et al., 1996). The average width of the ALL in the lumbar spine in 25 cadaveric specimens was measured to be 37.1 mm with a mean cross-sectional area of 32.4 mm^2 and a range from 10.6 to 52.5 mm^2 (Pintar et al., 1992).

The ALL consists of numerous collagen fibers that are densely packed and form three distinct layers: superficial, intermediate, and deep (Bannister et al., 1996; Bogduk, 1997; Lang, 1993). The superficial fibers are the longest, spanning anywhere from three to five vertebrae, whereas the intermediate fibers span between two and three vertebrae, and the deep fibers span from one vertebral body to the next, connecting adjacent vertebrae (Bannister et al., 1996; Lang, 1993). These longitudinal fibers attach strongly to the IV discs and the anterior margins of the vertebral bodies (Bannister et al., 1996; Bogduk, 1997; Dickman et al., 1999). These fibers form looser, secondary attachments to the midportion of the vertebral bodies, filling their concave surfaces and flattening the appearance of anterior surface of the vertebral column (Bogduk, 1997). At this point, the deep fibers of the ALL blend with the periosteum, whereas the more superficial fibers bridge the concavity (Bogduk, 1997). The fibers from the ALL also blend with the external surface of the anulus fibrosus, resulting in anatomist proposing varying opinions on the origins of these fibers (Bogduk, 1997). While some authors believe these fibers are to be part of the anulus fibrosus, others feel they constitute a "disc capsule," but Bogduk (1997) demonstrated that the deep fibers of the ALL should not be considered part of the anulus fibrosus due to differences in the embryological origin of these two structures. Accordingly, the fibers of the ALL have attachments to cortical bone, which is always the case with these ligaments (Bogduk, 1997). Bogduk (1997) demonstrated that the anulus fibrosus does not attach to cortical bone but rather to the vertebral end plate. In this demonstration, Bogduk (1997) also illustrated some key differences in ALL structure at varying regions of the vertebral column, such as the thoracic region, which was the only location where the ALL was not associated with any of the prevertebral muscles and, therefore, stood alone. Another distinction was made in the lumbar spine at the point where the crura of the diaphragm attached to the first three lumbar vertebrae (Bogduk, 1997). In this region, the tendons of the crura extend caudally beyond the three vertebrae and form much of what is described as the ALL in this region

Surgical anatomy of the lateral transpsoas approach to the lumbar spine. https://doi.org/10.1016/B978-0-323-67376-1.00009-4

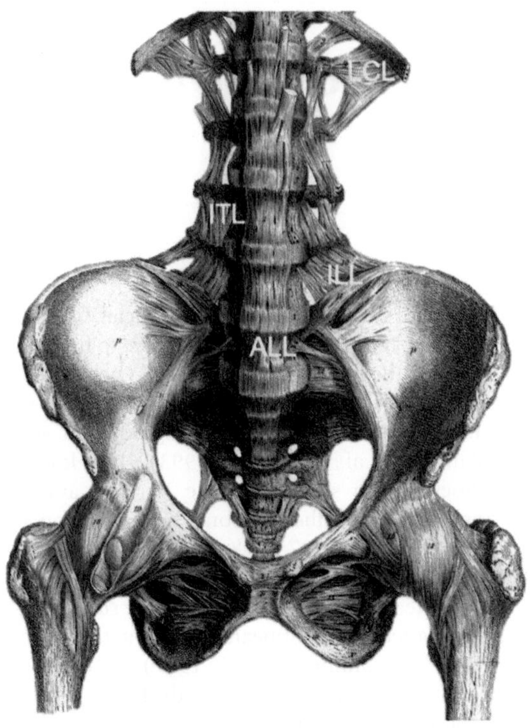

FIG. 9.1 Drawing of an anterior view of the lumbar vertebrae and their associated ligaments. Note the lumbocostal ligament (LCL), intertransverse ligament (ITL), iliolumbar ligament (ILL), and anterior longitudinal ligament (ALL).

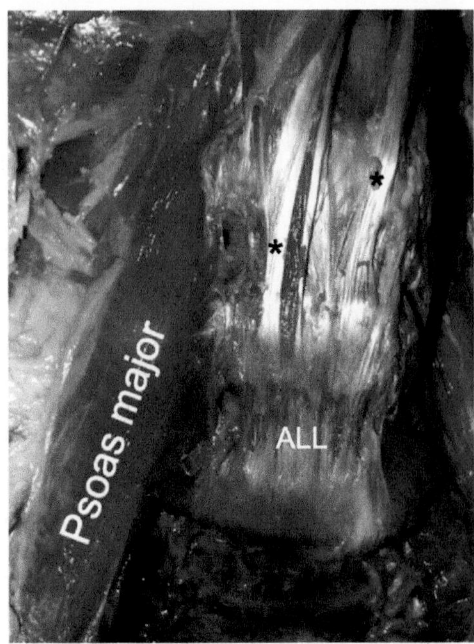

FIG. 9.2 Cadaveric view of the anterior lumbar spine. Note the left and right diaphragmatic crura (asterisks) and anterior longitudinal ligament (ALL).

(Fig. 9.2) (Bogduk, 1997). This peculiarity has led Bogduk to suggest that the ALL may, to some extent, be a continuation of a tendon attachment in addition to its ligamentous nature (Bogduk, 1997).

Biomechanics

The ALL primarily functions to maintain the stability of the vertebral column by restricting the motion of the spinal segments during extension (Bogduk, 1997; Moore et al., 2010). There are varying opinions on what causes the ALL to function. Neumann et al. (1992) suggested that the ALL functions during extension, lateral bending, and axial rotation, whereas Zander et al. (2004) believed that the ALL is only loaded during extension and is unloaded during other movements of the spinal column. The ALL is the strongest and largest of the spinal ligaments and is the only one that limits extension; the remaining IV ligaments limit flexion movements (Moore et al., 2010; Neumann et al., 1992; Zander et al., 2004). In a study conducted by Neumann et al. (1992), they found the ALL to have a significantly greater stiffness than that of the posterior spinal ligaments. They also noted that the ALL strength decreased slightly in subjects between the ages of 21 and 43 years (Neumann et al., 1992). In a subsequent study, Neumann et al. (1993) found the mean failure loads of bone-ALL-bone complexes to be 802 N (N). This result is drastically different from other studies, in which the mean values ranged from 330 to 473 N (Neumann et al., 1993). Neumann and colleagues explained this difference by the properties of the specimens used in their study; they suggested that the difference was due to using specimens from younger and presumably, less sedentary specimens, whereas other studies used ALL specimens from older subjects (Neumann et al., 1993). They also found that younger ALL specimens were more than twice as strong as older specimens (Neumann et al., 1993). They proposed, however, that bone mineral content tends to be a more accurate predictor of bone-ligament-bone structural properties opposed to age, due to the fact that there is a linear increase in ultimate force, stiffness, and energy of this complex with increasing bone density (Neumann et al., 1993). Pintar et al. (1992) reported the mean stiffness value for the ALL in the lumbar spine to be 33.0 N/mm with a margin of 15.7 N/mm. The highest values of energy to failure were observed for the ALL and the supraspinous ligament (SSL), with values ranging from 0.82 to 8.68 J (J) for the ALL and

3.18–11.64 J for the SSL (Pintar et al., 1992). According to Paniabi et al. (1982), failure results from these ligaments needing to withstand functionally more force and deformation. Failure stresses were found to be similar between the ALL and posterior longitudinal ligament (PLL), at 8.2–16.1 MPa and 7.2–28.4 MPa, respectively (Pintar et al., 1992). The values of stress and strain at failure reported by Pintar et al. (1992) were similar to the values reported by Chazal et al. (1985).

POSTERIOR LONGITUDINAL LIGAMENT

Anatomy

The PLL (Figs. 9.3 and 9.4) is a band of longitudinal fibers that runs within the vertebral canal along the posterior aspect of the vertebral bodies (Bannister et al., 1996; Bogduk, 1997; Dickman et al., 1999; Lang, 1993). Rostrally, the PLL is continuous with the

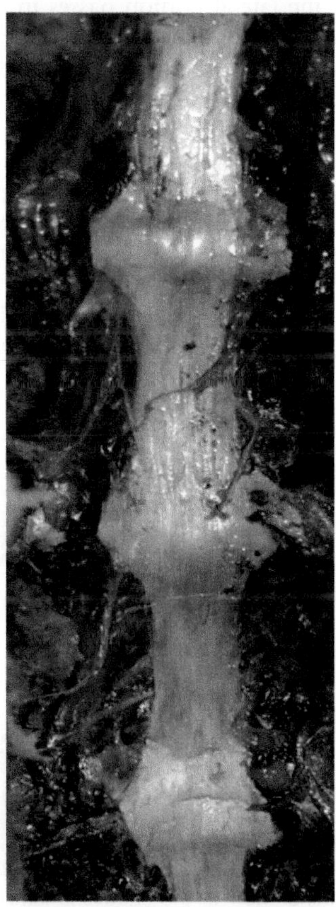

FIG. 9.3 Cadaveric view of the posterior longitudinal ligament (PLL) of the lumbar spine. Also note the regional vertebral venous plexus.

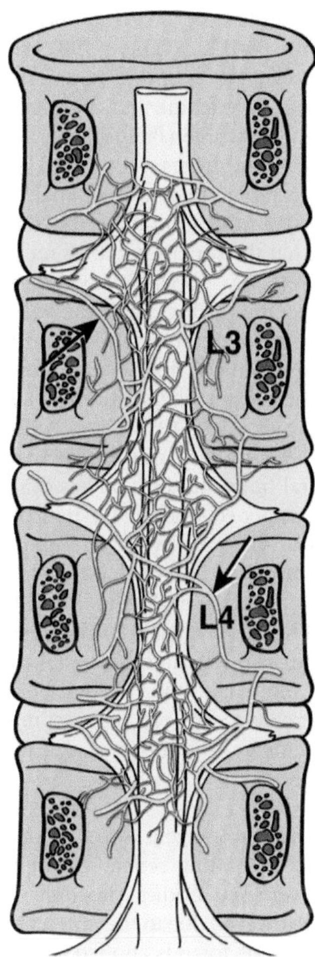

FIG. 9.4 Schematic drawing of the lumbar posterior longitudinal ligament and overlying nerve plexus contributed to by the recurrent meningeal nerves (arrows).

tectorial membrane, and in the upper lumbar region, the PLL takes on a caudal direction. Attaching to the tip of the vertebral body below, the lateral deep fibers at this level take a horizontal path and extend out to the IV foramen, covering the lower half of the anulus fibrosus and attaching at its lateral opening (Lang, 1993). The average width of the PLL in the lumbar spines of 21 cadaveric specimens was 33.3 mm, with a mean cross-sectional area of 5.2 mm^2 (Pintar et al., 1992).

The fibers of the PLL are more compact than those of the ALL (Dickman et al., 1999). Between the ligamentous fibers lay the basivertebral veins and the venous rami that drain them into anterior internal vertebral plexuses (Bannister et al., 1996). Early studies also describe an abundance of free and encapsulated nerve endings within the PLL (Lang, 1993). Similar to the ALL, the superficial fibers of the PLL can span anywhere from three to five vertebrae and the deepest fibers between adjacent vertebrae (Bannister et al., 1996; Bogduk, 1997). These layers, however, become more pronounced in the immediate postnatal years (Bannister et al., 1996). Further examination of the layers of the PLL showed that the superficial fibers measure a length of 0.5–1.0 cm (Lang, 1993). The fibers of the PLL attach more firmly to the IV discs than the vertebral bodies, with deep fibers fused to the annuli fibrosi in the adult spine and the superficial fibers being more easily separable from the deeper fibers when over the vertebral bodies (Bannister et al., 1996; Lang, 1993). The deep layer of the PLL forms a narrow ligament at the middle of the vertebral body, but as it travels caudally and approaches the upper edge of the IV space, it diverges toward the lip of the next lower vertebral body, as well as a portion of the pedicle of that next lower vertebral body (Lang, 1993). As per Bogduk (1997), the deep fibers of the PLL not only fuse with the fibers of the anulus fibrosus but also penetrate through them to attach to the posterior margins of the vertebral bodies (Bogduk, 1997). In this way, these deep fibers act much like "paravertebral ligaments" (Bannister et al., 1996).

Biomechanics

The PLL functions to prevent hyperflexion of the vertebral column by resisting separation of the posterior ends of the vertebral bodies (Bogduk, 1997; Moore et al., 2010). However, due to the polysegmental nature of this ligament, its force is applied over several interbody joints as opposed to just one (Bogduk, 1997). The PLL also functions to prevent posterior herniation of the nucleus pulposus (Moore et al., 2010). It contains nociceptive nerve endings and is the source of pain from IV disc herniation as the anulus fibrosus impinges on the ligament (Moore et al., 2010). Pintar et al. (1992) reported that the PLL has the smallest cross-sectional area, with a mean of 5.2 mm^2, compared with the other lumbar spinal ligaments. This ligament also had the lowest value of energy to failure, at a range of 0.07–0.33 J, as well as the least strain at failure, ranging between 11.3% and 16.2%. Failure stresses were found to be similar between the ALL and PLL at 8.2–16.1 MPa and 7.2–28.4 MPa, respectively (Pintar et al., 1992). Similar values for stress and strain at failure were reported by Chazal et al. (1985) (Pintar et al., 1992). The mean stiffness value for the PLL in the lumbar spine was 20.4 ± 11.9 Nmm^{-1} (Pintar et al., 1992).

LIGAMENTUM FLAVUM

Anatomy

The ligamenta flava (LF) (Figs. 9.5–9.7) are a series of ligaments that connect the lamina of adjacent vertebrae to form alternating sections of the posterior wall of the vertebral canal (Bannister et al., 1996; Bogduk, 1997; Dickman et al., 1999; Moore et al., 2010). The LF are present bilaterally at each vertebral level, converging in the midline (Bogduk, 1997; Moore et al., 2010). This ligament's perpendicular fibers attach to the anterior surface of the lower edge of the lamina above, as well as the inferior aspect of the pedicle, and proceed to descend down to the posterior surface of the upper edge of the lamina below (Bannister et al., 1996; Bogduk, 1997; Dickman et al., 1999; Moore et al., 2010; Yong-Hing et al., 1976). As this ligament descends inferiorly, it divides into medial and lateral portions (Bogduk, 1997). The medial portion passes to the back of the next lower lamina where it attaches to the rough area on the upper quarter of the dorsal surface of the lamina, and the lateral portion passes in front of the zygapophyseal joint formed by two vertebrae to which the ligament connects (Bogduk, 1997). Inferiorly, the lateral portion of each ligament extends to the midpoint between two pedicles and forms the anterior capsule of the zygapophyseal joint, as it attaches to the anterior aspects of the inferior and superior articular processes of the zygapophyseal joint (Bannister et al., 1996; Bogduk, 1997; Yong-Hing et al., 1976). In fact, the most lateral fibers extend along the root of the superior articular process as far as the next lower pedicle to which they are attached (Bogduk, 1997). From where the posterior margins of the ligament meet as the ligament's

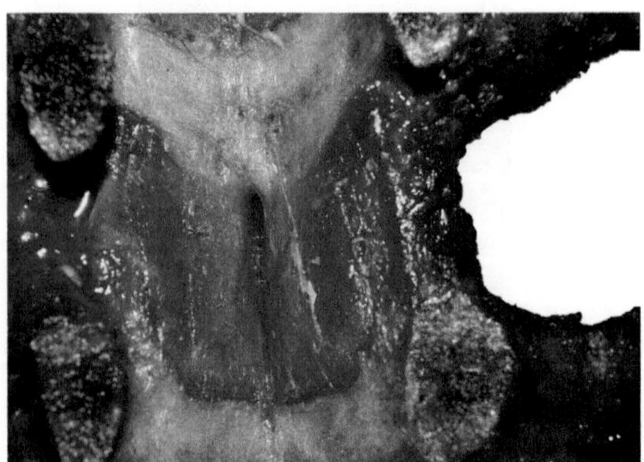

FIG. 9.5 Anterior view of the cadaveric lumbar ligamenta flava. Note the gap between the two ligaments in this specimen.

attachments extend from the zygapophyseal capsule to where the laminae fuse to form spines, the ligament is only partially united, with intervals being left for veins connecting the internal to posterior external posterior vertebral venous plexus (Bannister et al., 1996). Pintar et al. (1992) measured the lumbar LF in 22 cadaveric specimens and found that, on average, the LF measures 15.2 mm in length with a mean cross-sectional area of 84.2 mm^2. In the cervical region, the LF are thin and broad but thicken as they descend caudally, with the thickest ligaments found in the lumbar region (Bannister et al., 1996; Moore et al., 2010). The average thickness of the LF, both at midline and laterally, was noted to be 2–3 mm by Yong-Hing et al. (1976).

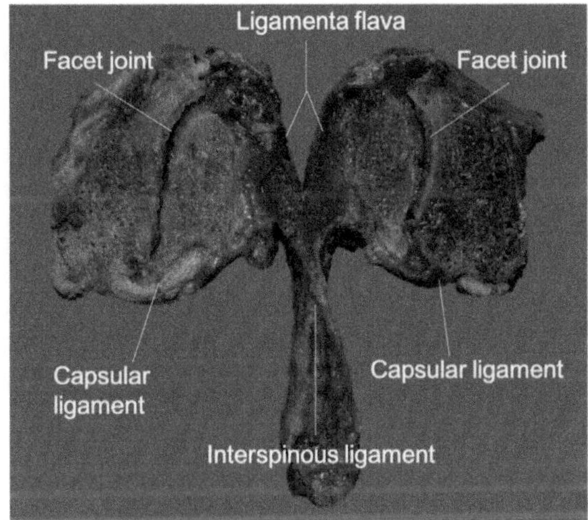

FIG. 9.6 Axial cut through a lumbar vertebra and related ligaments. Note that the interspinous ligament is confluent with the ligamenta flava.

Recently, they concluded that the ligamentum flavum and interspinous ligaments (ISLs) in the lumbar region are confluent and are not two separate entities (Fig. 9.7) (Iwanaga et al., 2019).

Biomechanics

The LF functions to oppose separation of the vertebral laminae during spinal flexion (Bannister et al., 1996; Bogduk, 1997; Dickman et al., 1999; Moore et al., 2010). This is accomplished by arresting abrupt flexion and aiding in restoring the vertebral column to an erect posture, thereby preserving the normal curvature of spine and protecting the IV discs from injury (Bannister et al., 1996; Bogduk, 1997; Dickman et al., 1999; Moore et al., 2010; Yahia et al., 1990). The elastic nature of this ligament plays an important role in achieving this function, as a collagenous ligament would be able to resist separation but would buckle when the laminae were approximated (Bogduk, 1997). On average, it is composed of 80% elastin and 20% collagen with the elastic fibers being oriented parallel to the long axis of the ligament (Bannister et al., 1996; Paniabi et al., 1982; Panjabi et al., 1991). Yong-Hing and colleagues, in 1976, obtained 51 specimens, which were stained with Gomori's aldehyde fuchsin stain to measure the elastin (stained purple) and collagen (stained green) content of these ligaments (Panjabi et al., 1991). In these specimens, they found that the ligaments' composition consisted of 50%–80% elastin and 20%–50% collagen (Panjabi et al., 1991). While anteriorly the ligament is thin due to the elastic fibers, the posterior capsule of each posterior joint is thicker due to the collagenous content (Panjabi et al., 1991). A study on the ultrastructure of the ligament demonstrated that the LF contains two morphologically different types of

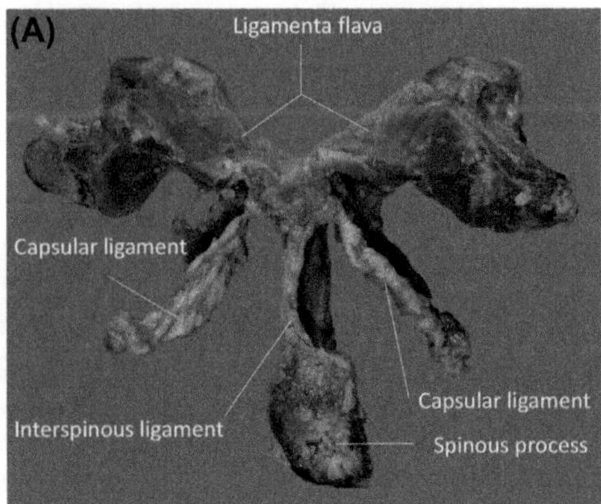

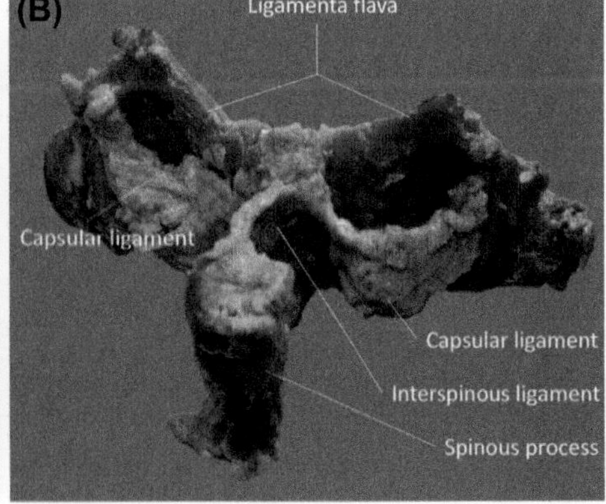

FIG. 9.7 Two views **(A** and **B)** of the relationships between the ligamenta flava of a lumbar vertebra and the associated capsular and interspinous ligaments.

elastin fibers: elastic and elaunin fibers (Paniabi et al., 1982). While the elastic fibers proper were found throughout the ligament, though mainly in the central region, the elaunin fibers, which are composed of few elastin deposits interspersed with microtubules, were more prominent along the bony attachments of the ligaments (Bannister et al., 1996; Paniabi et al., 1982). Very few spindle-shaped fibroblasts were also associated with the ligament (Paniabi et al., 1982). The LF differs from all other ligaments of the lumbar spine, as it is the only ligament consisting of predominately elastic fibers as opposed to collagen (Bannister et al., 1996). The LF are also noted to retain their elastin content with increasing age (Panjabi et al., 1991). It was previously postulated that the elastin content of the ligament decreases and the ligament becomes more rigid in patients with spondylosis, but Yong-Hing and colleagues found no evidence to support this claim; therefore, they noted that there is no correlation between elastin content and age, duration of symptoms of low back or leg pain, or the presence of degenerative spondylosis (Panjabi et al., 1991). They also noted that there is no evidence that, with increasing age, any hypertrophy, hyperplasia, or degeneration of elastin takes place (Panjabi et al., 1991).

Buckling is minimal with an elastic ligament, which allows the contents of the spinal canal to be protected from damage (Bogduk, 1997). The elastic nature of this ligament aids in restoring a flexed lumbar spine to its extended position, whereas the lateral division of the ligament will prevent the anterior capsule of the zygapophyseal joint from being nipped within the joint capsule during movement (Bogduk, 1997). The LF exerts a disc pressure of 0.7 kg/cm^2 and serves to prestress the IV disc; however, the biological significance of this is unknown (Bogduk, 1997). The lateral portion of the ligament prevents injury to the anterior capsule of the zygapophyseal joint during movement (Bogduk, 1997). While some believe that the LF assists in extension of the spine with the help of the erector spinae muscles, Bogduk (1997) questions the importance of this ligament in producing extension movements (Yong-Hing et al., 1976). Pintar et al. (1992) reported that the LF exhibited the greatest cross-sectional area compared with the other lumbar spinal ligaments, with a mean area of 84.2 ± 17.9 mm^2, similar to the values reported by Panjabi et al. (1991). The LF had the lowest overall failure stresses at 1.3–4.1 MPa, with findings similar to those reported by Nachemson and Evans (1968) (Pintar et al., 1992). Similar values for stress and strain at failure were reported by Chazal et al. (1985) (Pintar et al., 1992). Panjabi et al. (1991) reported the LF lengths ranging from 11.6 to 16.0 mm, which is, again, similar to the range (13.0–18.0 mm) reported by Pintar et al. (1992). The mean stiffness value for the LF was 27.2 ± 9.2 Nmm^{-1} (Pintar et al., 1992).

There have been no reported disabilities in patients with LF excised at single or multiple sites; this is most likely due to the location rather than the function of the ligament, as the ligament lies immediately behind the vertebral canal and is, therefore, immediately adjacent to nervous structures within the canal (Bogduk, 1997). The lateral extensions of the LF have elasticity of medial and anterior capsule of the posterior joints that balances the elasticity of the intervertebral disc (Yong-Hing et al., 1976).

We recently described a midline ligament (Figs. 9.8 and 9.9) found just anterior to the LF. This small vertical ligament, to our knowledge, has not been previously mentioned in the literature.

SUPRASPINOUS LIGAMENT

Anatomy

The SSL (Figs. 9.10–9.12) is composed of a strong fibrous cord connecting the tips of spinous processes of the vertebral column (Bannister et al., 1996; Bogduk, 1997; Dickman et al., 1999; Moore et al., 2010). Fibrocartilage has been noted to be present where the ligament attaches to the spinous process (Dickman et al., 1999). There are inconsistencies in the description of the SSL among anatomists, with many anatomists describing the SSL as beginning at the seventh cervical

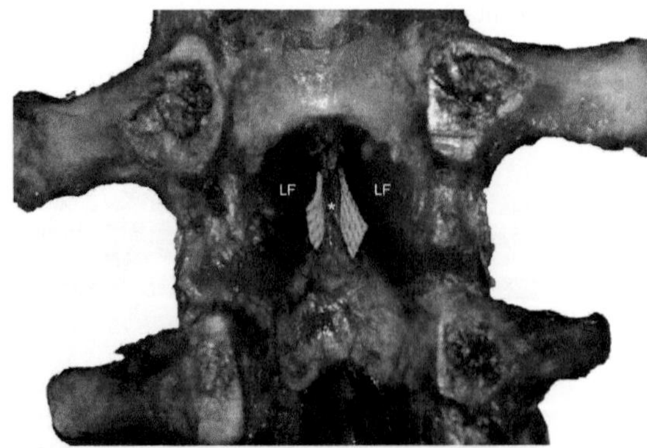

FIG. 9.8 Anterior cadaveric view of a ligament described by our group. Here, the ligamenta flava (LF) are seen laterally and just anterior to these structures and in the midline is the ligament called by us the median interlaminar ligament (asterisk).

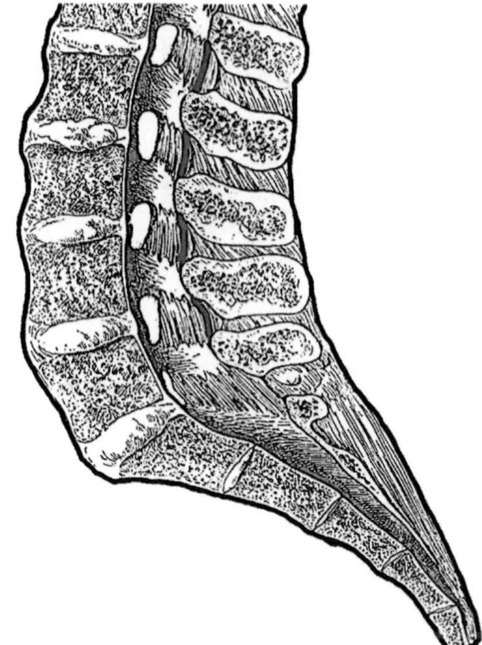

FIG. 9.9 Schematic drawing with the position of the ligament shown in Fig. 9.8 highlighted in blue.

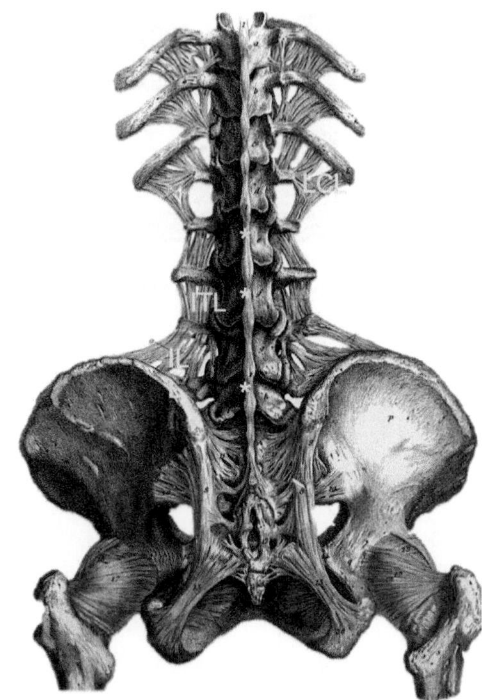

FIG. 9.10 Posterior view of the ligaments related to the lumbar spine. Note the lumbocostal ligament (LCL), intertransverse ligament (ITL), iliolumbar ligament (ILL), and supraspinous ligaments (asterisks).

vertebra, where it then merges with the nuchal ligament to extend to the occipital protuberance and extending in a caudal direction along the length of the vertebral column to the sacrum (Bannister et al., 1996; Dickman et al., 1999; Moore et al., 2010). As this ligament passes caudally, it will thicken and become broader in the lumbar region where it will blend intimately with the neighboring fascia (Bannister et al., 1996). While there is no disagreement about where the ligament begins cranially, Parke (1975), Heylings (1978), and Bogduk (1997) all suggest that the SSL extends caudally only as far as the fifth lumbar vertebra (Bannister et al., 1996). According to Bogduk (1997), the SSL bridges the L4–L5 interspace in only 5% of individuals. He suggests that the ligament ends at the third lumbar spinous process in 22% of individuals and at L4 in the remaining 73% (Bogduk, 1997). Caudal to L5, the SSL is replaced by medial tendons of the erector spinae muscle (Heylings, 1978). The average length of the SSL in the lumbar spine is 25.2 mm with a mean cross-sectional area of 25.2 mm^2 based on a study of 22 cadaveric specimens (Pintar et al., 1992).

The SSL consists of three layers: superficial, middle, and deep (Bogduk, 1997). Similar to the ALL, the superficial fibers are composed of longitudinally oriented collagen fibers and extend over three to four spinous processes (Bannister et al., 1996; Bogduk, 1997). This layer ranges in size, from a few thin bundles of fibers to very thick bundles measuring 5–6 mm wide and 3–4 mm thick, with the majority ranging somewhere between these extremes (Bogduk, 1997). Deep to this layer comes the middle layer, which spans two to three spinous processes, has a thickness of 1 mm, and is composed of fibers of the dorsal layer of the thoracolumbar fascia (Fig. 9.13) and the aponeurosis of the longissimus thoracis muscle (Bogduk, 1997). The deepest layer of SSL connects adjacent spinous processes and consists of strong tendinous fibers of the aponeurosis of the longissimus thoracis muscle (Bogduk, 1997). This layer is reinforced by the tendon of the multifidus muscle (Bogduk, 1997). Given the tendinous nature of the middle and deep layers of the SSL, Bogduk (1997) questions the validity of the SSL as a true ligament (Bogduk, 1997).

Biomechanics

The SSL functions to limit flexion but provides little resistance to separation of the spinous processes (Bogduk, 1997; Heylings, 1978). Heylings (1978) suggests that

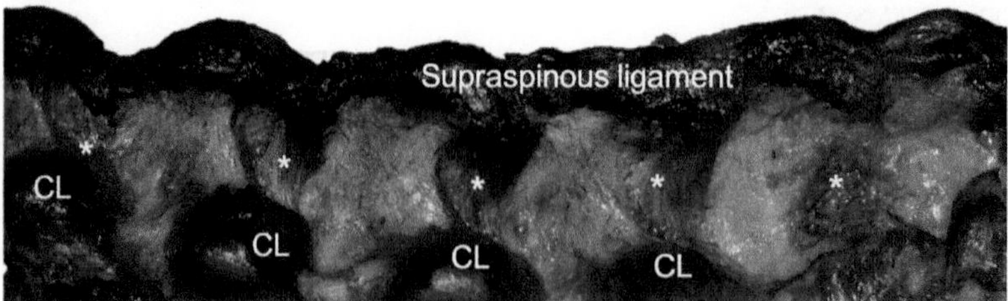

FIG. 9.11 Lateral cadaveric view of the supraspinous ligament, interspinous ligaments (asterisks), and capsular ligaments (CL) of the lumbar spine.

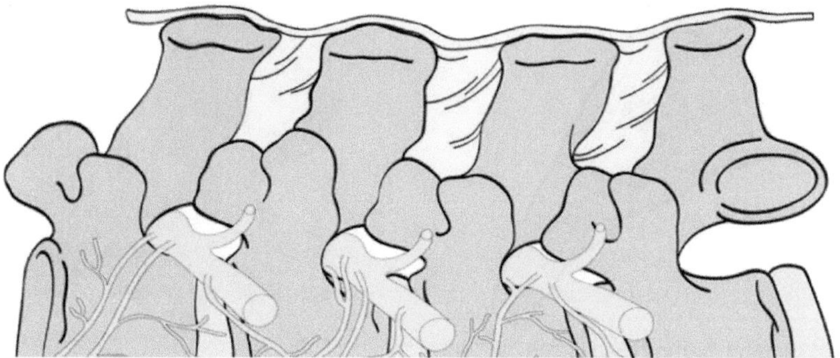
FIG. 9.12 Schematic view of the lumbar supraspinous and interspinous ligaments and their relationship to the facet joints and intervertebral foramina.

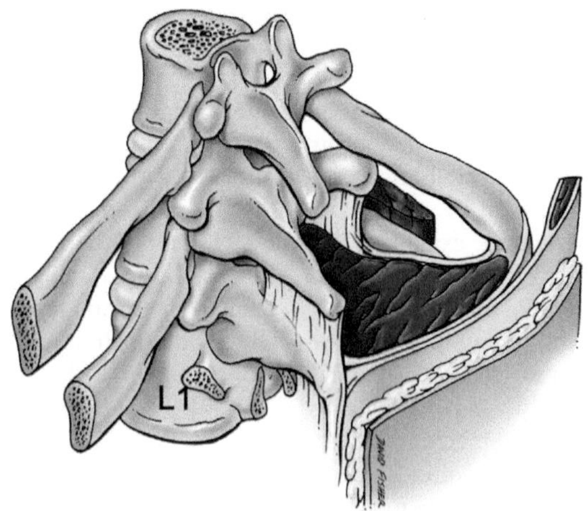

FIG. 9.13 Schematic, posterolateral view of the thoracolumbar junction noting the relationship of the supraspinous ligament to the thoracolumbar fascia and related muscles.

the absence of the SSL at the lumbosacral junction may account for the increased mobility of the spine in this region. He also suggests that this absence may play a role in the etiology of low back pain and the musculoskeletal disorders that often affect the lumbosacral junction (Heylings, 1978). Gudavalli and Triano (1999) used computer modeling to assess the lumbar spinal ligaments and found that the SSL carries the greatest load during flexion, followed by the LF, capsular ligament, and the intertransverse and ISLs. They also found that the SSL undergoes the greatest increase in length (Gudavalli and Triano, 1999). Hindle et al. (1990) found that the supraspinous and ISLs carried very little load during the first half of flexion but resisted a much greater load toward the end of flexion. They suggest that while these ligaments are useful in limiting passive flexion when acting in concert with other support structures, they lack much mechanical function when isolated (Hindle et al., 1990). Due to its continuous nature, the SSL was found to have one of the greatest original lengths, next to the ALL and PLL, when compared with other spinal ligaments (Pintar et al., 1992). The highest values of energy to failure were observed for the ALL and the SSL, with values ranging from 0.82 to 8.68 J and 3.18–11.64 J, respectively (Pintar et al., 1992). Pintar et al. (1992) also reported the SSL as having the highest strain at failure (70.6%–115.0%). The mean stiffness value reported for the SLL was $23.7 \pm 10.9\ \text{Nmm}^{-1}$ (Pintar et al., 1992).

INTERSPINOUS LIGAMENT

Anatomy

The ISL (Figs. 9.11 and 9.12) is a thin and almost membranous ligament connecting adjacent vertebral spinous processes (Bannister et al., 1996; Bogduk, 1997; Dickman et al., 1999; Moore et al., 2010). Its attachments extend from the root to apex of each spinous process, meeting the SSL dorsally and the LF ventrally (Bannister et al., 1996; Dickman et al., 1999; Moore et al., 2010). The ISL is poorly developed in the neck, elongated and narrow in the thoracic region, and thicker and broader in the lumbar region (Bannister et al., 1996; Dickman et al., 1999). There are many inconsistencies in the description of the fibers of the ISL (Heylings, 1978). With regard to the cervical bundles, some anatomists describe these bundles of the ISL as part of the ligamentum nuchae, whereas others describe them as distinct interspinous fascicles (Bannister et al., 1996). Also, major discrepancies exist regarding the lumbar supraspinous and ISLs in humans (Heylings, 1978). Many anatomists describe these fibers as crossing the interspinous space in a posterocaudal direction (Bannister et al., 1996; Parke, 1975; Spalteholz, 1943). However, Heylings (1978), Rissanen (1976), Grant, and Bogduk (1997) describe the fibers as traversing in a posterocranial direction, especially in the lumbar spine where, anteriorly, the ISL is essentially a paired structure with ligaments on each side, split by a midline cavity filled with fat (Agur and Dalley, 2005). This cavity, however, is not present more posteriorly (Bogduk, 1997). Pintar et al. (1992) reported the average length of the ISL in the lumbar spine of 18 studied specimens as 16 mm with a standard deviation of 3.2 mm and a mean cross-sectional area of 35.1 mm^2 with a standard deviation of 15.0 mm^2 (Pintar et al., 1992).

Heylings (1978) postulated that to allow the ligament to maintain a physiologically desirable degree of tensile control throughout the movement from extension to flexion while still being stable enough to bring this movement to a halt, the ligaments needed to be directed almost radially with respect to the axis of movement, as seen in the collateral ligaments of the joints in the limbs (Heylings, 1978). The fibers that cross the interspinous space in a posterocranial direction fulfill these criteria, but if the fibers were running in the posterocaudal direction, they would limit flexion too early, or if the fibers ran a straight course between their attachments, they would be so lax in extension that the ligament would be useless in controlling in the spine except in the movement of flexion (Heylings, 1978).

Biomechanics

The ISL functions along with the LF and SSL to provide protection and stability to the vertebral joints and to store muscular energy during movement (Yahia et al., 1990). It functions weakly to limit flexion especially in the lumbar spine; the ISL also serves to resist separation of the spinous processes because the fibers run almost perpendicular to the direction of separation of the spinous processes (Bogduk, 1997; Heylings, 1978). Hindle et al. (1990) found that the supraspinous and interspinous ligaments carried very little load during the first half of flexion but resisted a greater load toward the end of flexion. They suggest that while these ligaments are useful in limiting passive flexion, when acting in concert with other support structures, they lack much mechanical function when isolated (Hindle et al., 1990). They also noted that when the SSL was removed, the ISL resisted 75% of the load on its own (Hindle et al., 1990). The ISL is the only spinal ligament that is not loaded during lateral bending (Zander et al., 2004). When compared with the other lumbar ligaments, this ligament was recorded to exhibit the lowest overall stiffness, at a value of 11.5 ± 6.6 Nmm^{-1}, with the joint capsule giving the highest stiffness at a value of 33.9 ± 10.7 Nmm^{-1} as well as the lowest stress value, ranging between 1.8 and 5.9 MPa (Pintar et al., 1992).

INTERTRANSVERSE LIGAMENT

Anatomy

The intertransverse ligament (ITL) (Figs. 9.1, 9.10 and 9.14) is a complicated ligament, interpreted in a variety of ways. It consists of sheets of connective tissue that extend from the superior border of one transverse process to the inferior border of the transverse process above (Bannister et al., 1996; Bogduk, 1997; Dickman et al., 1999; Moore et al., 2010). In the cervical region, this ligament consists of a few irregular and scattered fibers interspersed and within and largely replaced by the intertransverse muscles (Bannister et al., 1996; Moore et al., 2010). The ITL is composed of rounded fibrous cords in the thoracic region intimately blended with adjacent muscles and thin, membranous fibers in the lumbar region (Bannister et al., 1996; Dickman et al., 1999; Moore et al., 2010). Thus, Bogduk (1997) states that the ITL is not a true ligament but rather, a membranous continuation of muscular fibers, with the medial and lateral continuations comprising part of a complex fascial system that separates certain paravertebral compartments. In fact, Bogduk (1997) states that the only true ligament in the intertransverse area is the ligament

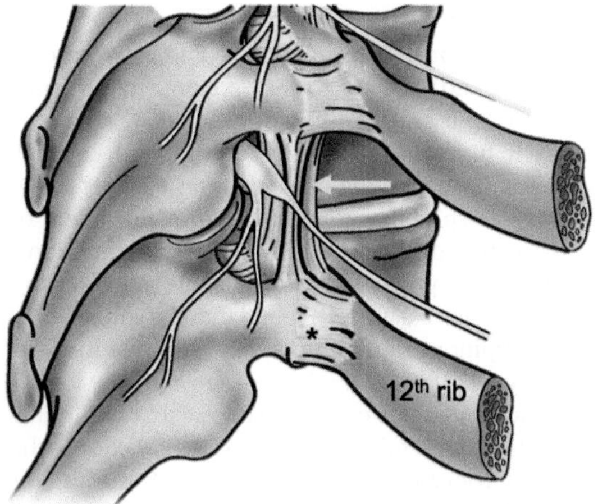

FIG. 9.14 Posterolateral view of the thoracolumbar junction demonstrating the relationship between the exiting nerve root branches and the intertransverse ligament (arrow). Also note the 12th rib's attachment to the transverse process of the adjacent thoracic vertebra via the lateral transverse costal ligament (asterisk).

of Bourgery; this ligament connects the base of the transverse process to the mammillary process below.

The ITL is not considered a true ligament, as it lacks distinct medial and lateral borders, and its collagen fibers are not as densely packed nor are they as regularly oriented as the fibers of true ligaments (Bogduk, 1997; Jiang et al., 1994). An additional reason for why this ligament has been questioned as a true ligament is due to its fibrous fascicles between the transverse processes of the adjacent vertebrate not directly attaching to the upper and lower transverse processes, as Jiang et al. (1994) described, using a study of 32 human cadavers. This study suggested that the ligament actually consisted of tendinous fascicles of the semispinalis thoracis muscle and tendons of the levatores costarum longi muscle with the former fascicles arising from the transverse process and inserting via tendons into the spinous process and the latter fascicles arising from the ends of the transverse process and passing obliquely downward and laterally until, eventually, inserting into the outer surface of the rib caudal to the vertebrae from which it originated (Jiang et al., 1994). This hypothesis was corroborated by these fascicular fibers, though thought to be ligamentous fibers, being inseparable from the muscular fibers during dissection of the 32 human cadavers (Jiang et al., 1994). These features suggest that the ITL resembles a membrane, rather than a ligament with its ligamentous appearance produced by the interweaving of muscle tendons between adjacent transverse processes (Jiang et al., 1994).

In the lumbar spine, the ITL forms a septum dividing the anterior musculature from the posterior musculature in the intertransverse spaces (Bogduk, 1997). Laterally, the ligament divides into two layers: an anterior layer of thoracolumbar fascia that covers the front of the quadratus lumborum muscle and a posterior layer that blends with the transverse abdominus aponeurosis to form the middle layer of the thoracolumbar fascia (Bogduk, 1997). Medially, the ITL splits into dorsal and ventral leaves (Bogduk, 1997). The dorsal leaf extends medially and attaches to the lateral margin of the lamina of the vertebra lying opposite to the intertransverse space, while inferiorly blending with the capsule of the adjacent facet joint (Bogduk, 1997). Meanwhile, the ventral leaf curves forward and extends over the lateral surface of vertebral bodies and blends with lateral margins of the ALL (Bogduk, 1997). By covering the lateral aspect of the vertebral column, the ventral leaf forms a membranous sheet that closes the outer end of the interventricular foramen (Bogduk, 1997). As such, this ventral leaf has two noted perforations that transmit structures into and out of the IV foramen (Bogduk, 1997). Running through the superior opening are nerve branches to the psoas muscle, and running through the inferior opening are the ventral rami of spinal nerves, as well as spinal branches of lumbar arteries and veins (Bogduk, 1997). Sandwiched between the dorsal and ventral leaves is a wedge-shaped space called the superior articular recess that serves to accommodate movements of the subadjacent facet joint (Bogduk, 1997). This recess is filled with fat that is continuous with the intraarticular in the joint below, via the foramen in the superior capsule (Bogduk, 1997).

Biomechanics

Similar to most of the other ligaments of the subaxial spine, the ITL is loaded during flexion (Zander et al., 2004). The ITL and ALL carry the highest load during lateral bending movements of the vertebral column (Zander et al., 2004). The ITL, however, is the only ligament that is not loaded during torsion. Gudavalli and Triano (1999) assessed ligament loads using a computer model and concluded that the SSL undergoes the maximum increase in length during torsion, followed by the ISL, LF, facet capsular ligament, and, finally, the ITL.

FACET CAPSULAR LIGAMENT

Anatomy

The facet capsular ligament (Figs. 9.6 and 9.7) fully encases the facet joint by covering the joint from a rostral to caudal direction with a nonuniform thickness

(Jaumard et al., 2011). The lumbar facet capsule has been reported to be approximately 2.0 mm thick in the posterior region while being as much as 3.2 mm thick in the anterior region (Jaumard et al., 2011). The superior and inferior regions of the capsule have been reported to be approximately 2.4 mm thick (Jaumard et al., 2011). *Gray's Anatomy* identifies three distinct types of intracapsular structures: adipose tissue fat pads (anterosuperior, posteroinferior or a combination of the two), fibroadipose meniscoids (located at the superior or inferior pole or at both poles of the capsule), and connective tissue rims (either anterior or posterior or both) (Bannister et al., 1996). While the fat pads of the facet capsules are similar to those found in many other joint capsules, the connective tissue rims of the zygapophyseal joint are representative of the capsular ligament (CL) (Bannister et al., 1996). Each joint is surrounded by a thin, loose CL, which attaches to the margins of the articular processes of adjacent vertebrae (Dickman et al., 1999; Moore et al., 2010). The average length of the CL in the lumbar spine in 24 individuals' capsular ligaments was measured to be 16.4 mm (±2.9) and an average cross-sectional area of 43.8 mm^2 (±28.3) (Pintar et al., 1992).

Biomechanics

Together with other accessory ligaments of the vertebral column, the capsular ligaments help stabilize the vertebral column and its joints. In the cervical region, the loose nature of this ligament allows for a wide range of movement (Moore et al., 2010). In the sacral spine, however, the CL functions to prevent the lumbar vertebra from sliding anteriorly down the incline of the sacrum (Moore et al., 2010). This arises as the facets on S1 face posteromedially and interlock with the anterolateral facing inferior facets of the L5 vertebra (Moore et al., 2010).

Due to the makeup of the facet capsular ligament, it can only provide mechanical resistance when the two adjacent vertebrae articulating in the zygapophyseal joint undergo movement relative to one another (Jaumard et al., 2011). The role of the ligament was demonstrated in studies using C3–C7 cadaveric spine segments subjected to 100 N of compression with either 2 nm (nm) of sagittal bending or 5 nm of axial torsion, before and after graded bilateral removal of the capsular ligament (Jaumard et al., 2011). After removal of 50% of the facet capsule, axial rotation increased by 19% when torsion was applied, while the vertical distance between the C4 and C6 spinous processes increased by 5% under flexion (Jaumard et al., 2011). The extent of axial torsion and posterior displacement increased by 25% and 32%, respectively, after 75% of the facet capsule was removed (Jaumard et al., 2011). The increases in the range of motion observed after capsular transection or removal supports the hypothesis that the facet capsular ligament provides a substantial contribution to constraining vertebral motion, particularly flexion and lateral bending/torsion (Jaumard et al., 2011).

ILIOLUMBAR LIGAMENT

Anatomy

The iliolumbar ligament (Figs. 9.1, 9.10 and 9.15) is attached to the tip of anteroinferior aspect of the L5 transverse process bilaterally, as well as the L4 transverse process in some cases, and radiates laterally to attach to the pelvis (Bannister et al., 1996; Bogduk, 1997). The iliolumbar ligament begins to radiate as it passes laterally from the transverse process and splits into two bands, upper and lower, to attach to the pelvis (Bannister et al., 1996). The lower bands (the lumbosacral portion of the iliolumbar ligament) originate from the inferior aspect of the L5 transverse process and travel to the anterosuperior lateral surface of the sacrum and eventually blend in with the anterior sacroiliac ligament (Bannister et al., 1996). The upper bands traverse laterally and attach to the inner lip of the iliac crest just anterior to the sacroiliac articulation, with the superior portion of the upper bands becoming continuous with the lumbodorsal fascia (Bannister et al., 1996; Bogduk, 1997). The psoas major muscle surrounds the iliolumbar ligament anteriorly, while the muscles

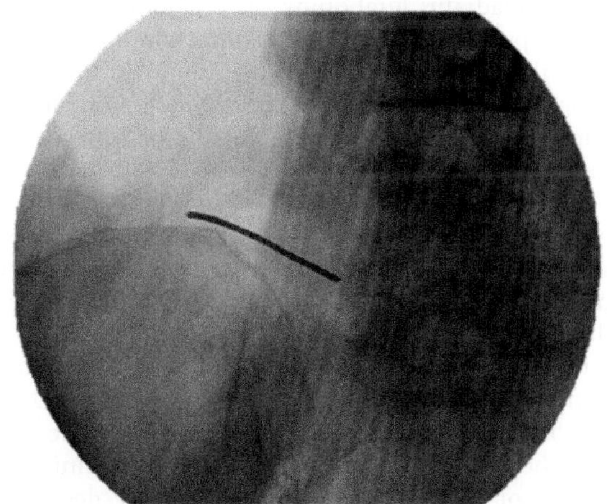

FIG. 9.15 Anterior view of the right iliolumbar ligament with metal wire applied to it.

occupying the vertebral groove surround the iliolumbar ligament posteriorly and superiorly by the quadratus lumborum (Bannister et al., 1996).

Early anatomists postulated that the iliolumbar ligament consisted of five parts (Bogduk, 1997). The anterior part was a well-developed ligamentous band whose fibers span the entire anteroinferior border of the L5 transverse process (from the border of L5 vertebral body to the tip of the L5 transverse process) (Bogduk, 1997). As the fibers from the medial end of the L5 transverse process pass laterally, they begin to cover the fibers arising from the lateral end and the tip of the L5 transverse process, such that all the fibers become continuous as the band leaves the transverse process and passes posterolaterally to attach to the ilium (Bogduk, 1997). The upper surface of this anterior bundle of the iliolumbar ligament forms the site of attachment of the ligament to the inferior portion of the quadratus lumborum muscle (Bogduk, 1997). The superior bundle of the iliolumbar ligament is thought to be formed from the anterior and posterior thickenings of the fascia that surround the base of the quadratus lumborum muscle; these thickenings will attach to the anterosuperior border of the L5 transverse process near the lateral tip (Bogduk, 1997). As this bundle travels laterally, it separates to pass in front of and behind the quadratus lumborum muscle and ultimately attach to the ilium superiorly and inferiorly blend with the anterior ligament to form a channel from which the quadratus lumborum muscle arises (Bogduk, 1997). The posterior bundle of the iliolumbar ligament originates from the tip and posterior border of the L5 transverse process and inserts into the ligamentous area of the ilium behind the origin of the quadratus lumborum; on a unique side note, the deepest fibers of the longissimus lumborum arise from the posterior bundle of the iliolumbar ligament (Bogduk, 1997). The fourth part of the iliolumbar ligament is the inferior bundle, which arises from the lower border of the transverse process and the body of L5 vertebra (Bogduk, 1997). These fibers pass downward and laterally across the surface of the anterior sacroiliac ligament to attach to the superoposterior part of the iliac fossa (Bogduk, 1997). To distinguish these fibers from the anterior sacroiliac ligament, one must observe the oblique orientation of the inferior bundle of the iliolumbar ligament (Bogduk, 1997). The final portion of the iliolumbar ligament is the vertical bundle, which arises from the anteroinferior border of the L5 transverse process and descends almost vertically to attach to the posterior end of the iliopectineal line of the pelvis (Bogduk, 1997). The significance of this bundle lies in its formation of the lateral margin of the channel through which the L5 ventral ramus enters the pelvis (Bogduk, 1997).

According to Bogduk (1997), a recent study confirmed the presence of anterior and posterior parts of the iliolumbar ligament but denied the existence of the superior part. Moreover, this study made no comment on the inferior and vertical part. This study stated that superior part of the iliolumbar ligament is actually the anterior fascia of the quadratus lumborum muscle and, as such, lacks the characteristic features of a true ligament, which include the oriented collagen fibers passing directly from one bone to another (Bogduk, 1997). The vertical and inferior bundles of the iliolumbar ligament were overlooked as part of the ventral sacroiliac ligament because these bundles attach to the lumbar portion and ilium and not to the sacrum and ilium as previously thought; thus, these bundles are now thought to deserve the name "iliolumbar ligament" and not "ventral sacroiliac ligament" (Bogduk, 1997).

Hanson et al. (1998) found that the mean length of the iliolumbar ligament in Caucasians was approximately 33.2 mm while the length in African Americans was approximately 61.8 mm. These differences were also observed to hold true in both sexes, i.e., African American females had iliolumbar ligaments that were longer than those of Caucasian females (Hanson et al., 1998).

Thus, the numerous insertions and fiber directions of the iliolumbar ligament suggest a diversity of biomechanical functions for the iliolumbar ligament (Pool-Goudzwaard et al., 2001).

Biomechanics

The iliolumbar ligament is the most important ligament for restraining excess movement and in maintaining stability at the lumbosacral junction (Luk et al., 1986; Pool-Goudzwaard et al., 2001). The iliolumbar ligament is composed of two bands, an anterior and a posterior band, both of which serve different functions (Luk et al., 1986). While its overall function is multifocal, the iliolumbar ligament, as a whole, is thought to be a ligament that prevents forward sliding of the L5 vertebrae onto the sacrum (Bogduk, 1997). The anterior band of the iliolumbar ligament is thought to be responsible for "squaring" the L5 vertebrae on the sacrum and preventing the tilt of the vertebrae in the coronal plane, as well as for preventing lateral bending; conversely, the posterior band is thought to prevent anterior slipping of the L5 vertebrae over the sacrum during weight-bearing movements and to help to resist forward bending (Bogduk, 1997; Luk et al., 1986; Sims and Moorman, 1996). Together with the strong intervertebral disc, the iliolumbar ligament helps stabilize the lumbosacral junction and may play a significant role in maintaining the lumbosacral stability in patients with lumbosacral pathology (Bogduk, 1997; Luk et al., 1986).

During flexion, the iliolumbar ligament will significantly limit anterior displacement of L5 vertebra (Sims and Moorman, 1996). When the iliolumbar was divided bilaterally, there was a 77.5% increase noted in anterior flexion of L5, with the posterior bands accounting for the majority, approximately 61.2%, of the increase and the anterior bands contributing only a small amount to the anterior stability of the L5 (Sims and Moorman, 1996). Meanwhile, during extension, a 20.41% increase in flexion of L5 was noted after bilateral division of the ligament; in this case, however, it was the anterior band that contributed to all of the stability during extension (Sims and Moorman, 1996). Lateral bending with bilateral division of the ligament did result in a dramatic increase of 141.7% in flexion of L5 during contralateral bending, with much of this increase being attributed to the anterior bands (Sims and Moorman, 1996). During torsion of the L5 vertebrae, division of the iliolumbar ligament did not produce much change in the flexion of L5, but both bands together did restrict torsion by 5.3% (Sims and Moorman, 1996). These results by Sims and Moorman (1996) suggest that the iliolumbar ligament plays a very insignificant role in limiting the displacement of L5 onto the sacrum during torsion, thus further suggesting that other structures are primarily responsible for limiting this displacement during torsion. Sims and Moorman (1996) used these data to create the theory that the iliolumbar ligament is the probable cause of a majority of chronic low back pain.

Yamamoto et al. (1990) performed in vitro studies on four fresh cadavers of males aged 25–45 years (total of eight ligament specimens) to evaluate the biomechanical function of the iliolumbar ligament, both intact and after transection of the ligament. This study involved applying a load of 10 Nm to the intact iliolumbar ligament, a right transected iliolumbar ligament, and bilateral transected iliolumbar ligaments, with the movements of the vertebral column tested before and after the transaction (Yamamoto et al., 1990). Flexion increased by 0.9° or approximately 12% after removal of right iliolumbar ligament and by 1.7° or approximately 23% after bilateral iliolumbar ligament removal (Yamamoto et al., 1990). Extension increased by 0.6° (11%) with right iliolumbar ligament transection and by 1.1° (20%) with bilateral iliolumbar ligament transaction (Yamamoto et al., 1990). Iliolumbar ligaments significantly restricted the motion of the vertebral column to the contralateral side when under torsional load (Yamamoto et al., 1990). Thus, bilateral iliolumbar ligaments significantly restrict the movements of the lumbosacral junction in the directions of flexion and extension, with a slight increase in destabilization seen with unilateral transection and a statistically significant increase in destabilization seen with bilateral transection (Yamamoto et al., 1990). However, when comparing all the movements of flexion, extension, right and left lateral bending, and right and left axial rotation, the iliolumbar ligament seems to be most effective in resisting lateral bending of the vertebral column (Yamamoto et al., 1990).

In addition to stabilizing the lumbosacral junction, the iliolumbar ligament may play an important role in also stabilizing the sacroiliac joint by restraining excess movement and thus possibly helping to prevent onset of low back pain (Pool-Goudzwaard et al., 2001, 2003). In his study, Pool-Goudzwaard et al. (2003) defined stability as the ability of a joint to bear loading forces without allowing any uncontrolled displacements. He states that the ligaments of this lumbopelvic and sacroiliac region contribute to stability by controlling the relative positions of the joint, thus restricting the joint to only those positions that the joint can handle when loading forces are applied (Pool-Goudzwaard et al., 2003). The existence of the sacroiliac part of the iliolumbar ligament, verified by MRI and cryosectioning of the pelvis in coronal and transverse plane, reinforces the idea that the iliolumbar ligament has a direct restraining effect on movements in the sacroiliac joints (Pool-Goudzwaard et al., 2001). In 2001, Pool-Goudzwaard et al. studied 12 human specimens and applied incremental moment to the sacroiliac joint to induce rotation in the sagittal plane (Pool-Goudzwaard et al., 2001, 2003). The results of this study indicated that the sacroiliac joint mobility in the sagittal plane increased monumentally after the total transection of both iliolumbar ligaments, with most of the increase seen after cutting the ventral band of the ligament (Pool-Goudzwaard et al., 2003). This suggests that the iliolumbar ligaments restrict sacroiliac joint mobility in the sagittal plane with the ventral band of the iliolumbar ligament contributing to most of this restriction (Pool-Goudzwaard et al., 2003). Strangely, the locality of the ventral band of the iliolumbar ligament seems to draw skepticism as to how this band is able to restrict the sacroiliac joint's mobility in the sagittal plane (Pool-Goudzwaard et al., 2003). Pool-Goudzwaard et al. (2003), however, offered an explanation in his study that postulated that this phenomenon could be due to the orientation of the auricular surfaces of the sacroiliac joint with respect to the fiber direction of the ventral band of the iliolumbar ligament. The shape of the sacrum is a wedge with the ventral (anterior) aspect of the sacrum being larger than the dorsal (posterior) aspect of the sacrum (Pool-Goudzwaard et al., 2003). With the auricular surfaces of sacroiliac joint being oriented dorsomedially and ventrolaterally, one would expect most of the restriction from the ligaments during sagittal rotation of the sacroiliac joint to be parallel to this orientation of the auricular surfaces (Pool-Goudzwaard et al., 2003). Since the most ventral fibers of the ventral band of the iliolumbar ligament are arranged more parallel to the auricular surfaces of the sacroiliac joint compared with the fibers of the iliolumbar ligament's other components, loading of the ventral band of the iliolumbar ligament is likely to be stimulated by sacroiliac rotation in the sagittal plane (Pool-Goudzwaard et al., 2003).

Several recent studies of the lumbopelvic region have demonstrated support for the following hypothesis: loss of the stability of the sacroiliac joints is crucial in the etiology of nonspecific low back pain (Pool-Goudzwaard et al., 2003). However, in addition to the loss of ligamentous support, it is now believed that a variety of factors, such as a decrease in muscle forces and the dysfunction of the mechanoreceptors in the ligamentous system of the lumbosacral area that are important in activating the muscles necessary for posture control, all contribute to the development of nonspecific low back pain (Pool-Goudzwaard et al., 2003).

Lastly, short segmental bands of connective tissue that cross near the intervertebral foramina have been termed the transforaminal ligaments (Fig. 9.16). Although the function of such ligaments is uncertain, they can occupy space and potentially compress structures entering and leaving the intervertebral foramen.

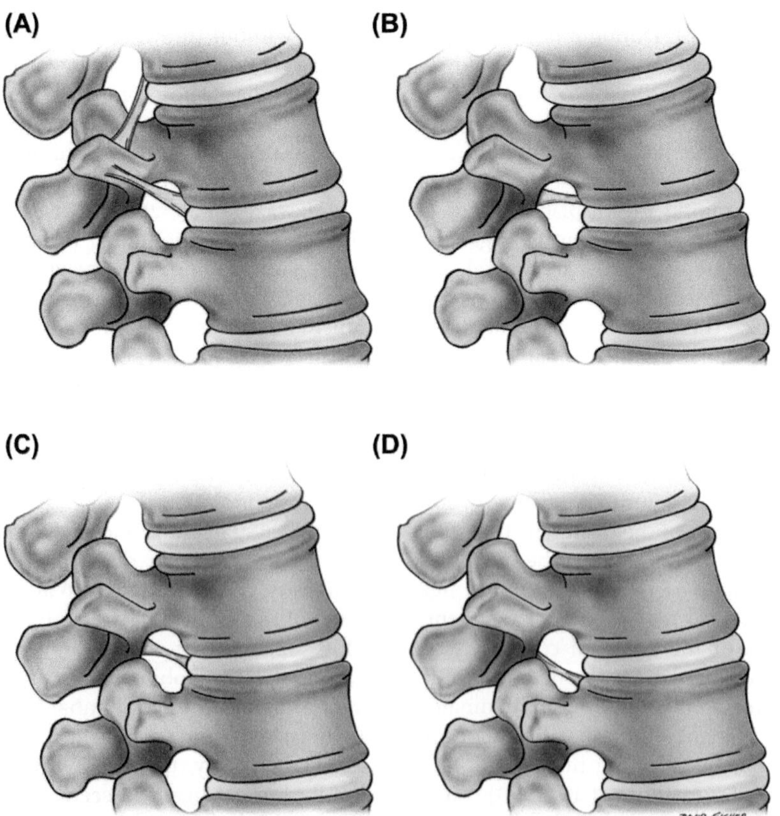

FIG. 9.16 Schematic drawings **(A–D)** of the various ligaments associated with the intervertebral foramina.

REFERENCES

Agur, A.M.R., Dalley, A.F., 2005. Grant's Atlas of Anatomy, eleventh ed. Lippincott Williams and Wilkins, Baltimore.

Bannister, L.H., Berry, M.M., Collins, P., Dyson, M., Dussek, J.E., Ferguson, M.W.J. (Eds.), 1996. Gray's Anatomy, 38th edn. Churchill Livingston, New York.

Bogduk, N., 1997. Clinical Anatomy of the Lumbar Spine and Sacrum, third ed. Churchill Livingston, New York.

Chazal, J., Tanguy, A., Bourges, M., Gaurel, G., Escande, G., Guillot, M., Vanneuville, G., 1985. Biomechanical properties of spinal ligaments and a histological study of the supraspinal ligament in traction. J. Biomech. 18 (3), 167–176.

Dickman, C.A., Rosenthal, D.J., Perin, N.I., 1999. Thoracoscopic Spine Surgery. Thieme Medical Publishers, New York.

Gudavalli, M.R., Triano, J.J., 1999. An analytical model of lumbar motion segment in flexion. J. Manip. Physiol. Ther. 22, 201–208.

Hanson, P., Magnusson, S.P., Sorensen, H., Simonsen, E.B., 1998. Differences in the iliolumbar ligament and the transverse process of the L5 vertebra in young white and black people. Acta Anat. 163 (4), 218–223.

Heylings, D.J.A., 1978. Supraspinous and interspinous ligaments of the human lumbar spine. J. Anat. 125 (1), 127–131.

Hindle, R.J., Pearcy, M.J., Cross, A., 1990. Mechanical function of the human lumbar interspinous and supraspinous ligaments. J. Biomed. Eng. 12, 340–344.

Iwanaga, J., et al., 2019. The lumbar ligamentum flavum does not have two layers and is confluent with the interspinous ligament: anatomical study with application to surgical and interventional pain procedures. Clin. Anat. https://doi.org/10.1002/ca.23437 (in press).

Jaumard, N.V., Welch, W.C., Winkelstein, B.A., 2011. Spinal facet joint biomechanics and mechanotransduction in normal, injury and degenerative conditions. J. Biomech. Eng. 133 (7), 071010.

Jiang, H., Raso, J.V., Moreau, M.J., Russell, G., Hill, D.L., Bagnall, K.M., 1994. Quantitative morphology of the lateral ligaments of the spine: assessment of their importance in maintaining lateral stability. Spine 19 (23), 2676–2682.

Lang, J., 1993. Clinical Anatomy of the Cervical Spine. Thieme Medical Publishers, New York.

Luk, K.D.K., Ho, H.C., Leong, J.C.Y., 1986. The iliolumbar ligament: a study of its anatomy, development, and clinical significance. J. Bone Joint Surg. 68, 197–200.

Moore, K.L., Dalley, A.F., Agur, A.M.R., 2010. Clinically Oriented Anatomy, sixth ed. Lippincott Williams & Wilkins, Baltimore.

Nachemson, A.L., Evans, J.H., 1968. Some mechanical properties of the third human lumbar interlaminar ligament (*Ligamentum flavum*). J. Biomech. 1 (3), 211–220.

Neumann, P., Keller, T.S., Ekstrom, L., Perry, L., Hansson, T.H., Spengler, D.M., 1992. Mechanical properties of the human lumbar anterior longitudinal ligament. J. Biomech. 25 (10), 1185–1194.

Neumann, P., Keller, T., Ekstrom, L., Hult, E., Hansson, T., 1993. Structural properties of the anterior longitudinal ligament. Spine 18 (5), 637–645.

Paniabi, M.M., Goel, V.K., Takata, K., 1982. Physiologic strains in the lumbar spinal ligaments. Spine 7 (3), 192–203.

Panjabi, M.M., Greenstein, G., Duranceau, J., Nolte, L.P., 1991. Three-dimensional quantitative morphology of lumbar spinal ligaments. J. Spinal Disord. 4 (l), 54–62.

Parke, W.W., 1975. The Spine, vol. 1. W. B. Saunders Co, Philadelphia, London, Toronto.

Pintar, F.A., Yoganandan, N., Myers, T., Elhagediab, A., Sances Jr., A., 1992. Biomechanical properties of human lumbar spine ligaments. J. Biomech. 25 (11), 1351–1356.

Pool-Goudzwaard, A.L., Kleinrensink, G.J., Snijders, C.J., Entius, C., Stoeckart, R., 2001. The sacroiliac part of the iliolumbar ligament. J. Anat. 199, 457–463.

Pool-Goudzwaard, A.L., Hoek van Dijke, G., Mulder, P., Spoor, C., Snijders, C.J., Stoeckart, R., 2003. The iliolumber ligament: its influence on stability of the sacroiliac joint. Clin. Biomech. 18 (2), 99–105.

Rissanen, P.M., 1976. The surgical anatomy and pathology of the supraspinous and interspinous ligaments of the lumbar spine, with special reference to ligament ruptures. Acta Orthop. Scand. (Suppl. 46), 1–100.

Sims, J.A., Moorman, S.J., 1996. The role of the iliolumbar ligament in low back pain. Med. Hypotheses 46, 511–515.

Spalteholz, W., 1943. Hand Atlas of Human Anatomy, seventh ed., vol. 1. JB Lippincott Co, Philadelphia, London.

Yahia, L.H., Garzon, S., Strykowski, H., Rivard, C.H., 1990. Ultrastructure of the human interspinous ligament and ligamentum flavum: a preliminary study. Spine 15 (4), 262–268.

Yamamoto, I., Panjabi, M.M., Oxland, T.R., Crisco, J.J., 1990. The role of the iliolumbar ligament in the lumbosacral junction. Spine 15, 1138–1141.

Yong-Hing, K., Reilly, J., Kirkaldy-Willis, W.H., 1976. The ligamentum flavum. Spine 1 (4), 226–234.

Zander, T., Rohlmann, A., Bergmann, G., 2004. Influence of ligament stiffness on the mechanical behavior of a functional spinal unit. J. Biomech. 37 (7), 1107–1111.

FURTHER READING

Alderink, G.J., 1991. The sacroiliac joint: review of anatomy, mechanics, and function. J. Orthop. Sports Phys. Ther. 13 (2), 71–84.

DonTigny, R.L., 1985. Function and pathomechanics of the sacroiliac joint: a review. Phys. Ther. 65 (1), 35–44.

Goode, A., Hegedus, E., Sizer Jr., P., Brismee, J.M., Linberg, A., Cook, C.E., 2008. Three-dimensional movements of the sacroiliac joint: a systematic review of the literature and assessment of clinical utility. J. Man. Manip. Ther. 16 (1), 25–38.

Hammer, N., Steinke, H., Slowik, V., Josten, C., Stadler, J., Bohme, J., Spanel-Borowski, K., 2009. The sacrotuberous and the sacrospinous ligament – a virtual reconstruction. Ann. Anat. 191 (4), 417–425.

McGrath, C., Nicholson, H., Hurst, 2009. The long posterior sacroiliac ligament: a histological study of morphological relations in the posterior sacroiliac region. Joint Bone Spine 76 (1), 57–62.

Morris, C.E., 2005. Low Back Syndromes: Integrated Clinical Management. McGraw-Hill, New York.

Onan, O.A., Heggeness, M.H., Hipp, J.A., 1998. A motion analysis of the cervical facet joint. Spine 23 (4), 430–439.

Serhan, H.A., Varnavas, G., Dooris, A.P., Patwardhan, A., Tzsermiadonis, M., 2007. Biomechanics of the posterior lumbar articulating elements. Neurosurg. Focus 22 (1), E1.

Sturesson, B., Selvik, G., Uden, A., 1989. Movements of the sacroiliac joints: a roentgen stereophotogrammetric analysis. Spine 14, 162–165.

Vleeming, A., Stoeckart, R., Snijders, C.J., 1989. The sacrotuberous ligament: a conceptual approach to its dynamic role in stabilizing the sacroiliac joint. Clin. Biomech. 4 (4), 201–203.

Vleeming, A., Van Wingerden, J.P., Snijders, C.J., Stoeckart, R., Stijnen, T., 1989. Load application to the sacrotuberous ligament; influences on sacroiliac joint mechanics. Clin. Biomech. 4 (4), 204–209.

Wilder, D.G., Pope, M.H., Frymoyer, J.W., 1980. The functional topography of the sacroiliac joint. Spine 5 (6), 575–579.

Willard, F.H., Carreiro, J.E., Manko, W., 1998. The long posterior interosseous ligament and the sacrococcygeal plexus. In: Procedings of the Third Interdisciplinary World Congress on Low Back and Pelvic Pain, pp. 207–209.

CHAPTER 10

The Lumbar Intervertebral Foramina

DARIUS ANSARI • R. SHANE TUBBS

INTRODUCTION

Intervertebral foramina (IVF) (Fig. 10.1) are the apertures through which the vertebral canal and extraspinal structures communicate that provide a conduit for a multitude of structures at every level of the vertebral column, including, but not limited to, the spinal nerves and related vessels. Their contents' delicacy, together with the potential for modification of bony architecture in pathologic states, confers substantial physiological and clinical significance on the IVF. Therefore, a thorough understanding of their anatomy is of paramount interest to the surgeon, who must be confident in diagnosing disorders of this structure, as well as performing appropriate intervention, as precise knowledge of the course of the nerve roots is essential to prevent nerve injury.

ANATOMY

Boundaries

The surrounding bony architecture determines the IVF's shape and cross-sectional area, in which the neighboring vertebrae's respective pedicles constitute the superior and inferior borders. The intervertebral disc's posterolateral aspect and the body of the inferior vertebra's posterolateral part form the IVF's ventral aspect, whereas the facet synovial joint's capsule and the ligamentum flavum's ventral aspect form the dorsal boundary (Standring, 2016).

In the lumbar vertebrae, the inferior vertebral notch is deeper than the superior and confers a teardrop shape to the foramen overall with a large vertical axis. Quantitatively, the lumbar IVF's vertical diameter ranges from 12 to 19 mm, whereas the sagittal diameter can be as little as 7 mm. These anatomical features of the foramina not only confer protection but also make them susceptible to encroachment by neighboring structures. For example, a nerve may be spared completely in the case of a complete disc collapse (because of the large vertical axis) but could be compressed in pathologic states that compromise the foramen's sagittal diameter (Garfin et al., 2018).

The IVF's dimensions vary based on the spine's movement and position. Maximum flexion of the spine maximizes all of the IVF's diameters, as the pedicles move apart from one another and the disc is least convex in this position. Conversely, when the spine is extended, the pedicles move closer together and all IVF diameters are at a minimum, which can lead to a 20% reduction in foraminal height (Gkasdaris and Kapetanakis, 2015). Maintenance of the foramen's height is important, as this protects the exiting nerves from the ascension of the inferior articular processes during normal extension movements, as well as from pathologic processes, for example spondylolisthesis, generalized disc protrusion, or facet joint osteoarthritis.

Contents

A foramen contains a segmental mixed spinal nerve and its sheaths, from two to four recurrent meningeal (sinuvertebral) nerves, spinal ganglia, foraminal ligaments, variable numbers of spinal arteries, and plexiform venous connections between the internal and external vertebral venous plexuses (Figs. 10.2 and 10.3). At the lumbar segments, the total area of the neurovascular bundle itself is estimated at 20%–50% of the total foraminal area (Panjabi et al., 1983).

Arteries

Paired branches of the descending aorta supply the vertebral column in the thorax and abdomen. On each side in the lumbar region, the main trunk of the lumbar artery passes around the vertebral body, giving off primary periosteal and equatorial branches to the body anteriorly, and then a major dorsal branch posteriorly. Before supplying the facet joints, laminae, overlying musculature, and skin, the major dorsal branch gives off a spinal branch that enters the IVF either as a single vessel or may protrude from the dorsal segmental branch as numerous separate vessels (Garfin et al., 2018).

Surgical anatomy of the lateral transpsoas approach to the lumbar spine. https://doi.org/10.1016/B978-0-323-67376-1.00010-0

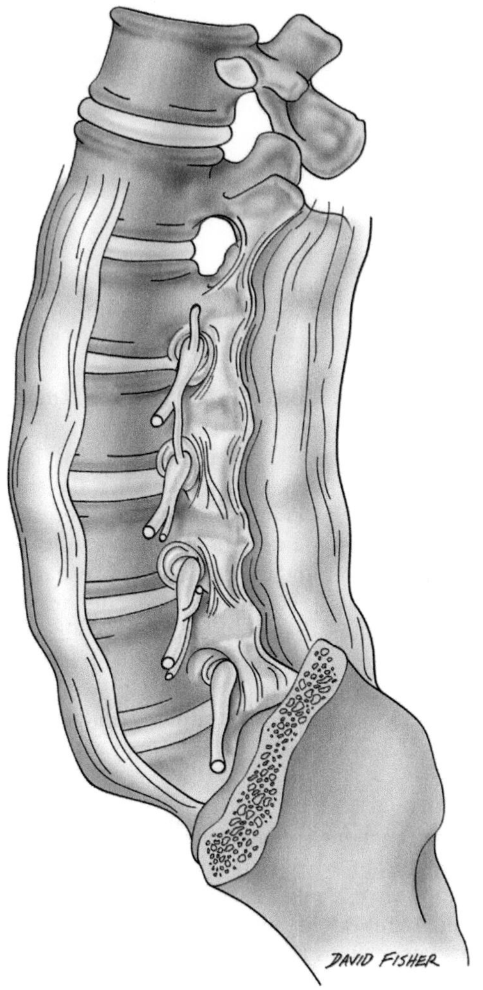

FIG. 10.1 Lateral view of the lumbar spine noting the intervertebral foramina, some with exiting nerve roots.

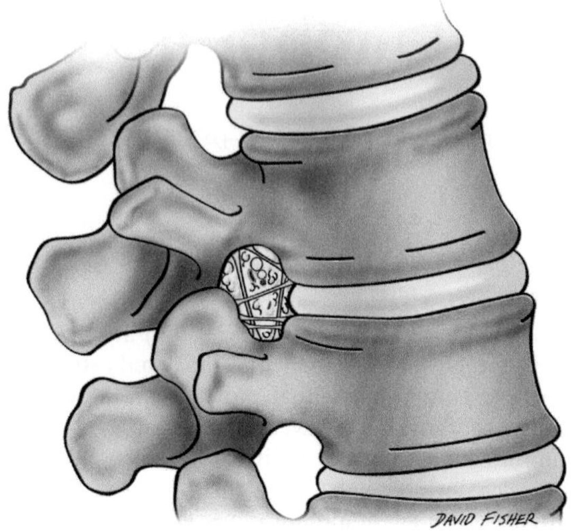

FIG. 10.2 Contents of a lumbar intervertebral foramen. Note the segmental nerves, vessels, and ligaments within the foramen.

Regardless, it divides into postcentral, prelaminar, and radicular branches ultimately.

The postcentral branches are the primary arterial supply to the vertebral bodies and periphery of the intervertebral discs, and within the posterior longitudinal ligament, they anastomose with the vertebral bodies' postcentral branches directly superior and inferior. The prelaminar branches also form an anastomosis on the vertebral canal's posterior wall and supply the vertebral arch, dura and epidural tissues, and the ligamentum flavum. In their radiographic study, Demondion et al. (2012) found that anterior and posterior radicular vessels bifurcate from the radicular branch and generally enter the foramen anterior to their respective nerve roots (i.e., anterior and posterior roots).

Veins

An internal and external venous plexus drains the vertebral column and, in general, parallels the arterial supply's distribution. The internal plexuses, embedded in collagenous fibers and epidural fat, are divided further into anterior and posterior plexuses. On the vertebral arches and ligamenta flava's ventral surfaces, posterior internal plexuses form anastomoses with the posterior external plexuses. The anterior internal plexuses are located on the vertebral bodies' posterior surfaces on the posterior longitudinal ligament's lateral edges. Notably, these internal plexuses receive the basivertebral sinuses that drain the vertebral bodies and are connected to the anterior interior plexuses via transverse vessels. Anterior and posterior internal plexuses are joined via the retrocorporal veins to form intervertebral veins that traverse the IVF together with the spinal nerves and drain craniocaudally along the spine. In the lumbar region, these veins join with ascending lumbar veins in front of the vertebrae's transverse processes or proceed anterior to the vertebral bodies and drain into the inferior vena cava.

External plexuses also are classified into anterior and posterior divisions: they are found anterior to the

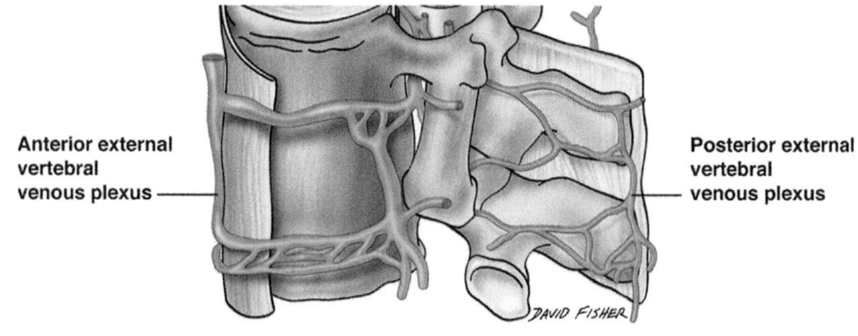

FIG. 10.3 Relationships of the vertebral venous plexus and lumbar intervertebral foramen.

vertebral bodies and posterior to the laminae, with extensive anastomoses with each other and with the internal plexuses. These external plexuses receive the internal veins' draining segmental tributaries through the IVF and communicate ultimately with the caval and azygos system's lumbar tributaries.

Nerves

The IVF is the route through which spinal nerves exit the spinal canal to communicate with the external environment. As the average adult spinal cord terminates at the first lumbar vertebra's body, lumbar spinal nerve roots originate from the T10 to L1 vertebral levels. A spinal nerve is comprised by a ventral root that originates from the cord's anterolateral aspect and a dorsal root from the posterolateral aspect, both of which are continuous with the spinal cord. They travel through the subarachnoid space and dura mater as separate roots and then unite either within or just proximal to the IVF to form a single spinal nerve. Cerebrospinal fluid (CSF) envelops each root via a separate arachnoid sheath. As they pass through the IVF, fine meningovertebral ligaments tether the root sheaths to the foramina's walls.

The ventral and dorsal roots are not equivalent in morphology: dorsal spinal roots exhibit spinal ganglia characterized by oblong swellings just before they join their associated ventral root at, or within, the IVF itself (Fig. 10.4) (Standring, 2016; Gkasdaris and Kapetanakis, 2015). At the low lumbar levels, the dorsal root ganglion tends to be within the spinal canal proximal to the foramina (Vetter et al., 2017). In a magnetic resonance imaging study, Hasegawa et al. (1996) found that the L5–S1 foramen is the smallest of the lumbar IVF and that at this segment, the spinal dorsal root ganglion occupies the largest proportion of the IVF.

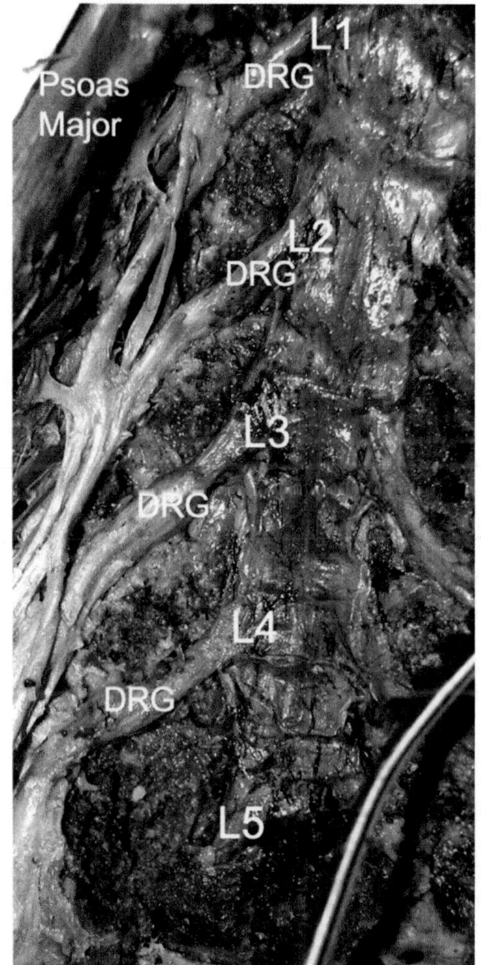

FIG. 10.4 Coronal dissection through the lumbar intervertebral foramina. Note the relationships between the dorsal root ganglia at each level.

During development, the vertebral column lengthens more rapidly than does the spinal cord, culminating in progressive disparity between the levels at which spinal nerves originate and the levels at which they exit. Consequently, nerve roots become longer and directed more obliquely in the lower lumbar region. This is in stark contrast to the cervical region, in which the nerve roots exit the vertebral column at the same level at which they originate within the spinal cord (Garfin et al., 2018).

The nerve root is related to the vertebra's pedicle; Ebraheim et al. (1997) reported that, in the lumbar spine, the pedicles' distance averages 1.5 mm from the inferior nerve root, 5.3 mm from the superior nerve root, and 1.5 mm from the medial pedicle wall to the dura. Generally, nerve roots exit the dural sac approximately one vertebral level superior to their respective IVF and then course caudally and laterally to enter the IVF. Upon reaching the foraminal border, the spinal nerves travel anterolaterally about the pedicles and transverse processes' bases.

The distance between the nerve root and lumbar disc at the IVF is not the same at each level, and it is important to be aware of this variation to assess the risk of injury. At the IVF's medial line, the disc-root distance increases gradually from L1–L2 to L5–S1. Similarly, Garfin et al. (2018) found that from L1–L2 to L5–S1, the foramen's lateral line increases in distance from the intersection between the nerve root's medial edge and the disc's superior edge. This has clinical consequences in cases of foraminal lumbar disc herniations; although these are less common than posterolateral disc herniations, they remain a cause of low back pain encountered frequently. The compression of the dorsal root ganglion causes the pain's radicular character in part. According to Arslan et al. (2012), as the nerve roots are near the intraforaminal disc space, they are at risk of injury during surgical treatment to remove the herniated disc. Because the L1, L2, and L3 nerve roots are farther from the discs (compared with the lower levels), they are at lower risk of injury during such procedures as transforaminal percutaneous endoscopic discectomy.

Ligaments

Numerous ligaments, such as the longitudinal ligaments, ligamenta flava, and others, support the spine's joints, but those most relevant are the transforaminal ligaments (TFLs) found in approximately 80% of the lumbar IVF. TFLs are subdivided classically into five different types: the superior and inferior transforaminal, the superior and inferior corporotransverse, and the midtransforaminal (Vetter et al., 2017). These ligaments form separate compartments within the IVF that the spinal nerves, vasculature, and lymphatics occupy.

Some theorize that the space the TFLs occupy compresses the foraminal contents (e.g., the nerves), resulting in back pain related to lumbar stenosis. However, this association is unclear, as it has been proposed recently that foraminal stenosis attributable to TFLs' compression is uncommon and, on the contrary, they may serve a protective function for the nerves coursing out of the vertebrae (Zhao et al., 2016).

Fat

Epidural fat is distributed around and within the IVF (Garfin et al., 2018). It is firm, plays a mechanically supportive role for the nerves and vasculature spanning the foramen, and extends along the exiting spinal nerves on their ventral and inferior aspects. The fat separates the nerve roots from the foramen's inferior border (i.e., the inferior vertebral body and pedicles' superior aspects). Functionally, it buffers the nerve from caudal and ventral distraction that occurs during regular spine and lower limb movements.

Triangular Working Zone

With minimally invasive and percutaneous spinal procedures' increasing popularity, surgeons have continued to identify safe working areas to minimize damage to the spinal nerves that exit the IVF. Of these, one of the surgical corridors for endoscopic microdiscectomy described best is through Kambin's triangle.

Kambin's triangular working zone, described first in 1988, is bordered anteriorly by the exiting nerve root, inferiorly by the lower lumbar segment's proximal plate, medially by the dural sac, and posteriorly by the superior articular process of the inferior vertebra's lateral edge (Gkasdaris and Kapetanakis, 2015). This forms a right-triangular space in which the spinal nerve is the hypotenuse. The average triangular safe zone's dimensions were determined to be 18.9 mm wide, 12.3 mm high, and 23.0 mm at the hypotenuse. However, radiological measurements are recommended before an endoscopic discectomy procedure, including spinal root axial, coronal angle, and foraminal areas (Mirkovic et al., 1995). The triangle is accessed by making an incision 8–9 cm from the midline with a 35 degree converging angle into the foramen, which averts the need for a facetectomy to identify the nerve root. It has been found that angles smaller than 35 degrees carry a significant risk of damaging the exiting nerve.

Many percutaneous endoscopic discectomy techniques incorporate this approach, as it offers favorable outcomes for soft disc herniation. This relatively safe route also has been used for steroid injections, biopsies, and nerve root blocks (Tumialán et al., 2019). Because of the substantially larger angle available to reach around the IVF's superior border compared with its inferior border, endoscopic instruments can access the spinal canal's upper portion readily, for example, to remove disc material that has migrated cephalad. Caudally migrated disc herniations are less suitable for removal via this approach, as the foramen's inferior boundary limits transforaminal access to the spinal canal's inferior portions. This is clinically significant, as a cannula positioned improperly could potentially compress the spinal nerve and precipitate neural injury or pain in the associated extremity.

A brief discussion of the use of the term "Kambin's triangle" in its application to fusion surgery is included here for clarification. Before transforaminal lateral interbody fusion (TLIF) emerged in the 1980s, Kambin's triangle was relatively unpopular among anyone other than endoscopic surgeons and certain interventionalists. The surgical corridor for TLIF Harms defined originally has the exact same boundaries as those Kambin defined; however, the difference exists in the angles of insertion: Harm's technique uses a 15–20 degrees perspective, in contrast to the characteristic 35 degrees angle Kambin described. However, this subtle distinction is essential, as the former necessitates a complete facetectomy to visualize the traversing nerve root (Tumialán et al., 2019). However, since TLIF proliferated and became incorporated into the fusion literature, the term "Kambin's triangle" has been used interchangeably for these techniques. As these are distinct entities, each with their own specific indications, Tumialán et al. (2019) proposed the term "expanded transforaminal corridor" recently to refer to a TLIF procedure in which the facet, lamina, and pars interarticularis are removed.

REFERENCES

Arslan, M., et al., 2012. Nerve root to lumbar disc relationships at the intervertebral foramen from a surgical viewpoint: an anatomical study. Clin. Anat. 25 (2), 218–223.

Demondion, X., et al., 2012. Radiographic anatomy of the intervertebral cervical and lumbar foramina (vessels and variants). Diagn. Interv. Imaging 93 (9), 690–697.

Ebraheim, N.A., et al., 1997. Anatomic relations between the lumbar pedicle and the adjacent neural structures. Spine 22 (20), 2338–2341.

Garfin, S.R., et al., 2018. Rothman-Simeone and Herkowitz's the Spine, seventh ed. Elsevier, Inc., Philadelphia.

Gkasdaris, G., Kapetanakis, S., 2015. Clinical anatomy and significance of the lumbar intervertebral foramen: a review. J. Anat. Soc. India 64 (2), 7.

Hasegawa, T., et al., 1996. Morphometric analysis of the lumbosacral nerve roots and dorsal root ganglia by magnetic resonance imaging. Spine 21 (9), 1005–1009.

Mirkovic, S.R., Schwartz, D.G., Glazier, K.D., 1995. Anatomic considerations in lumbar posterolateral percutaneous procedures. Spine 20 (18), 1965–1971.

Panjabi, M.M., Takata, K., Goel, V.K., 1983. Kinematics of lumbar intervertebral foramen. Spine 8 (4), 348–357.

Standring, S., 2016. Gray's Anatomy: The Anatomical Basis of Clinical Practice, 41st ed. Elsevier Limited, New York.

Tumialán, L.M., et al., 2019. The history of and controversy over Kambin's triangle: a historical analysis of the lumbar transforaminal corridor for endoscopic and surgical approaches. World Neurosurg. 123, 402–408.

Vetter, M., Oskouian, R.J., Tubbs, R.S., 2017. 'False' ligaments: a review of anatomy, potential function, and pathology. Cureus 9 (11), e1853.

Zhao, Q., et al., 2016. The morphology and clinical significance of the intraforaminal ligaments at the L5-S1 levels. Spine J. 16 (8), 1001–1006.

CHAPTER 11

Sectional Anatomy for the Lateral Transpsoas Approach to the Lumbar Spine: A Pictorial Guide

BEOM SUN CHUNG

INTRODUCTION

For performing lateral transpsoas approaches to the lumbar spine, the anatomy of the region should be well understood, and conventional cadaveric dissection is still considered the best method for viewing this anatomy (Banagan et al., 2011). However, sectional anatomy of the region is necessary for a more concrete understanding of the spatial relationship. After grasping the sectional anatomy, surgeons can avoid possible iatrogenic injuries and interpret magnetic resonance images (MRIs) and computed tomography images (CTs) more accurately (De Barros et al., 2001).

As mentioned above, the best material for learning this anatomy is sectioned cadaveric high-resolution images. Influenced by the Visible Human project (Ackerman, 1998), the Visible Korean project was launched to produce sectioned images of the whole male cadaver using 24 bits color and a voxel size of 0.2 × 0.2 × 0.2 mm (Park et al., 2005). On the sectioned images, 937 anatomical structures were manually segmented. The sectioned images and segmented images were put into a browsing software, which shows sectional anatomy in the horizontal plane (Shin et al., 2011). The sectioned images and segmented images were also made into volume models, which show sectional anatomy in the sagittal, coronal, and oblique planes (Chung and Park, 2019). The segmented images are made into surface models, which are helpful for learning stereoscopic anatomy (Shin et al., 2012). The segmented images thus enable the identification of various anatomical structures in great detail (Fig. 11.1).

The purpose of this chapter is to elucidate the sectional anatomy for the lateral transpsoas approach to the lumbar spine using the images and models produced by the Visible Korean project. Both the bony and soft tissue anatomy of the retroperitoneum will be observed. To fully experience this project, it is recommended that the reader experience interactive virtual anatomy with the images and models that can be downloaded from anatomy.co.kr for free.

ANATOMY

The following figures show sectional anatomy of the lumbar region in horizontal, sagittal, coronal, and oblique planes. The horizontal plane was achieved first by serial sectioning, whereas the sagittal, coronal, and oblique planes were produced from the volume model. Simple head shapes are drawn for orientation of the various planes. The positions of the images are indicated using yellow lines for the different planes (Figs. 11.2–11.5). So as to learn sectional anatomy efficiently, proper planes should be selected for each structures. For instance, to observe the proximal portion of the iliohypogastric and ilioinguinal nerves, which run laterally, the sagittal plane is appropriate (Fig. 11.3C). On the other hand, to observe the distal portion of the nerves that run anteriorly, the coronal plane is more appropriate (Fig. 11.4C). The horizontal, sagittal, and coronal planes are adequate for grasping the spatial relationship between the anatomical structures, whereas the oblique plane is most similar to the actual view seen at surgery i.e., lateral transpsoas approach.

For the lateral transpsoas approach, the first step is to determine the entry point in the anterolateral abdominal wall usually between the 12th rib and iliac crest. The three muscle layers (external oblique, internal oblique, and transversus abdominis) can be distinguished in the horizontal and coronal planes. The distal part of the iliohypogastric and ilioinguinal nerves can be

Surgical anatomy of the lateral transpsoas approach to the lumbar spine. https://doi.org/10.1016/B978-0-323-67376-1.00011-2

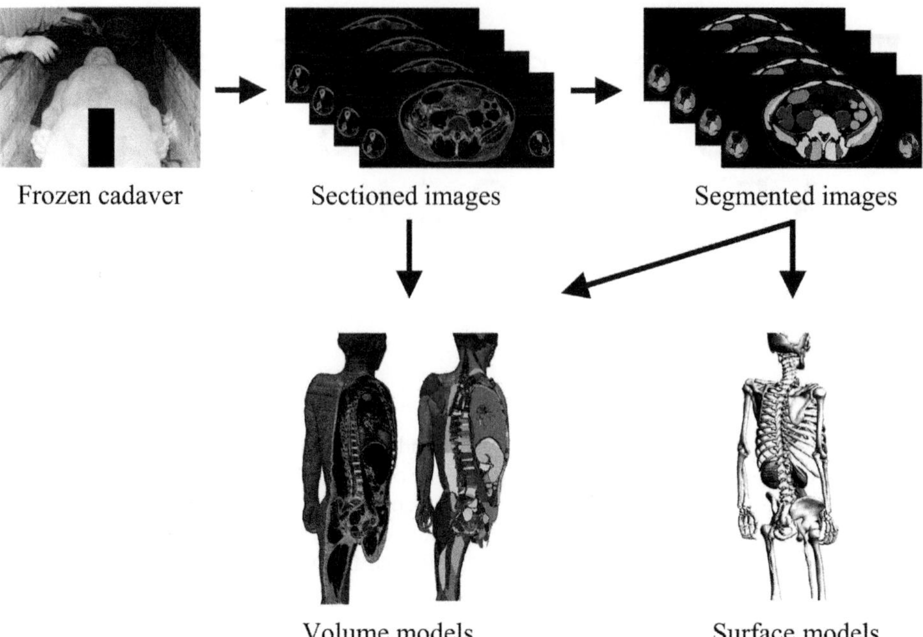

FIG. 11.1 Production process from frozen cadaver to two-dimensional and three-dimensional images for showing sectional anatomy.

identified within the anterolateral abdominal wall (Figs. 11.2 and 11.4).

For the overall course through the retroperitoneal space, Fig. 11.2D can be referenced. After passing through the abdominal wall muscles, the extraperitoneal fat will be encountered. Regarding the layers, external to the fat is the transversalis fascia, whereas internal to the fat is the parietal peritoneum. One should proceed posterior to the ascending colon without piercing the parietal peritoneum. For confirming the insertion of instruments into the retroperitoneal space, the surgeon's finger can be inserted to dissect within the correct plane (Ozgur et al., 2006).

After locating the most distinct structures of the retroperitoneal space, the kidney, and the quadratus lumborum, one should proceed between the two. The proximal parts of the iliohypogastric and ilioinguinal nerves should be avoided (Fig. 11.3C) (Uribe et al., 2010; Dakwar et al., 2011). One should identify the boundary between the quadratus lumborum and the psoas major, which can be considered as the posterior border of the psoas major. At the posteromedial border of the psoas major, small structures such as the iliolumbar artery and ventral ramus of the fifth lumbar nerve are found (Fig. 11.2F). The kidney should be retracted to locate the anterior border of the psoas major. During the procedure, one should appreciate the nearby ureter (Fig. 11.2E).

As the next step, the surgeon will penetrate the psoas major that contains nerves including the ventral rami of lumbar nerves at its posterior portion; among them, the ventral rami of the third, fourth, and fifth lumbar nerves innervate the muscle. The muscle's superficial part is attached to the 12th thoracic vertebra (Fig. 11.4B). The ventral rami of lumbar nerves are covered by this superficial part. Additionally, at the level of the fifth lumbar vertebra, the psoas major contains tendinous tissue at its posteromedial side (Fig. 11.2E and F) (Santaguida and McGill, 1995).

For the procedure, the origin of the psoas major should be appreciated as well as its attachment to the vertebral bodies and intervertebral discs (Fig. 11.4A). Neighboring structures such as the diaphragm and inferior vena cava should be recognized (Fig. 11.3E and F). The intervertebral discs are in contact with the anterior and posterior longitudinal ligaments, and the relationship between the ventral rami of the lumbar nerves and the intervertebral discs must be appreciated (Fig. 11.2) (Papanastassiou et al., 2011). By comparing the sectioned images and surface models at anatomy.co.kr, a better stereoscopic understanding can be had (Fig. 11.6).

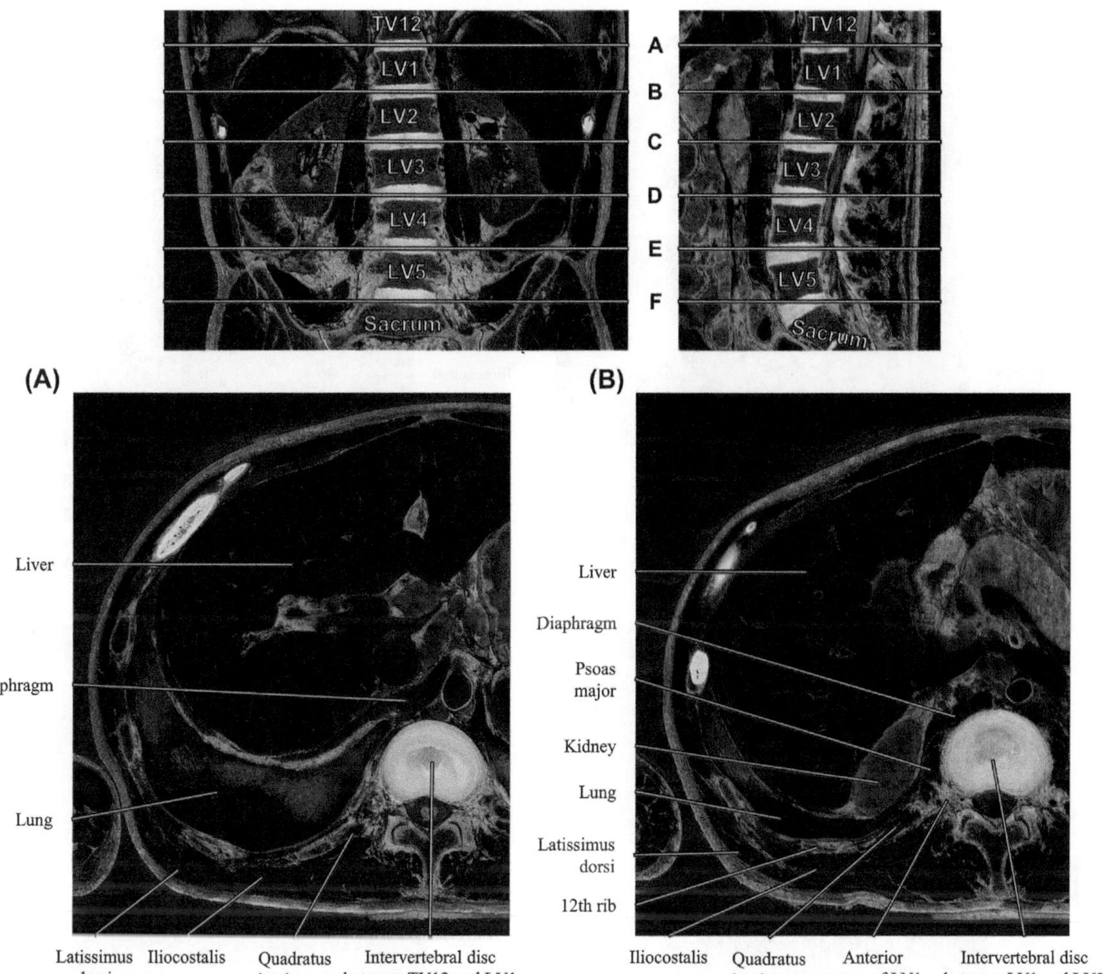

FIG. 11.2 Horizontally sectioned cadaveric images of the lumbar region. LV, lumbar vertebra; LN, lumbar nerve.

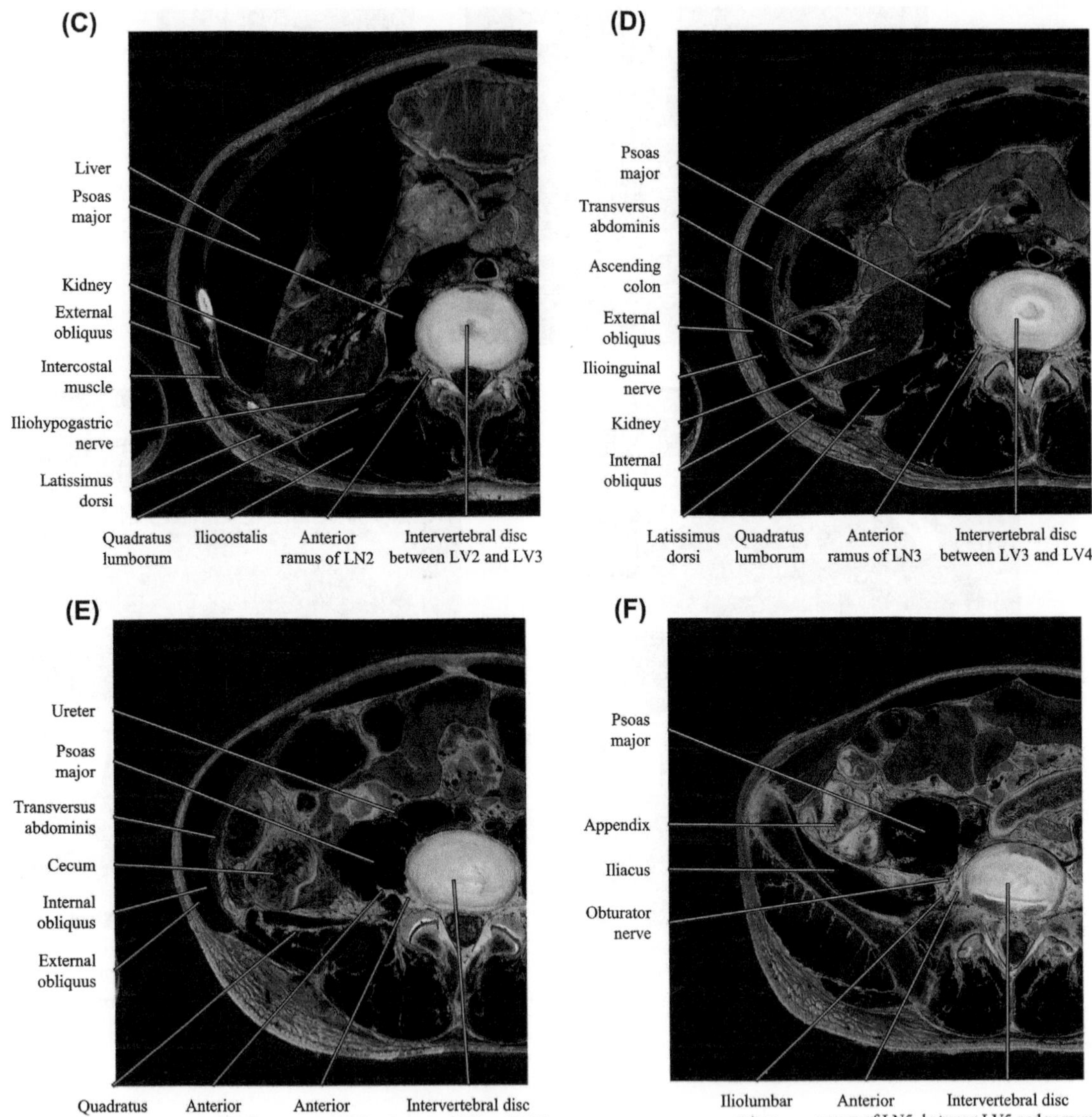
(C)
Liver
Psoas major
Kidney
External obliquus
Intercostal muscle
Iliohypogastric nerve
Latissimus dorsi
Quadratus lumborum
Iliocostalis
Anterior ramus of LN2
Intervertebral disc between LV2 and LV3
(D)
Psoas major
Transversus abdominis
Ascending colon
External obliquus
Ilioinguinal nerve
Kidney
Internal obliquus
Latissimus dorsi
Quadratus lumborum
Anterior ramus of LN3
Intervertebral disc between LV3 and LV4
(E)
Ureter
Psoas major
Transversus abdominis
Cecum
Internal obliquus
External obliquus
Quadratus lumborum
Anterior ramus of LN3
Anterior ramus of LN4
Intervertebral disc between LV4 and LV5
(F)
Psoas major
Appendix
Iliacus
Obturator nerve
Iliolumbar artery
Anterior ramus of LN5
Intervertebral disc between LV5 and sacrum

FIG. 11.2 cont'd.

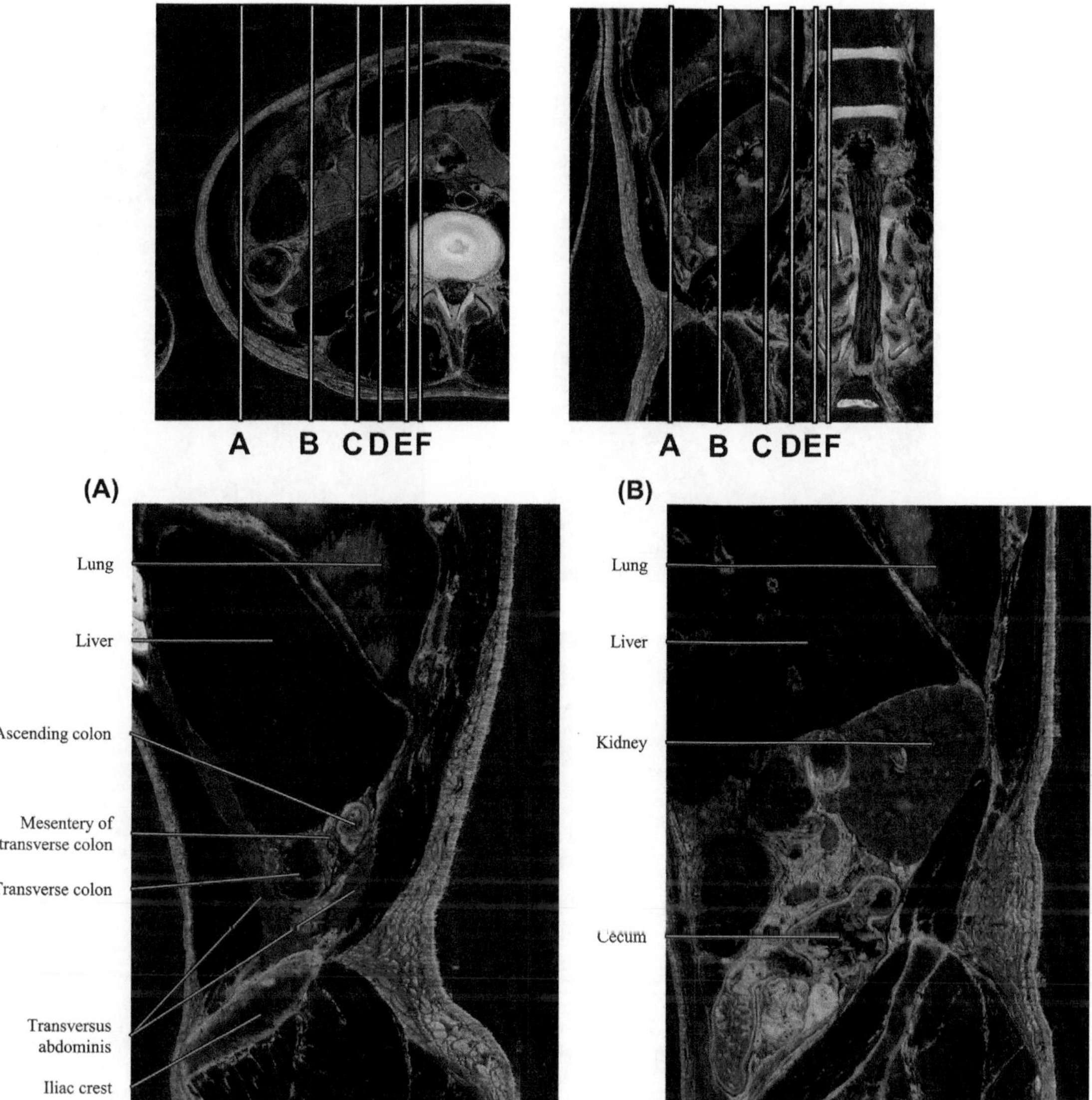

FIG. 11.3 Sagittal sectioned cadaveric images of the lumbar region.

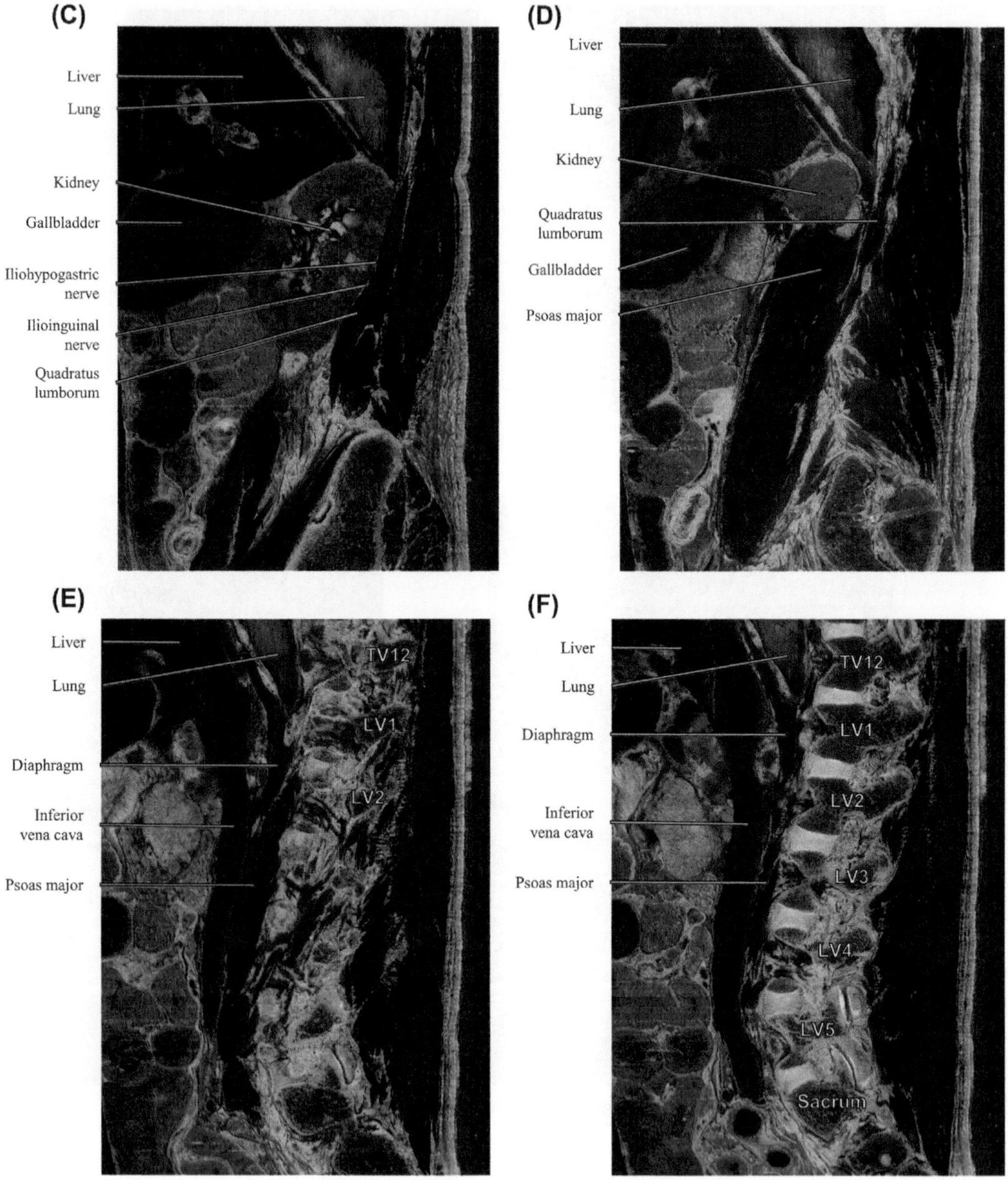

(C)

Liver
Lung
Kidney
Gallbladder
Iliohypogastric nerve
Ilioinguinal nerve
Quadratus lumborum

(D)

Liver
Lung
Kidney
Quadratus lumborum
Gallbladder
Psoas major

(E)

Liver
Lung
Diaphragm
Inferior vena cava
Psoas major
TV12
LV1
LV2

(F)

Liver
Lung
Diaphragm
Inferior vena cava
Psoas major
TV12
LV1
LV2
LV3
LV4
LV5
Sacrum

FIG. 11.3 cont'd.

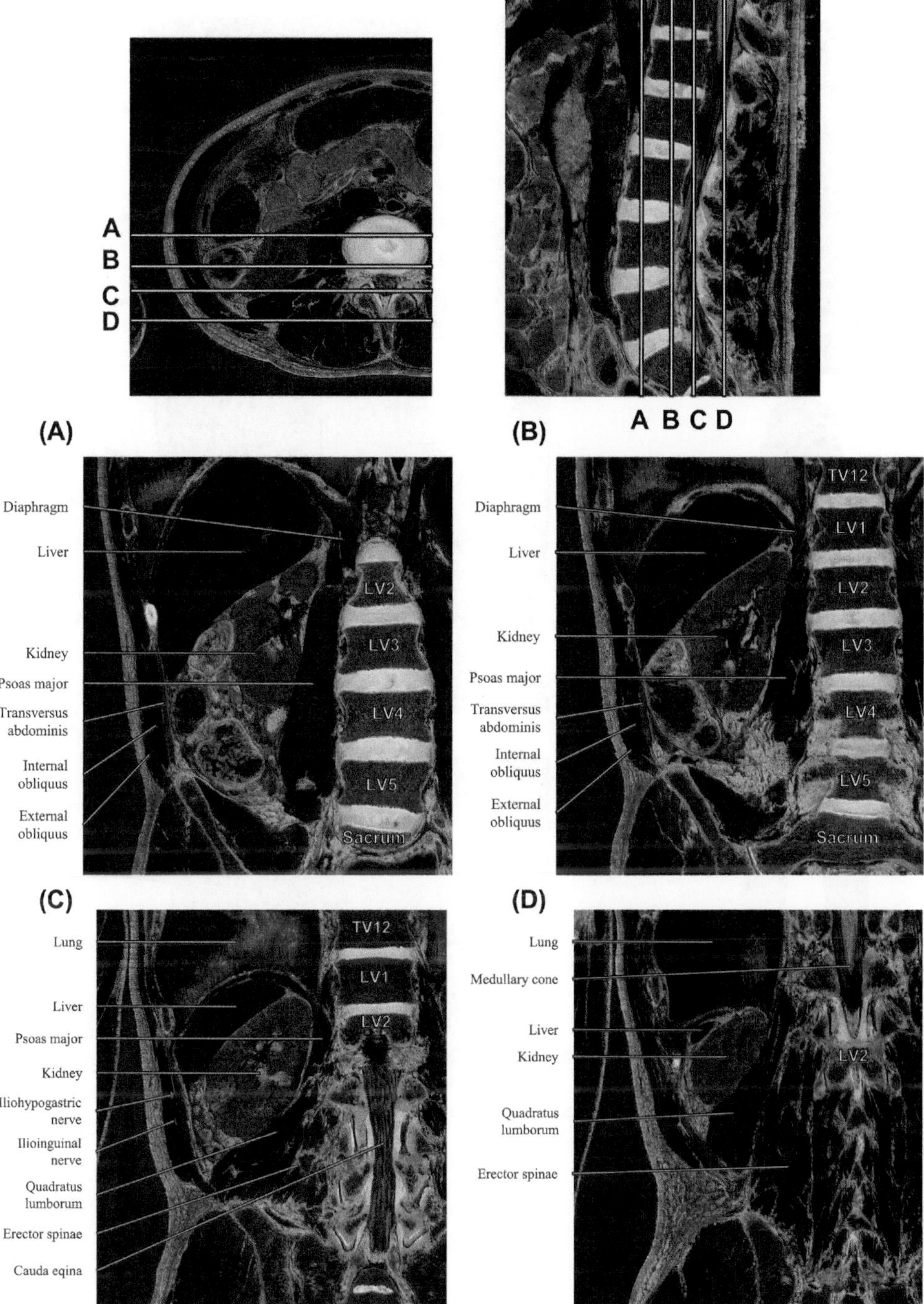

FIG. 11.4 Coronal sectioned cadaveric images of the lumbar region.

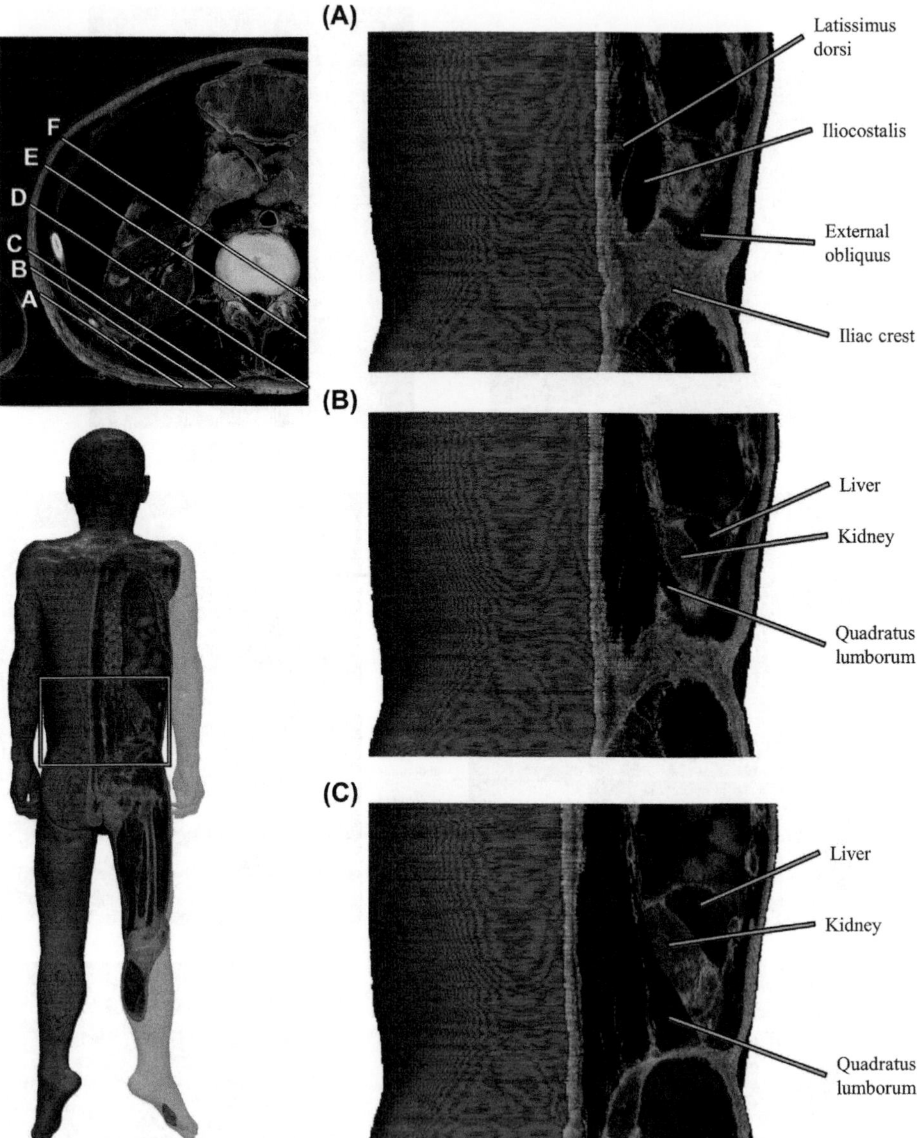

FIG. 11.5 Obliquely sectioned cadaveric images of the lumbar region.

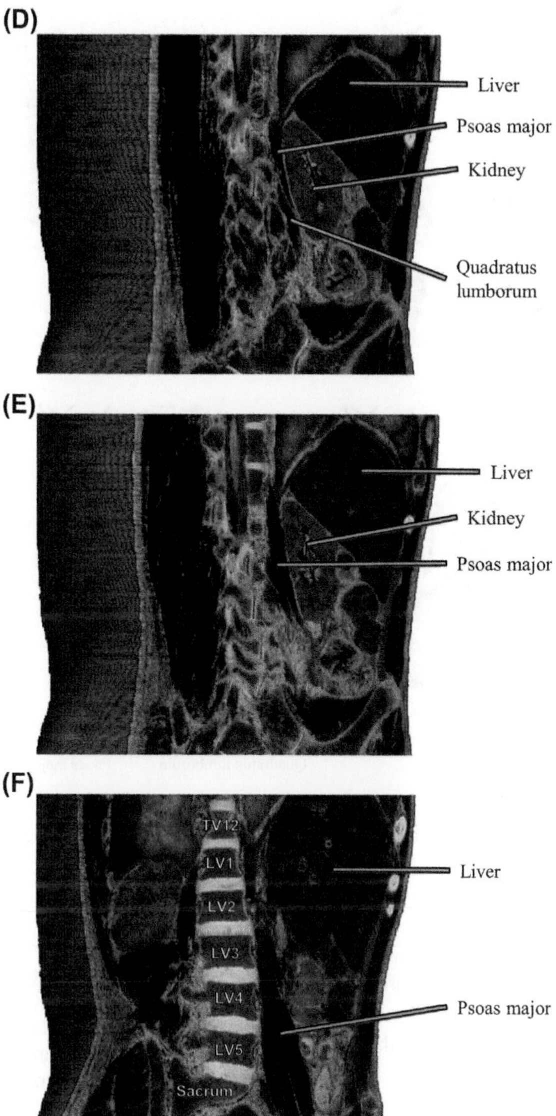
(D)
Liver
Psoas major
Kidney
Quadratus lumborum
(E)
Liver
Kidney
Psoas major
(F)
TV12
LV1
LV2
LV3
LV4
LV5
Sacrum
Liver
Psoas major

FIG. 11.5 cont'd.

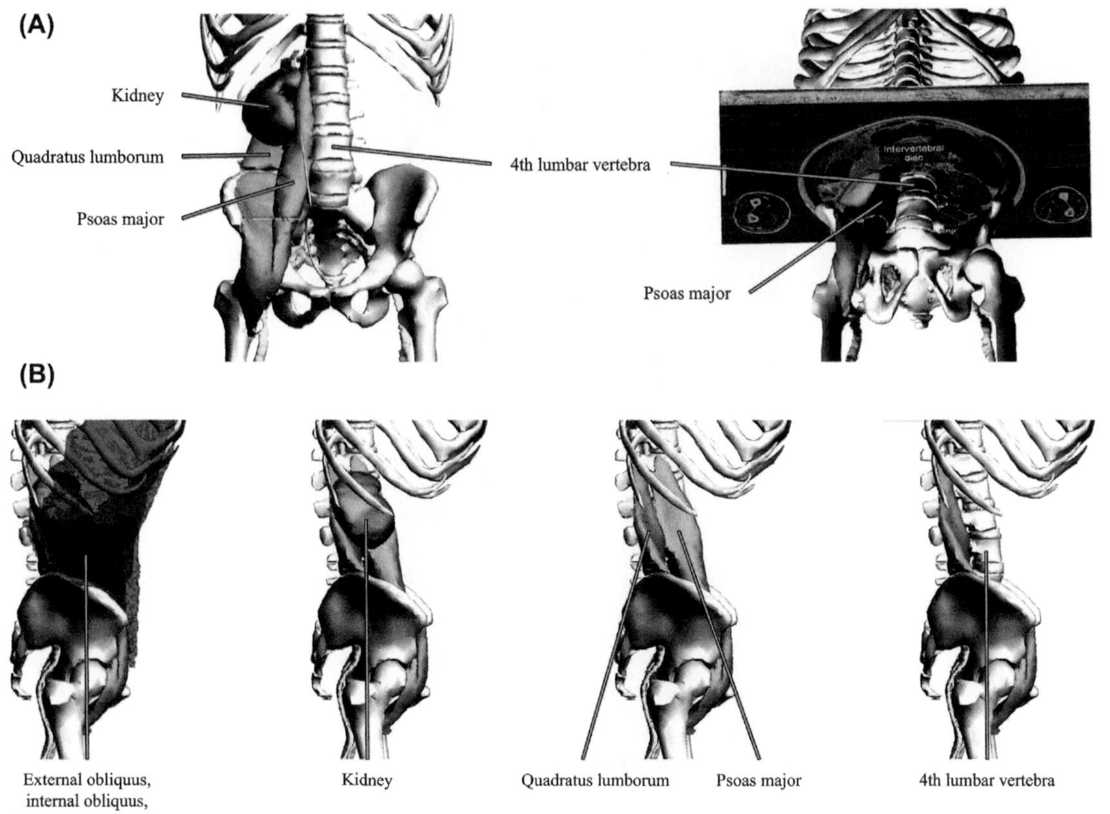

FIG. 11.6 Surface models showing the lumbar region. Surface models are overlapped with original sectioned images (right upper).

CONCLUSIONS

As a detailed understanding of the retroperitoneal anatomy is a prerequisite for the spine surgeon performing lateral transpsoas approaches, the images provided in this chapter will be useful in demonstrating this complex anatomy.

REFERENCES

Ackerman, M.J., 1998. The visible human project. Proc. IEEE 86 (3), 504–511.

Banagan, K., Gelb, D., Poelstra, K., Ludwig, S., 2011. Anatomic mapping of lumbar nerve roots during a direct lateral transpsoas approach to the spine: a cadaveric study. Spine 36 (11), E687–E691.

Chung, B.S., Park, J.S., 2019. Real-color volume models made from real-color sectioned images of visible Korean. J. Korean Med. Sci. 34 (10), e86.

Dakwar, E., Vale, F.L., Uribe, J.S., 2011. Trajectory of the main sensory and motor branches of the lumbar plexus outside the psoas muscle related to the lateral retroperitoneal transpsoas approach. J. Neurosurg. 14 (2), 290–295.

De Barros, N., Rodrigues, C.J., Rodrigues Jr., A.J., De Negri Germano, M.A., Cerri, G.G., 2001. The value of teaching sectional anatomy to improve CT scan interpretation. Clin. Anat. 14 (1), 36–41.

Ozgur, B.M., Aryan, H.E., Pimenta, L., Taylor, W.R., 2006. Extreme lateral interbody fusion (XLIF): a novel surgical technique for anterior lumbar interbody fusion. Spine J. 6 (4), 435–443.

Papanastassiou, I.D., Eleraky, M., Vrionis, F.D., 2011. Contralateral femoral nerve compression: an unrecognized complication after extreme lateral interbody fusion (XLIF). J. Clin. Neurosci. 18 (1), 149–151.

Park, J.S., Chung, M.S., Hwang, S.B., Lee, Y.S., Har, D.H., Park, H.S., 2005. Visible Korean human: improved serially sectioned images of the entire body. IEEE Trans. Med. Imaging 24 (3), 352–360.

Santaguida, P.L., McGill, S.M., 1995. The psoas major muscle: a three-dimensional geometric study. J. Biomech. 28 (3), 339–345.

Shin, D.S., Chung, M.S., Park, H.S., Park, J.S., Hwang, S.B., 2011. Browsing software of the Visible Korean data used for teaching sectional anatomy. Anat. Sci. Educ. 4 (6), 327–332.

Shin, D.S., Chung, M.S., Park, J.S., Park, H.S., Lee, S., Moon, Y.L., Jang, H.G., 2012. Portable document format file showing the surface models of cadaver whole body. J. Korean Med. Sci. 27 (8), 849–856.

Uribe, J.S., Arredondo, N., Dakwar, E., Vale, F.L., 2010. Defining the safe working zones using the minimally invasive lateral retroperitoneal transpsoas approach: an anatomical study. J. Neurosurg. 13 (2), 260–266.

CHAPTER 12

The Sympathetic Trunk in the Abdomen

JOE IWANAGA • R. SHANE TUBBS

INTRODUCTION

Prior to the advent of the lateral approach to the spine, the anterior and posterior approaches were the mainstays of spine surgery (Basho and Chen, 2011; Knight et al., 2009). These techniques entailed many undesirable complications and became less favored when the minimally invasive lateral approach to the spine was introduced. The aim of this new procedure was to avoid the complications that arose from the anterior approach, such as injury to abdominal organs, and from the posterior approach, such as nerve root injury (Sofianos et al., 2012; Graham et al., 2014). The lateral approach is also advantageous in allowing for smaller incisions, less blood loss, and shorter operations (Graham et al., 2014). However, it has its own distinctive risks and possible complications. In this chapter, we review the lumbar sympathetic trunk and its potential complications following lateral approaches to spine.

SPINE APPROACHES AND THE SYMPATHETIC TRUNK

The main advantage of the lateral over the anterior approach is that it avoids exposing the abdominal viscera, the great vessels, and the sympathetic trunk (Pawar et al., 2015). The open anterior approach requires a larger incision, which can cause more injury to the abdominal wall, significant postoperative pain, morbidity, and ileus (Pawar et al., 2015; Brody et al., 2002). It also places the abdominal organs, vascular structures, and sympathetic trunk (Fig. 12.1) at risk (Sofianos et al., 2012; Graham et al., 2014), as it often requires these anatomical structures to be maneuvered to gain access to the lumbar spine. The lateral approach is advantageous because it uses a smaller incision, causing less abdominal wall injury. This leads to decreased operative times, shorter hospital stays, decreased postoperative pain, and a more rapid return to activities of daily living (Graham et al., 2014; Pawar et al., 2015; Guérin et al., 2012; Ozgur et al., 2006). These advantages have increased its popularity among both surgeons and patients (Ozgur et al., 2006). However, the smaller incision used in the lateral approach reduces the visual window, which can result in injuries to important structures if they are not observed and avoided (Guérin et al., 2012; Regev and Kim, 2014).

The location of the lumbar plexus and the sympathetic trunk (Figs. 12.1–12.6) are important factors to consider in lateral lumbar spine surgery. Ensuring that these structures are clearly visualized during surgical procedures can help to reduce postoperative complications. Bengalis et al. suggest that the lumbosacral plexus moves ventrally as you proceed caudally from the L1 to the L5 disc level and is at greatest risk during the lateral approach to the L4–L5 level.

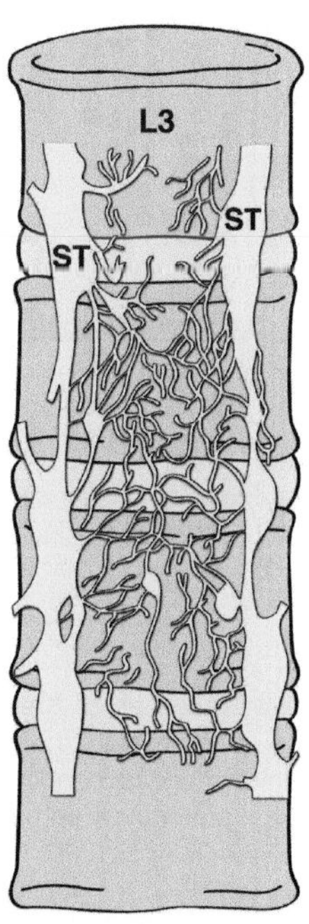

FIG. 12.1 Schematic drawing of the sympathetic trunk (ST) in the lumbar region. Note the intercommunicating fibers between left and right sides.

Surgical anatomy of the lateral transpsoas approach to the lumbar spine. https://doi.org/10.1016/B978-0-323-67376-1.00012-4

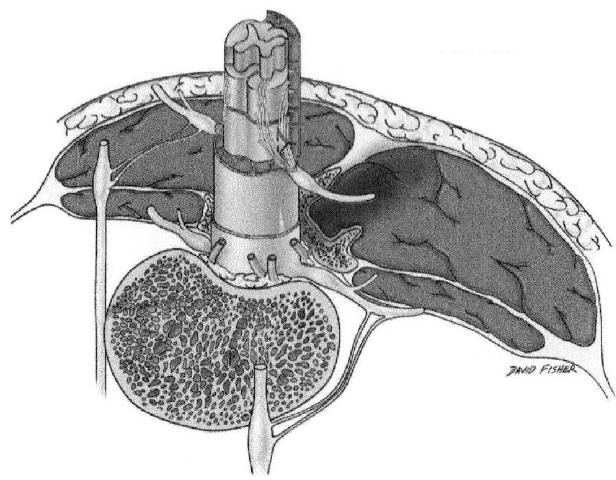

FIG. 12.2 Schematic view of the relationship of the sympathetic trunks in the lumbar region and communication to the upper lumbar spinal nerves (L1 and L2) via gray and white rami communicantes.

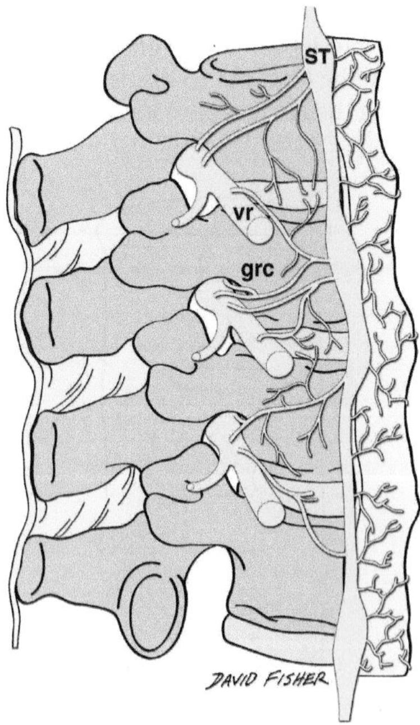

FIG. 12.3 Schematic drawings of the sympathetic trunk (ST) from a lateral perspective. Note the ventral ramus (vr) of the lumbar spinal nerve and its connection to the sympathetic trunk via a gray ramus communicans (grc).

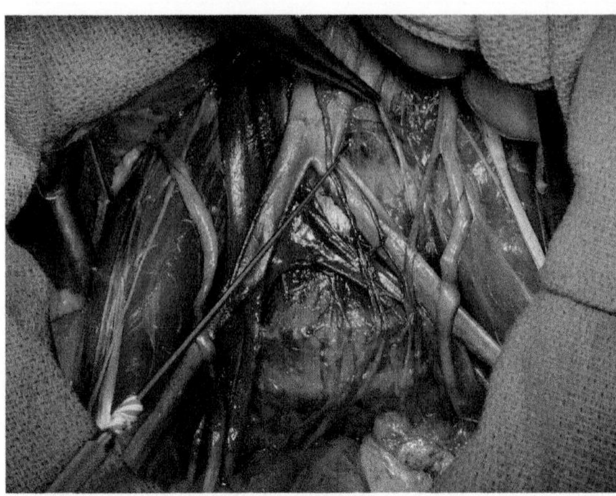

FIG. 12.4 Cadaveric dissection of the left sympathetic trunk shown here held with forceps. Note the relationship between this structure and the psoas major muscle.

Gu et al. studied the location of the lumbar plexus and sympathetic trunk as they relate to the superior border of the transverse process, and proposed a safe zone for performing discectomies, located between the lumbar plexus and sympathetic trunk, running along the anterior one-third of the vertebral bodies underneath the psoas muscle (Gu et al., 2001). One of the main risks of the lateral approach during psoas dissection is injury to the lumbar nerves exiting the neural foramen and running through the psoas to form the lumbosacral plexus (Knight et al., 2009; Sofianos et al., 2012; Graham et al., 2014; Guérin et al., 2012). Injury to the plexus, either directly during surgery or indirectly through compression during psoas muscle dilation, has been identified as the cause of postoperative motor and sensory deficits (Graham et al., 2014; Cummock et al., 2011). These deficits range from weakness in hip flexor and knee extensor muscles to paresthesias and dysesthesias (Knight et al., 2009; Sofianos et al., 2012; Graham et al., 2014; Cummock et al., 2011; Aichmar et al., 2013; Anand et al., 2010; Murray et al., 2015; Nunley et al., 2016). In most cases, the motor and sensory deficits are not permanent, and patients have reported improvements during follow-up (Knight et al., 2009; Sofianos et al., 2012; Graham et al., 2014; Cummock et al., 2011; Aichmar et al., 2013; Anand et al., 2010; Murray et al., 2015).

The anterior approach places the sympathetic nerves at increased risk (Sofianos et al., 2012; Graham et al., 2014; Pawar et al., 2015; Ozgur et al., 2006; Lieberman et al., 2000). It has been determined that disturbance of the superior hypogastric plexus during the anterior approach can lead to transient retrograde ejaculation (Ozgur et al., 2006; Lieberman et al., 2000). Lieberman et al. proposed the use of blunt techniques during dissection to mobilize autonomic structures and minimize injury. In the same study, transient peripheral

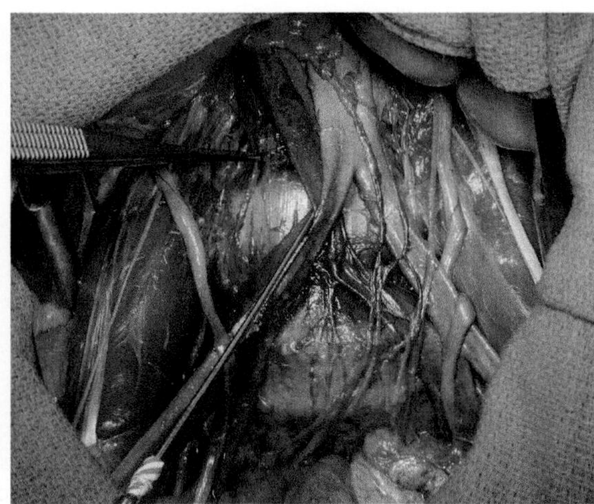

FIG. 12.5 Cadaveric dissection of the right sympathetic trunk shown here held with forceps. Note the inferior vena cava is retracted to the left.

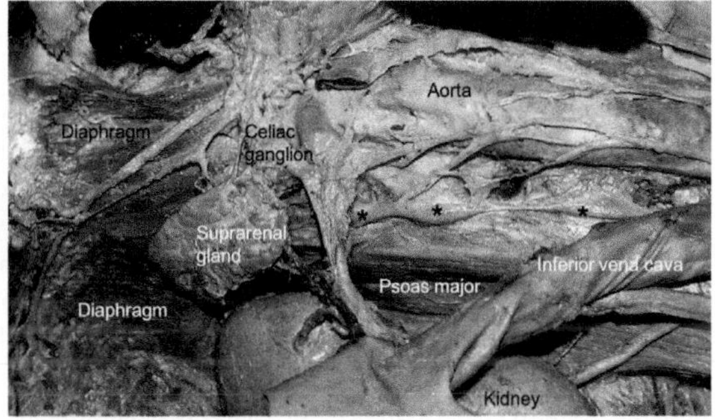

FIG. 12.6 Right lateral view of the sympathetic trunk and its ganglia (asterisks). Note the inferior vena cava has been transected and is retracted.

sympathetic vasomotor denervation occurred, which led to "warm leg." The authors attributed these sympathetic symptoms to neuropraxia rather than nerve division (Lieberman et al., 2000). In the study by Murray et al., there was one case of retrograde ejaculation, which was attributed to injury to the sympathetic plexus during the dissection of structures anterior to the anterior longitudinal ligament. In that case, the patient had completed three dissections and was the only patient in the study in whom the lateral access led to sympathetic injury. In general, the lateral approach is seen as safe, avoiding sympathetic nerve injury (Graham et al., 2014; Pawar et al., 2015; Brody et al., 2002; Ozgur et al., 2006). Brody et al. determined that the lateral laparoscopic exposure allows safe access to the disc space and avoids important structures such as the sympathetic trunk, ureter, and major blood vessels.

Lumbar sympathetic dysfunction (SD) is described as an increase in skin temperature, reduced perspiration, discoloration, dysesthesia, and swelling of the lower limb ipsilateral to the surgery. The incidence of sympathetic dysfunctions following anterior and lateral lumbosacral surgery varies. In a retrospective review by Hrabalek et al. of 431 patients who underwent ALIF at L5/S1, ALIF at T12–L5, and a lateral transpsoas approach at T12–L5, they found SD in 0.5%, 15%, and 4%, respectively. With respect to the lateral approach patients with SD, three of the patients had a lateral transpsoas approach at L4/5 and one at L5/6 (Hrabalek et al., 2015). The authors reported that the SD reduced the quality of life of two of the patients.

In a literature review by Regan et al. of 182 patients that had undergone anterior lumbar spine surgery, 16 patients (8.8%) reported experiencing a "warm leg." A warm leg is likely the ipsilateral side being warmer due to a lack of sympathetic vasoconstriction (Schulte et al., 2010). Rajaraman et al. and Kang et al. found rates of 6% and 10% for sympathetic dysfunction presenting as temperature variation, dysesthesias, discoloration, and swelling (Kang et al., 2009).

An oblique approach, anterior to the iliac crest and psoas major, has recently been introduced as a way to avoid potentially vital neural and visceral structures. In a review of 21 patients who underwent this approach, Gragnaniello and Seex (2016) reported one patient (5%) who had sympathetic dysfunction related to the mobilization of the sympathetic trunk.

In an anatomical study by Murata et al. looking at the number and location of lumbar sympathetic ganglia, they found that the L2/3 and L3/4 disc levels were the most common disc spaces with ganglia. Moreover, the zones having a greater than average number of ganglia were the L2 vertebral body, the L2–L3 disc space, and the L5 vertebral body.

In the posterior approach, the main concerns are extensive dissection and resection of the musculature, leading to ischemia and denervation, postoperative radiculitis, and incidental durotomies (Sofianos et al., 2012; Graham et al., 2014; Lieberman et al., 2000; Basho and Chen, 2011). The lateral approach avoids these complications but places the lumbar plexus and potentially the sympathetic trunk at greater risk (Graham et al., 2014; Guérin et al., 2012).

CONCLUSION

The lateral approach is seen as a safe and efficacious method for accessing the lateral spine (Brody et al., 2002). It eliminates the need for a general surgeon to establish access, there is minimal disturbance of the peritoneum and its contents, it avoids the sympathetic plexus and major vascular structures, and it significantly reduces surgical time (Graham et al., 2014; Pawar et al., 2015; Brody et al., 2002; Ozgur et al., 2006). These risks can be reduced with surgical experience, adequate visualization of the surgical field, and the use of neuromonitoring during surgery (Knight et al., 2009; Graham et al., 2014; Guérin et al., 2012; Ozgur et al., 2006; Aichmar et al., 2013). In neuromonitoring, an evoked electromyographic response is used to determine the proximity of the dilator to the lumbar plexus (Ozgur et al., 2006), but it provides no information about the proximity of the sympathetic trunk. Therefore, the anatomical position of the sympathetic trunk should be appreciated during surgery to avoid injury.

REFERENCES

Aichmar, A., Lykissas, M.G., Girardi, F.P., Sama, A.A., Lebl, D.R., Taher, F., Cammisa, F., Hughes, A.P., 2013. An institutional six-year trend analysis of the neurological outcome after lateral lumbar interbody fusion: a 6-year trend analysis of a single institution. Spine 38 (23), E1483–E1490. https://doi.org/10.1097/BRS.0b013e3182a3d1b4.

Anand, N., Rosemann, R., Khalsa, B., Baron, E.M., 2010. Mid-term to long-term clinical and functional outcomes of minimally invasive correction and fusion for adults with scoliosis. Neurosurg. Focus 28 (3), E6. https://doi.org/10.3171/2010.1.FOCUS09278.

Basho, R., Chen, J.H., 2011. Lateral interbody fusion: indications and techniques. Oper. Tech. Orthop. 21 (3), 204–207. https://doi.org/10.1053/j.oto.2011.06.005. ISSN 1048-6666.

Brody, F., Rosen, M., Tarnoff, M., Lieberman, I., 2002. Laparoscopic lateral L4-L5 disc exposure. Surg. Endosc. 16 (4) https://doi.org/10.1007/s00464-001-8195-6. Epub 2001 Dec 10.

Cummock, M.D., Vanni, S., Levi, A.D., Yu, Y., Wang, M.Y., 2011. An analysis of postoperative thigh symptoms after minimally invasive transpsoas interbody fusion. J. Neurosurg. Spine 15 (1), 11–18. https://doi.org/10.3171/2011.2.SPINE10374.

Gragnaniello, C., Seex, K., 2016. Anterior to psoas (ATP) fusion of the lumbar spine: evolution of a technique facilitated by changes in equipment. J Spine Surg 2 (4), 256–265. https://doi.org/10.21037/jss.2016.11.02.

Graham, R.B., Wong, A.P., Liu, J.C., 2014. Minimally invasive lateral transpsoas approach to the lumbar spine. Neurosurg. Clin. N. Am. 25 (2), 219–231. https://doi.org/10.1016/j.nec.2013.12.002.

Gu, Y., Ebraheim, N., Xu, R., Rezcallah, A., Yeasting, R., 2001. Anatomic considerations of the posterolateral lumbar disk region. Orthopedics 24, 56–58. https://doi.org/10.3928/0147-7447-20010101-20.

Guérin, P., Obeid, I., Bourghli, A., et al., 2012. The lumbosacral plexus: anatomic considerations for minimally invasive retroperitoneal transpsoas approach. Surg. Radiol. Anat. 34 (2), 151–157. https://doi.org/10.1007/s00276-011-0881-z.

Hrabalek, L., Sternbersky, J., Adamus, M., 2015. Risk of sympathectomy after anterior and lateral lumbar interbody fusion procedures. Biomed. Pap. Med. Fac. Univ. Palacky Olomouc Czech. Repub. 159 (2), 318–326. https://doi.org/10.5507/bp.2013.083.

Kang, B.U., Choi, W.C., Lee, S.H., Jeon, S.H., Park, J.D., Maeng, D.H., Choi, Y.G., 2009. An analysis of general surgery-related complications in a series of 412 minilaparotomic anterior lumbosacral procedures. J. Neurosurg. Spine 10 (1), 60–65. https://doi.org/10.5507/bp.2013.083.

Knight, R.Q., Schwaegler, P., Hanscom, D., Roh, J., 2009. Direct lateral lumbar interbody fusion for degenerative conditions: early complication profile. J. Spinal Disord. Tech. 22 (1), 34–37. https://doi.org/10.1097/BSD.0b013e3181679b8a.

Lieberman, I.H., Willsher, P.C., Litwin, D.E.M., Salo, P.T., Kraetschmer, B.G., 2000. Transperitoneal laparoscopic exposure for lumbar interbody fusion. Spine 25, 509–514. PMID: 10707399.

Murray, G., Beckman, J., Bach, K., Smith, D.A., Dakwar, E., Uribe, J.S., 2015. Complications and neurological deficits following minimally invasive anterior column release for adult spinal deformity: a retrospective study. Eur. Spine J. 24 (Suppl. 3), 397–404. https://doi.org/10.1007/s00586-015-3894-1.

Nunley, P., Sandhu, F., Frank, K., Stone, M., 2016. Neurological complications after lateral transpsoas approach to anterior interbody fusion with a novel flat-blade spine-fixed retractor. BioMed Res. Int. 2016, 8450712. https://doi.org/10.1155/2016/8450712.

Ozgur, B.M., Aryan, H.E., Pimenta, L., Taylor, W.R., 2006. Extreme Lateral Interbody Fusion (XLIF): a novel surgical technique for anterior lumbar interbody fusion. Spine J. 6 (4), 435–443. https://doi.org/10.1016/j.spinee.2005.08.012. ISSN 1529-9430.

Pawar, A., Hughes, A., Girardi, F., Sama, A., Lebl, D., Cammisa, F., 2015. Lateral lumbar interbody fusion. Asian Spine J. 9 (6), 978–983. https://doi.org/10.4184/asj.2015.9.6.978.

Regev, G.J., Kim, C.W., 2014. Safety and the anatomy of the retroperitoneal lateral corridor with respect to the minimally invasive lateral lumbar intervertebral fusion approach. Neurosurg. Clin. N. Am. 25 (2), 211–218. https://doi.org/10.1016/j.nec.2013.12.001. ISSN 1042-3680.

Schulte, T.L., Adolphs, B., Oberdiek, D., Osada, N., Liljenqvist, U., Filler, T.J., Marziniak, M., Bullmann, V., 2010. Approach-related lesions of the sympathetic chain in anterior correction and instrumentation of idiopathic scoliosis. Eur. Spine J. 19 (9), 1558–1568. https://doi.org/10.1007/s00586-010-1455-1.

Sofianos, D.A., Briseño, M.R., Abrams, J., Patel, A.A., 2012. Complications of the lateral transpsoas approach for lumbar interbody arthrodesis: a case series and literature review. Clin. Orthop. Relat. Res. 470 (6), 1621–1632. https://doi.org/10.1007/s11999-011-2088-3.

FURTHER READING

Benglis, D.M., Vanni, S., Levi, A., Benglis, D.M., Vanni, S., Levi, A.D., 2009. An anatomical study of the lumbosacral plexus as related to the minimally invasive transpsoas approach to the lumbar spine. J. Neurosurg. Spine 10 (2), 139–144. https://doi.org/10.3171/2008.10.SPI08479.

CHAPTER 13

The Lumbosacral Trunk and Tunnel

HALLE E.K. BURLEY • FELIPE H. SANDERS • R. SHANE TUBBS

The lumbosacral trunk (Fig. 13.1) consists of the ventral rami of L5 and a portion of L4. Before it merges with the L4 component, the L5 ramus passes through the lumbosacral tunnel, a passageway of bone and ligament at the superolateral margin of the sacral ala that can occasionally be a source of extraforaminal L5 nerve entrapment. These elements of the lumbosacral plexus traverse the surgical field of the lateral approach, and a surgeon must take care to avoid them in order to prevent postoperative radicular complications.

THE LUMBOSACRAL JUNCTION AND THE LATERAL APPROACH

Degenerative spinal disease is the most common major group of illnesses in the aging population and it is increasingly prevalent. Most degenerative spinal disease occurs in the lumbosacral segment, especially at L4-5 and L5-S1. With advances in technology and anatomical knowledge, minimally invasive surgery is becoming mainstream practice for spinal disease. Alternatives to classical posterior approaches, such as the lateral transpsoas approach, have been described and are becoming standard care (Pawar et al., 2015; Silber et al., 2002; Skovrlj et al., 2015; Yuan et al., 2014).

The lateral approach to the lumbar spine is designed to be minimally invasive, through a smaller incision, sparing the paraspinal muscle's aggressive retraction and minimizing blood loss, allowing discectomies and interbody fusion to be performed. The most frequent complications are neural injuries, particularly affecting the lumbar and lumbosacral plexuses. Here we describe the anatomy of the lumbosacral trunk, which connects the lumbar and sacral plexuses.

THE L4 SPINAL NERVE

After exiting the foramen, the L4 ventral ramus trifurcates into an anterior division (forming part of the obturator nerve), a posterior division (forming part of the femoral nerve), and a caudal division (Fig. 13.2), which fuses with the L5 ventral ramus to form the lumbosacral trunk (Fig. 13.2). Damage to the L4 ventral ramus or one of its branches may result in weakness in thigh adduction, leg extension, or foot dorsiflexion; sensory impairment to the anterior thigh and medial leg; or dermatomal pain to the anterior thigh, knee, and medial leg.

A Note About the Furcal Nerve

The furcal nerve is an independent nerve typically arising alongside the L4 nerve from its own spinal rootlets and dorsal root ganglion. Like L4, it sends branches to the femoral nerve, lumbosacral trunk, and obturator nerve, acting as a bridge between the lumbar and sacral plexuses. Its name "furcal" derives from this forked configuration. The femoral nerve receives about 60% of its fibers, the lumbosacral trunk about 30%, and the obturator nerve about 10% (Kikuchi et al., 1986). The furcal nerve may be the source of atypical radiculopathies and should be considered when interpreting the results of diagnostic blockade, steroid injections, or imaging of the lumbar spine.

THE L5 SPINAL NERVE

As it traverses inferiorly along the sacrum, the L5 ventral ramus (Fig. 13.3) travels through the lumbosacral tunnel. The lumbosacral ligament, which forms the wall of the tunnel, attaches medially at the L5 vertebral body and/or transverse process and laterally at the sacral ala. In roughly half of cases, some of its fibers fuse with the neighboring iliolumbar ligament. The lateral superior margin of the sacral ala forms the dorsal wall of the tunnel. In addition to the L5 nerve and its sympathetics, the lumbosacral tunnel contains the iliolumbar artery and vein and a certain amount of fat. In most cases, the gray ramus communicans of the L5 nerve pierces the lumbosacral ligament on its way from the sympathetic trunk (Figs. 13.4 and 13.5) (Protas et al., 2017). After exiting the tunnel, the L5 nerve is joined by the L4 nerve, and together they form the lumbosacral trunk.

Surgical anatomy of the lateral transpsoas approach to the lumbar spine. https://doi.org/10.1016/B978-0-323-67376-1.00013-6

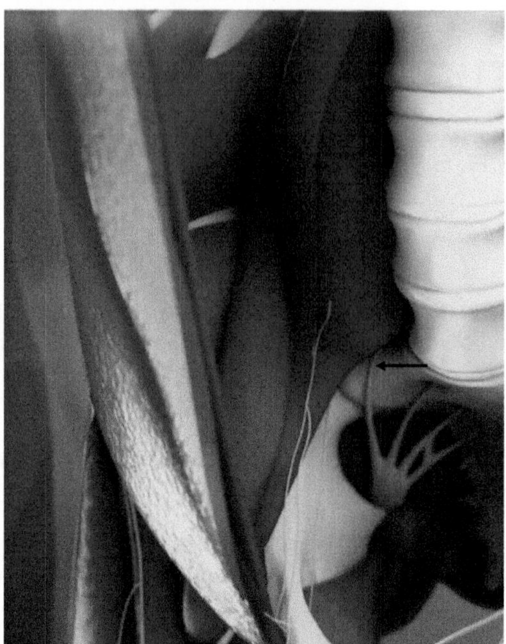

FIG. 13.1 Schematic drawing of the right lumbosacral trunk (black arrow) crossing the ala of the sacrum to join the S1 ventral ramus to form the lumbosacral plexus. Note the position of the lumbosacral trunk which is medial to the psoas major muscle.

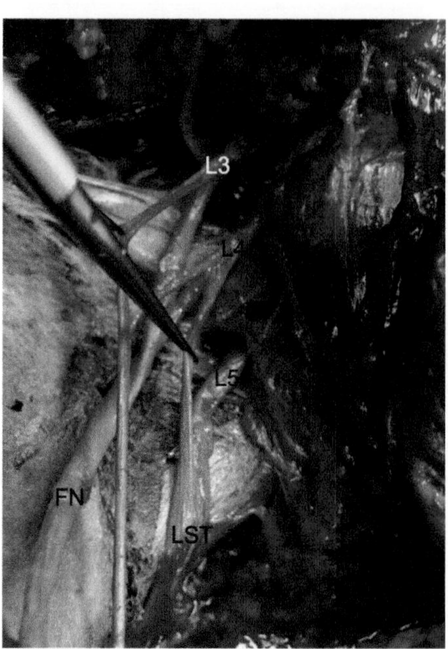

FIG. 13.2 The caudal part of the right L4 ventral ramus (held with forceps) is shown descending to join the L5 ventral ramus thus forming the lumbosacral trunk (LST). Note the femoral nerve (FN) and obturator nerve just medial to it. The ventral rami of L3-L5 are labeled.

Lumbosacral Tunnel Syndrome

Occasionally, narrowing of the lumbosacral tunnel will compress the L5 nerve against the sacrum, causing lumbosacral tunnel syndrome. Patients present with L5 radiculopathy with normal strength and no signs of muscle atrophy. The narrowing is most often caused by variations of width, shape, thickness, or origin of the lumbosacral ligament or by osteophytes of the lateral sacral ala or lateral margin of the L5 or S1 vertebrae. Sacral or pelvic rim fractures, tumors of the sacrum, soft-tissue irritation, or iliolumbar aneurysms have also been known to cause compression within the tunnel (Nathan et al., 1982; Pecina et al., 2001). Lumbosacral tunnel syndrome is most prevalent in the elderly population, but the average age of those affected has not been thoroughly established (Matsumoto et al., 2010).

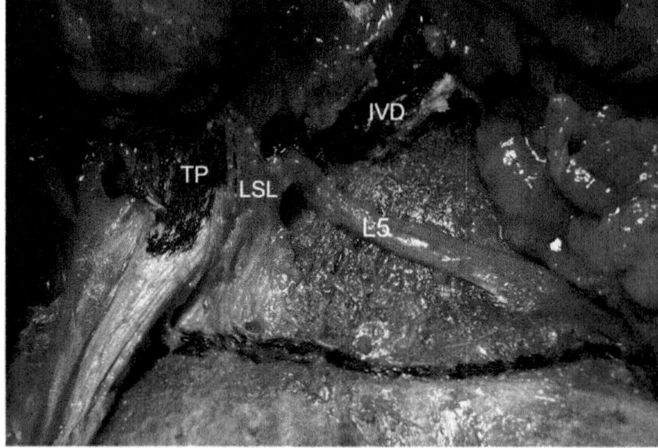

FIG. 13.3 Lateral view of the right L5 ventral ramus exiting posteromedial to the lumbosacral ligament (LSL) and lateral to the L5 disc (IVD and colored purple). The iliolumbar ligament is seen extending off the transverse process (TP and colored purple). The purple curvilinear line is the sacroiliac joint. Also, note that the L4 contribution to the L5 ventral ramus has been removed for clarity so that the distal L5 ventral ramus is actually the lumbosacral trunk.

THE LUMBOSACRAL TRUNK

The lumbosacral trunk (Fig. 13.6 A–C), comprised of a portion of the L4 ramus and all of the L5 ventral ramus, passes caudally over the sacral ala, crossing the sacroiliac joint about 2 cm below the pelvic brim. For the

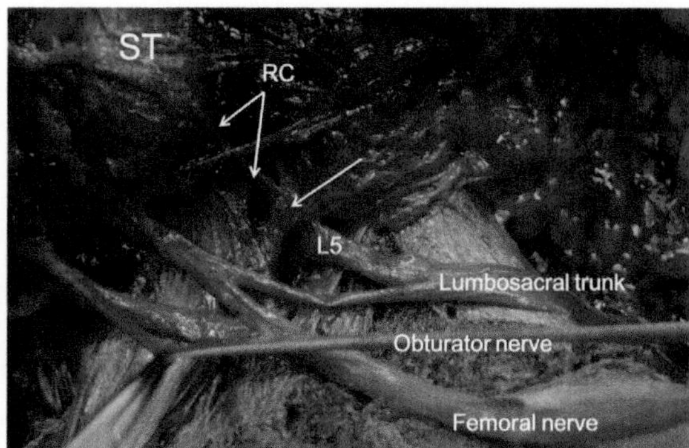

FIG. 13.4 Right lateral view of the lumbosacral ligament (arrow) with the ventral ramus of L5 exiting deep to it. A sympathetic ramus communicans (RC) is seen connecting the sympathetic trunk (ST) to the L5 ventral ramus by piercing the lumbosacral tunnel.

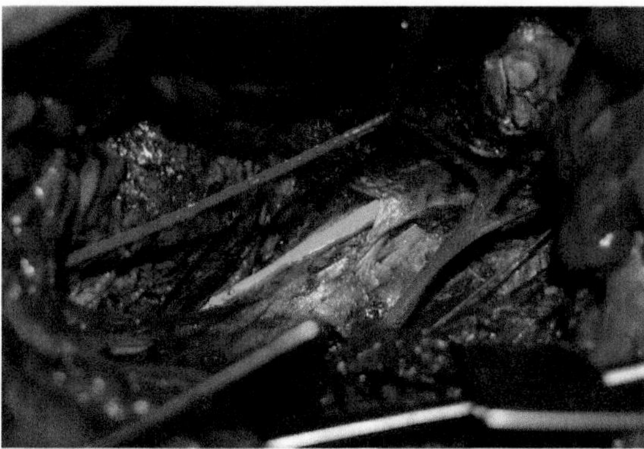

FIG. 13.5 Left lumbosacral junction. The L4 ventral ramus is seen here giving rise to the obturator nerve (orange) and femoral nerve (purple). The L5 ventral ramus (green) is seen exiting the lumbosacral tunnel.

(A) (B)

(C)

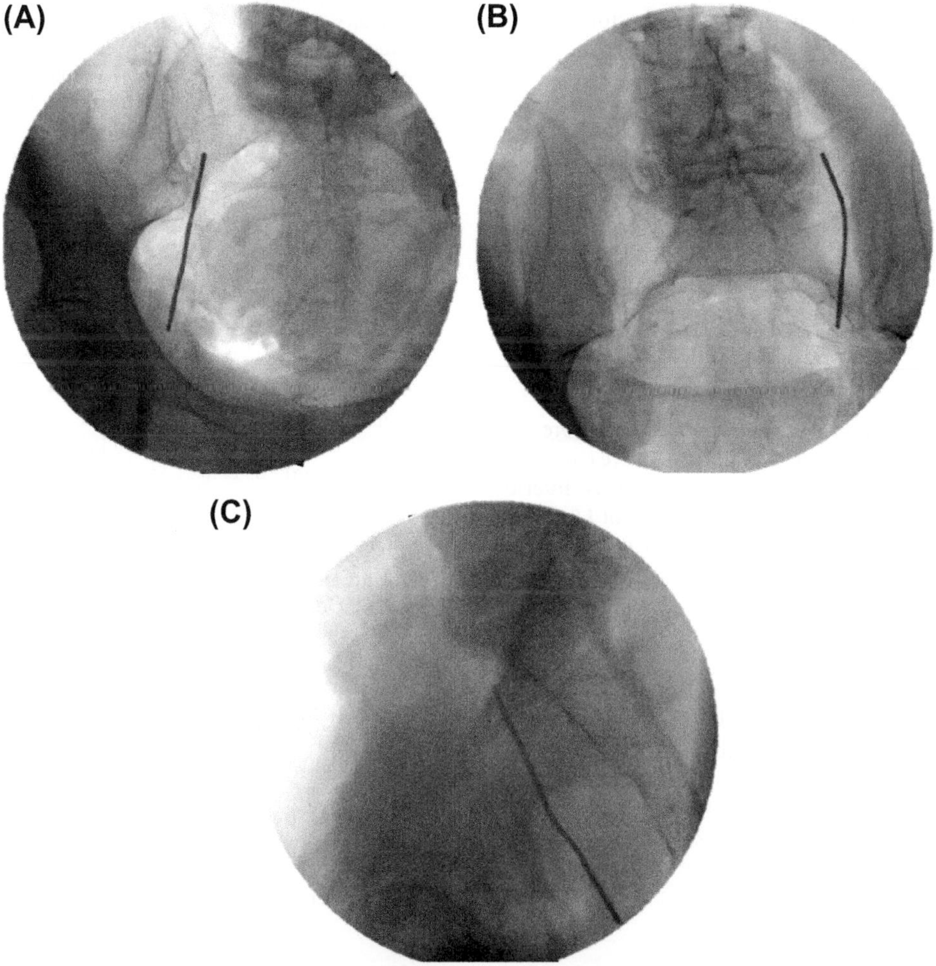

FIG. 13.6 Fluoroscopy of the right (A) and left (B) lumbosacral trunks with overlaid wire and lateral view of the right lumbosacral trunk, also with overlaid wire (C). Note that the trunk is variable in its proximal to distal formation depending on when L4 (furcal nerve) joins the L5 ventral ramus.

most part, the lumbosacral trunk is anchored to the sacral ala by fibrous connective tissue. It eventually joins the sacral plexus, forming the lumbosacral plexus. Most of the motor and sensory innervation to the peroneal division of the sciatic nerve is provided by the lumbosacral trunk.

Injury to the lumbosacral trunk manifests as foot drop (of the same clinical spectrum as a peroneal nerve palsy) along with more proximal weakness such as the posterior tibialis muscle innervated by the tibial nerve, and the gluteal muscles innervated by the superior and inferior gluteal nerves. Although the clinical presentation is similar, lumbosacral trunk injury can be differentiated from L5 nerve root radiculopathy through electrical testing and examining the paraspinal muscles for wasting, which occurs in L5 radiculopathy but not lumbosacral trunk injury. Prior diagnosis of lumbosacral trunk injury occurs mainly in obstetric patients, the newborn's head pressing against and injuring neural structures against the hip, or after hip fractures or hip surgeries.

Relation to the Psoas Major and Spinal Column

The lumbar plexus (drawing nerve fibers from T12-L4) courses within or posterior to the psoas, anterior to the transverse processes of the vertebrae, and posterior to the vertebral body center. As it extends caudally it also migrates ventrally, so that at the L4-5 level the nerve trunk is closer to the center of the disc space than more superior levels. The L5 nerve emerges medial to the psoas, immediately lateral to the posterior portion of the L5-S1 disc. On lateral fluoroscopy, the greatest concentration of nerves (and therefore the greatest risk of nerve injury and postoperative complications) is from the posteroinferior aspect of L4, inferior along the posterior one-third of the body of L5, to the level of the sacral promontory (Tubbs et al., 2017). The surgeon should take special care to avoid trauma to this area.

Plexus variants usually occur alongside variations of the vertebral column or psoas morphology. A teardrop-shaped psoas major, which is significantly thicker in the sagittal plane than the coronal plane, is associated with anterior migration of the lumbar plexus as well as posterolateral migration of the iliac vasculature. Psoas morphology can be assessed for preoperative planning on MRI (Louis et al., 2017). Sacralized lumbar vertebrae or lumbarized sacral vertebrae have also been associated with locational plexus variants.

Variants of nerve root contributions to the lumbar and lumbosacral plexuses are also well documented in the literature. In the prefixed, high form of the plexus, the lumbosacral trunk may draw fibers from the L3 level. Should the patient possess this particular variant, it would be reasonable to find L3-pattern deficits after lumbosacral trunk injury.

In some cases, the lumbosacral trunk may present as two ununited parallel trunks. It has also been found more superiorly than typical, medial to the psoas.

REFERENCES

Kikuchi, S., Hasue, M., Nishiyama, K., Ito, T., 1986. Anatomic features of the furcal nerve and its clinical significance. Spine 11, 1002–1007.

Louis, P.K., Narain, A.S., Hijji, F.Y., Yacob, A., Yom, K.H., Phillips, F.M., Singh, K., 2017. Radiographic analysis of psoas morphology and its association with neurovascular structures at L4-5 with reference to lateral approaches. Spine 42, E1386–E1392.

Matsumoto, M., Watanabe, K., Ishii, K., Tsuji, T., Takaishi, H., Nakamura, M., Toyama, Y., Chiba, K., 2010. Posterior decompression surgery for extraforaminal entrapment of the fifth lumbar spinal nerve at the lumbosacral junction. J. Neurosurg. Spine 12, 72–81.

Nathan, H., Weizenbluth, M., Halperin, N., 1982. The lumbosacral ligament (LSL), with special emphasis on the "lumbosacral tunnel" and the entrapment of the 5th lumbar nerve. Int. Orthop. 6, 197–202.

Pawar, A., Hughes, A., Girardi, F., Sama, A., Lebl, D., Cammisa, F., 2015. Lateral lumbar interbody fusion. Asian Spine J. 9, 978–983.

Pecina, M.M., Krmpotic-Nemanic, J., Markiewitz, A.D., 2001. Tunnel Syndromes: Peripheral Nerve Compression Syndromes, third ed. CRC Press, Boca Raton, pp. 199–200.

Protas, M., Edwards, B., Loukas, M., Oskouian, R.J., Tubbs, R.S., 2017. The lumbosacral tunnel: cadaveric study and review of the literature. Spine Scholar 1, 99–102.

Silber, J.S., Anderson, D.G., Hayes, V.M., Vaccaro, A.R., 2002. Advances in surgical management of lumbar degenerative disease. Orthopedics 25, 767–771 quiz 72-3.

Skovrlj, B., Gilligan, J., Cutler, H.S., Qureshi, S.A., 2015. Minimally invasive procedures on the lumbar spine. World J. Clin. Cases 3, 1–9.

Tubbs, R.I., Gabel, B., Jeyamohan, S., Moisi, M., Chapman, J.R., Hanscom, R.D., Loukas, M., Oskouian, R.J., Tubbs, R.S., 2017. Relationship of the lumbar plexus branches to the lumbar spine: anatomical study with application to lateral approaches. Spine J. 17, 1012–1016.

Yuan, P.S., Rowshan, K., Verma, R.B., Miller, L.E., Block, J.E., 2014. Minimally invasive lateral lumbar interbody fusion with direct psoas visualization. J. Orthop. Surg. Res. 9, 20.

FURTHER READING

Ahmadian, A., Deukmedjian, A.R., Abel, N., Dakwar, E., Uribe, J.S., 2013. Analysis of lumbar plexopathies and nerve injury after lateral retroperitoneal transpsoas approach: diagnostic standardization. J. Neurosurg. Spine 18, 289–297.

Bartynski, W.S., Kang, M.D., Rothfus, W.E., 2010. Adjacent double–nerve root contributions in unilateral lumbar radiculopathy. Am. J. Neuroradiol. 31, 327–333.

Bina, R.W., Zoccali, C., Skoch, J., Baaj, A.A., 2015. Surgical anatomy of the minimally invasive lateral lumbar approach. J. Clin. Neurosci. 22, 456–459.

Brailsford, J.F., 1929. Deformities of the lumbosacral region of the spine. Br. J. Surg. 16, 562–627.

Briggs, C.A., Chandraraj, S., 1995. Variations in the lumbosacral ligament and associated changes in the lumbosacral region resulting in compression of the fifth dorsal root ganglion and spinal nerve. Clin. Anat. 8, 339–346.

Ebraheim, N.A., Lu, J., Biyani, A., Huntoon, M., Yeasting, R.A., 1997. The relationship of lumbosacral plexus to the sacrum and the sacroiliac joint. Am J Orthop 26, 105–110.

Hashavardhana, N.S., Dabke, H.V., 2014. The furcal nerve revisited. Orthop. Rev. 6, 5428.

Houten, J.K., Alexandre, L.C., Nasser, R., Wollowick, A.L., 2011. Nerve injury during the transpsoas approach for lumbar fusion. J. Neurosurg. Spine 15, 280–284.

Jones 2nd, T.L., Hisey, M.S., 2012. L5 radiculopathy caused by L5 nerve root entrapment by an L5-S1 anterior osteophyte. Internet J. Spine Surg. 6, 174–177.

Katirji, B., 2007. Electromyography in Clinical Practice, a Case Study Approach. Mosby Elsevier, Philadelphia, pp. 81–97.

Mandelli, C., Colombo, E.V., Sicuri, G.M., Mortini, P., 2016. Lumbar plexus nervous distortion in XLIF® approach: an anatomic study. Eur. Spine J. 25, 4155–4163.

Matsumoto, M., Chiba, K., Nojiri, K., Ishikawa, M., Toyama, Y., Nishikawa, Y., 2002. Extraforaminal entrapment of the fifth lumbar spinal nerve by osteophytes of the lumbosacral spine: anatomic study and a report of four cases. Spine 27, 169–173.

Matsumoto, M., Chiba, K., Ishii, K., Watanabe, K., Nakamura, M., Toyama, Y., 2006. Microendoscopic partial resection of the sacral ala to relieve extraforaminal entrapment of the L-5 spinal nerve at the lumbosacral tunnel. J. Neurosurg. Spine 4, 342–346.

Mitchell, G.A.G., 1936. The lumbosacral Junction. J. Bone Jt. Surg. 16, 233–254.

Nathan, H., 1968. Compression of the sympathetic trunk by osteophytes of the vertebral column in the abdomen: an anatomical study with pathological and clinical consideration. Surgery 63, 609–625.

Olsewski, J.M., Simmons, E.H., Kallen, F.C., Mendel, F.C., 1991. Evidence from cadavers suggestive of entrapment of fifth lumbar spinal nerves by lumbosacral ligaments. Spine 16, 336–347.

Transfeldt, E.E., Robertson, D., Bradford, D.S., 1993. Ligaments of the lumbosacral spine and their role in possible extraforaminal spinal nerve entrapment and tethering. J. Spinal Disord. 6, 507–512.

Tubbs, R.S., Shoja, M.M., Loukas, M., 2016. Bergman's Comprehensive Encyclopedia of Human Anatomic Variation. John Wiley & Sons, Inc., Hoboken, pp. 1113–1127.

CHAPTER 14

Lateral Transpsoas Approaches to the Lumbar Spine and the Kidney, Ureter, and Colon

JOE IWANAGA • R. SHANE TUBBS

INTRODUCTION

The minimally invasive retroperitoneal approach to the lumbar spine was first described by Mayer in 1997 (Mayer, 1997; McAfee et al., 1998) followed by McAfee et al. (1998) and Pimenta, (2001) and (Ozgur et al. (2006), who first reported the extreme lateral lumbar interbody fusion procedure. This approach is a minimal invasive technique for lumbar fusion and approaches the lateral lumbar spine via the corridor between the 12th rib and highest point of the iliac crest to enter the retroperitoneal space and, through the psoas major muscle, reach the lumbar spine. This approach allows direct access to the intervertebral disc space with no disruption of the peritoneal space or posterior paraspinal musculature (Rodgers et al., 2010; Caputo et al., 2012; Malham et al., 2012; Patel et al., 2012; Formica et al., 2017).

According to (Kwon and Kim(2016), disadvantages of the lateral transpsoas approach to the lumbar spine include the learning curve associated with new surgical procedures and orientation of regional retroperitoneal anatomy, which is often unfamiliar to spine surgeons. Complications caused by this approach include neurologic deficits, injuries to abdominal organs, the ureters, or blood vessels (Uribe and Deukmedjian, 2015).

Kidneys

The kidneys are located lateral to the psoas major muscle with a superior border located at the level of the 12th thoracic vertebra and an inferior border at the level of the third to fourth lumbar vertebrae in the retroperitoneal space, making them vulnerable to injury during the lateral transpsoas approach (Figs. 14.1–14.3). This is especially true if there are anatomical variants or pathology involving the kidneys or if the operator is unfamiliar with the three-dimensional anatomy of the retroperitoneum.

In an anatomical study, we found that the closest distance from the wires for the disc space of L1/2, L2/3, and L3/4 to the kidney ranged from 13.2 to 32.9 mm (mean 21.1 mm), from 20.0 to 27.7 mm (mean 24.5 mm), and from 20.5 to 46.6 mm (mean 34.7 mm), respectively. The distance from the kidney to the disc space at L4/5 was not applicable because the distance was greater than 50 mm.

The surgical techniques and clinical outcomes of the extreme lateral transpsoas approach to the lumbar spine have been well documented (Caputo et al., 2012; Malham et al., 2012; Formica et al., 2017; Kwon and Kim, 2016). However, anatomical studies regarding this approach are scant (Alkadhim et al., 2015; Benglis et al., 2009; Hartl et al., 2016; Karsy et al., 2017; Voin et al., 2017). Most of these have focused on neurologic injury (Alkadhim et al., 2015; Benglis et al., 2009; Hartl et al., 2016; Karsy et al., 2017; Voin et al., 2017). To our knowledge, only three cases of iatrogenic renal injury during the extreme lateral transpsoas approach to the lumbar spine have been reported. Blizzard et al. (2016) reported a renal artery injury during the T12–L1 fixation, which was successfully identified and treated intraoperatively. Although the details were not included, Isaacs et al. (2010) reported injury of the kidney with a lateral transpsoas approach. Yuan et al. (2014) reported injury to the renal vein as a complication of the extreme lateral approach to the lumbar spine. In the present study, the closest distance to the kidney ranged from 13.2 to 46.6 mm, and for left and right sides, the kidney was nearest the operative field at the L1/2 level.

As the position of the kidneys is variable, preoperative imaging to localize their position might decrease

Surgical anatomy of the lateral transpsoas approach to the lumbar spine. https://doi.org/10.1016/B978-0-323-67376-1.00014-8

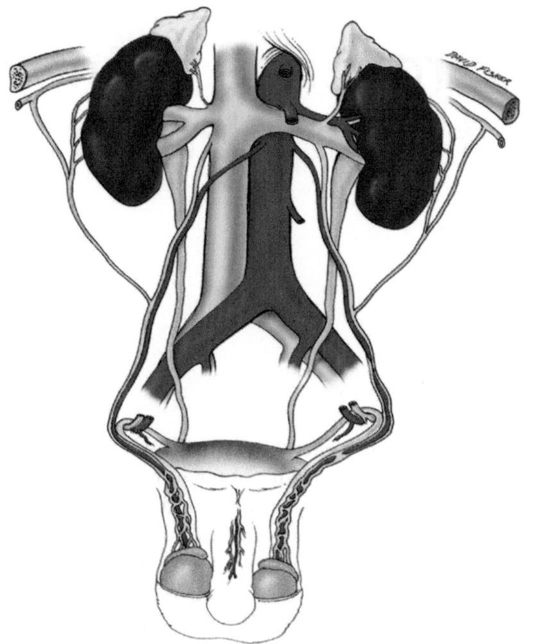

FIG. 14.1 Schematic drawing of the kidneys and surrounding anatomy. Note the relationships between the kidneys, renal vasculature, great vessels, and suprarenal glands. Also note the potential for drainage of the renal capsule into the subcostal veins.

the risks of iatrogenic injury during lateral approaches to the lumbar spine. Normally, the right kidney lies between the first and third lumbar vertebrae, and the left kidney is slightly lower than the right. Each kidney is approximately 11 cm in length, 6 cm in width, and 3 cm in its anteroposterior dimension. The left kidney is often slightly longer than the right kidney (Standring, 2015). However, the kidney is one of the most frequent organs to have variations in shape and position. Variants of the kidney such as a horseshoe kidney (Fig. 14.3), malrotation of the kidney, or an ectopic kidney often have aberrant renal arteries (Iwanaga et al., 2015, 2016; Boyan et al., 2007). Such variant renal vasculature might result in a greater risk of kidney injury with lateral spine approach. According to Satyapal et al. (2001), approximately 28% of kidneys have accessory renal arteries. Moreover, the course of additional arteries is unpredictable, as they can enter the renal hilum from either posteriorly or superiorly or enter directly into the renal parenchyma. Lastly, a retroaortic left renal vein is detected in approximately 2%–4% of the population (Davis and Lundberg, 1968; Karaman et al., 2007; Arslan et al., 2005) and brings the renal vein closer to the vertebral column and thus closer into the field of an extreme lateral approach to the lumbar spine.

Ureters

The ureters are 25–30 cm long and located anteriorly to the quadratus lumborum muscle and laterally to the psoas major muscle in the retroperitoneal space, making them vulnerable to injury during the transpsoas approach (Figs. 14.4–14.6). This is especially true if the surgeon is unfamiliar with retroperitoneal anatomy, or if there are anatomical variants or pathology involving the ureters. Several cases of injury of the ureter following transpsoas approaches have been reported.

In our earlier study (Voin et al., 2017), on lateral fluoroscopy, in the lumbar region, there was generally a posterior to anterior course of the left and right ureter with the right ureters being slightly shorter in length. From the direct lateral position and on all sides, the ureter was found to lie at or posterior to the anterior edge

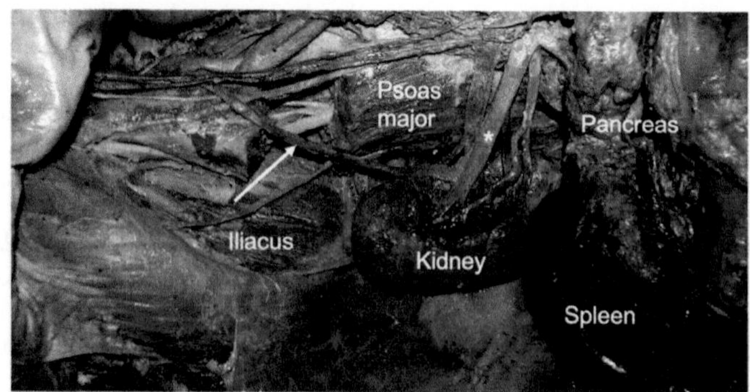

FIG. 14.2 Left kidney and its relationship to surrounding anatomy. Note the position lateral and slightly posterior to the psoas major. The ureter (arrow) is noted at the arrow. A piece of psoas major has been removed to show the close proximity to the lumbar plexus. An asterisk marks the renal vein, and the renal artery is seen to its right in this view.

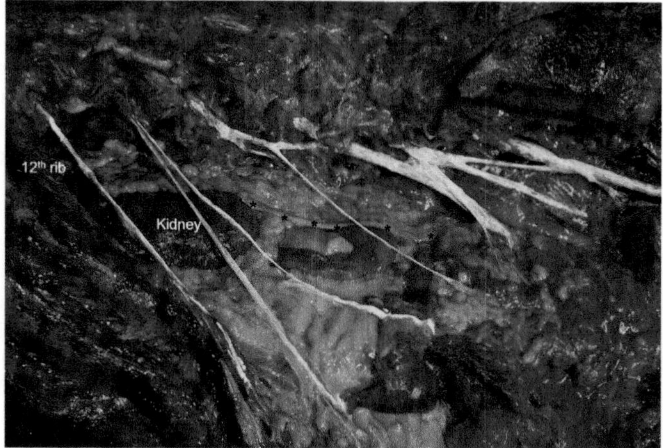

FIG. 14.3 Posterior view noting the close proximity of the left kidney and lumbar plexus. The ureter is marked with asterisks.

of the lumbar vertebral bodies, more so proximally. On two sides (12.5%), the right ureter was at or less than 1 cm anterior to the anterior border of the L2/L3 vertebrae. On 14 sides (87.5%), the ureter was on average 2.5 cm (range 2.0–3.2 cm) posterior to the anterior border of the vertebral bodies at L2, 3 cm posterior at L3, and 1.0 cm posterior at L4 and on the margin of the anterior vertebral bodies at L5. With the descent of the ureter, especially at L4 and L5, the ureter gradually moved anteriorly, i.e., closer to the anterior aspect of the vertebral body. In general, on all sides but two, the ureter, from a lateral perspective, crossed the posterior third of the upper lumbar vertebrae, approached the middle third at L3, and reached the anterior third at L4/L5 before descending into the pelvis. Roughly one half of the ureters made an acute directional change from the upper one half of the lumbar spine to the lower one half, whereas in the other one half, this transition was more gradual.

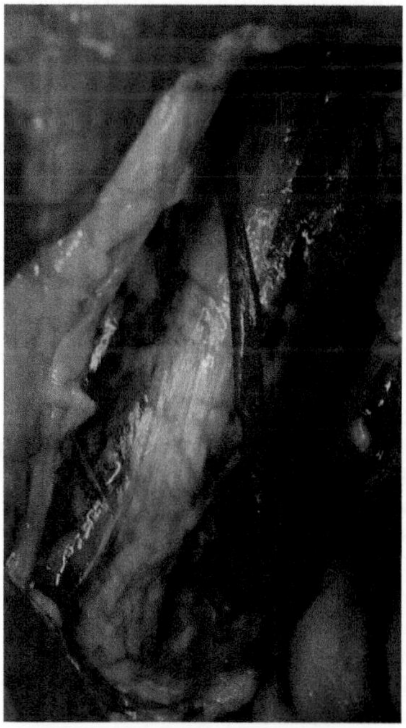

FIG. 14.4 Anterior view of the right ureter to the underlying psoas minor (white tendon) and psoas major.

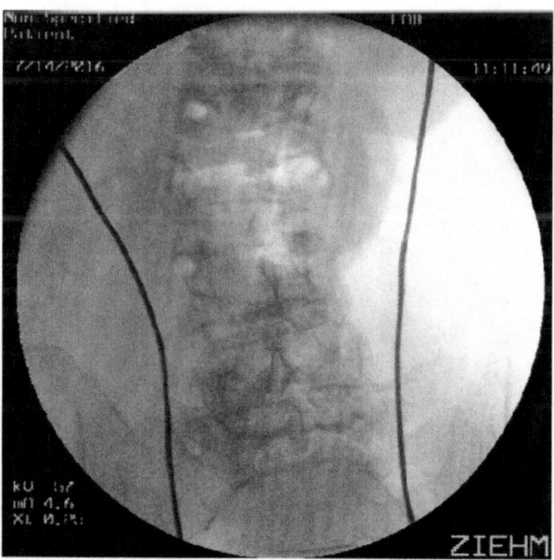

FIG. 14.5 Fluoroscopy of the left and right ureters with inserted wires and their relationship to the lumbar spine.

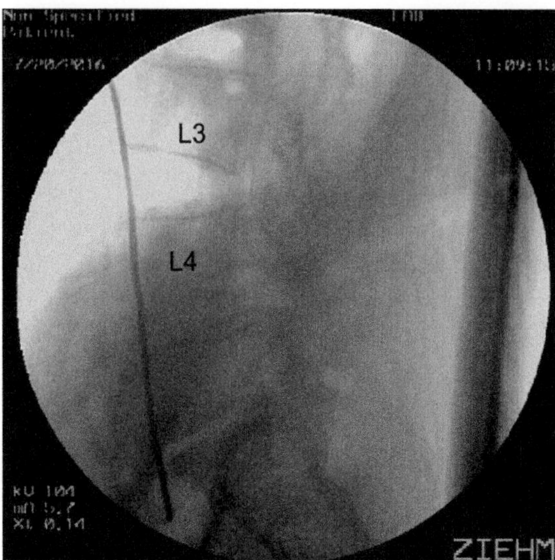

FIG. 14.6 Lateral fluoroscopy of the left ureter following lateral transpsoas discectomy at L3/L4.

Colon

To our knowledge, only a handful of cases of bowel injuries after lateral interbody fusion have been reported (Fig. 14.7). To prevent injury of peritoneal and retroperitoneal components, complete access to the retroperitoneal space is necessary. The muscle fibers have to be carefully spread, and dilators and retractors have to be placed through the space of the lateral border of the psoas major muscle. Careful removal of the retractor and ensuring that there are no obvious injuries to the bowel are crucial.

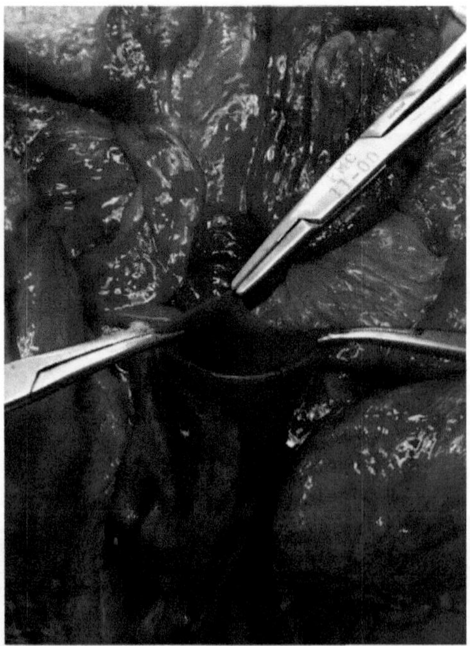

FIG. 14.7 Injury to the descending colon following lateral transpsoas approach to the lumbar spine in a cadaveric specimen by a senior spine surgeon.

In an earlier anatomical study, in the direct lateral position, we found the mean distance from the intervertebral disc space to the posterior edge of the ascending and descending colon was 23.2 mm (6.0–41.0 mm) at the L2/L3 level, 29.5 mm (14.0–45.0 mm) at the L3/L4 level and, 40.3 mm (20.0–60.0 mm) at the L4/L5 level. The L1/L2 level was above the colon on both sides.

CONCLUSIONS

Although uncommon, injury to the kidney, ureter, and colon can occur during lateral transpsoas approaches to the lumbar spine. Therefore, a good working knowledge of their anatomy in relation to this approach is very important for the spine surgeon.

REFERENCES

Alkadhim, M., Zoccali, C., Abbasifard, S., et al., 2015. The surgical vascular anatomy of the minimally invasive lateral lumbar interbody approach: a cadaveric and radiographic analysis. Eur. Spine J. 24 (Suppl. 7), 906–911.

Arslan, H., Etlik, Ö., Ceylan, K., et al., 2005. Incidence of retro-aortic left renal vein and its relationship with varicocele. Eur. Radiol. 15, 1717–1720.

Benglis, D.M., Vanni, S., Levi, A.D., 2009. An anatomical study of the lumbosacral plexus as related to the minimally invasive transpsoas approach to the lumbar spine. J. Neurosurg. Spine 10, 139–144.

Blizzard, D.J., Gallizzi, M.A., Isaacs, R.E., Brown, C.R., 2016. Renal artery injury during lateral transpsoas interbody fusion: case report. J. Neurosurg. Spine 25, 464–466.

Boyan, N., Kubat, H., Uzum, A., 2007. Crossed renal ectopia with fusion: report of two patients. Clin. Anat. 20, 699–702.

Caputo, A.M., Michael, K.W., Chapman Jr., T.M., et al., 2012. Clinical outcomes of extreme lateral interbody fusion in the treatment of adult degenerative scoliosis. Sci. World J. 2012, 680643.

Davis Jr., C.J., Lundberg, G.D., 1968. Retroaortic left renal vein: a relatively frequent anomaly. Am. J. Clin. Pathol. 50, 700–703.

Formica, M., Zanirato, A., Cavagnaro, L., et al., 2017. Extreme lateral interbody fusion in spinal revision surgery: clinical results and complications. Eur. Spine J. 26, 464–470.

Hartl, R., Joeris, A., McGuire, R.A., 2016. Comparison of the safety outcomes between two surgical approaches for anterior lumbar fusion surgery: anterior lumbar interbody fusion (ALIF) and extreme lateral interbody fusion (ELIF). Eur. Spine J. 25, 1484–1521.

Isaacs, R.E., Hyde, J., Goodrich, J.A., Rodgers, W.B., Phillips, F.M., 2010. A prospective, nonrandomized, multicenter evaluation of extreme lateral interbody fusion for the treatment of adult degenerative scoliosis: perioperative outcomes and complications. Spine 35 (26 Suppl. l), S322–S330.

Iwanaga, J., Saga, T., Tabira, Y., Watanabe, K., Yamaki, K., 2015. Contrast imaging study of the horseshoe kidney for transplantation. Surg. Radiol. Anat. 37, 1267–1271.

Iwanaga, J., Watanabe, K., Saga, T., Yamaki, K.-I., 2016. Bilateral malrotated kidney with major venous variant: a cadaver case report. Int. J. Acoust. Vib. 9.

Karaman, B., Koplay, M., Özturk, E., et al., 2007. Retroaortic left renal vein: multidetector computed tomography angiography findings and its clinical importance. Acta Radiol. 48, 355–360.

Karsy, M., Jensen, M.R., Cole, K., et al., 2017. Thoracolumbar cortical screw placement with interbody fusion: technique and considerations. Cureus 9, e1419.

Kwon, B., Kim, D.H., 2016. Lateral lumbar interbody fusion: indications, outcomes, and complications. J. Am. Acad. Orthop. Surg. 24, 96–105.

Malham, G.M., Ellis, N.J., Parker, R.M., Seex, K.A., 2012. Clinical outcome and fusion rates after the first 30 extreme lateral interbody fusions. Sci. World J. 2012, 246989.

Mayer, H.M., 1997. A new microsurgical technique for minimally invasive anterior lumbar interbody fusion. Spine 22, 691–699. Discussion 700.

McAfee, P.C., Regan, J.J., Geis, W.P., Fedder, I.L., 1998. Minimally invasive anterior retroperitoneal approach to the lumbar spine. Emphasis on the lateral BAK. Spine 23, 1476–1484.

Ozgur, B.M., Aryan, H.E., Pimenta, L., Taylor, W.R., 2006. Extreme lateral interbody fusion (XLIF): a novel surgical technique for anterior lumbar interbody fusion. Spine J. 6, 435–443.

Patel, V.C., Park, D.K., Herkowitz, H.N., 2012. Lateral transpsoas fusion: indications and outcomes. Sci. World J. 2012, 893608.

Pimenta, L., 2001. Lateral endoscopic transpsoas retroperitoneal approach for lumbar spine surgery. In: Paper Presented at: VIII Brazilian Spine Society Meeting.

Rodgers, W.B., Gerber, E.J., Patterson, J.R., 2010. Fusion after minimally disruptive anterior lumbar interbody fusion: analysis of extreme lateral interbody fusion by computed tomography. SAS J. 4, 63–66.

Satyapal, K.S., Haffejee, A.A., Singh, B., et al., 2001. Additional renal arteries: incidence and morphometry. Surg. Radiol. Anat. 23, 33–38.

Standring, S., 2015. Gray's Anatomy: The Anatomical Basis of Clinical Practice. Elsevier Health Sciences, London.

Uribe, J.S., Deukmedjian, A.R., 2015. Visceral, vascular, and wound complications following over 13,000 lateral interbody fusions: a survey study and literature review. Eur. Spine J. 24 (Suppl. 3), 386–396.

Voin, V., Kirkpatrick, C., Alonso, F., et al., 2017. Lateral transpsoas approach to the lumbar spine and relationship of the ureter: anatomic study with application to minimizing complications. World Neurosurg. 104, 674–678.

Yuan, P.S., Rowshan, K., Verma, R.B., Miller, L.E., Block, J.E., 2014. Minimally invasive lateral lumbar interbody fusion with direct psoas visualization. J. Orthop. Surg. Res. 9, 20.

CHAPTER 15

Lymphatics of the Abdomen

KARISHMA MEHTA • R. SHANE TUBBS

INTRODUCTION

Surgeons who operate within the retroperitoneum should have a good working knowledge of the general aspects of the regional lymphatics (Fig. 15.1). As the lateral transpsoas approach to the lumbar spine works within the retroperitoneum and in very close proximity to structures within the peritoneal cavity, spine surgeons using this approach need to know the basic anatomy of the lymphatics of these regions.

Specific to the abdomen, the lumbar lymph nodes include the preaortic, lateral aortic, and retroaortic subcategories; although depending on specialty and source, the terminology and exact anatomy of these various nodal groups varies.

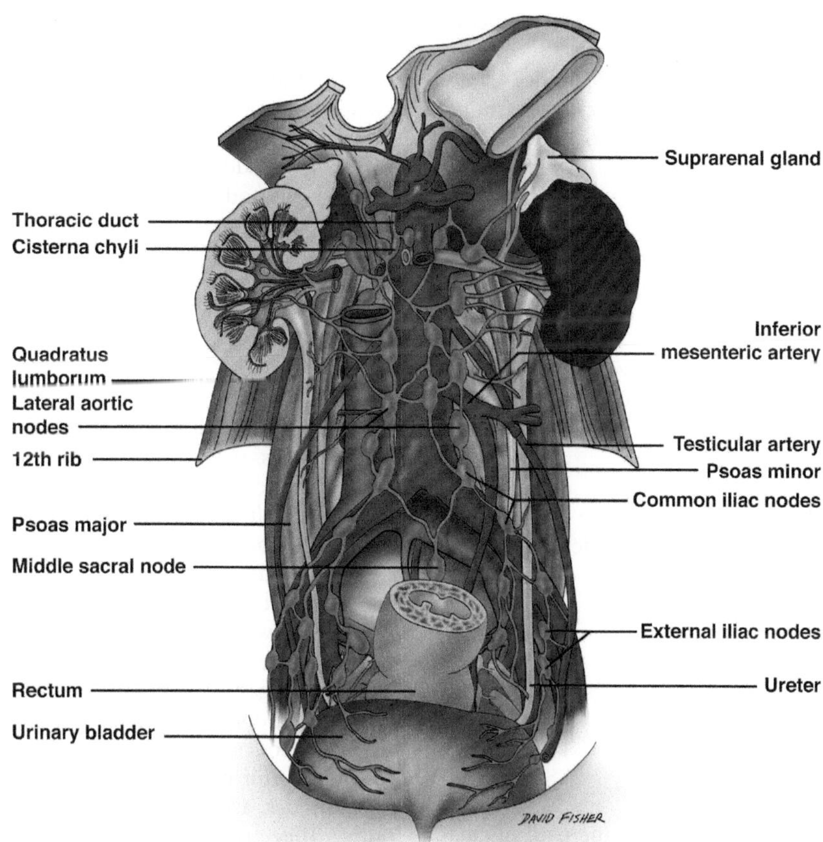

FIG. 15.1 Schematic drawing of the main lymphatic structures of the retroperitoneum.

Surgical anatomy of the lateral transpsoas approach to the lumbar spine. https://doi.org/10.1016/B978-0-323-67376-1.00015-X

The preaortic group of nodes is situated along the anterior surface of the aorta and contains the celiac, superior mesenteric, and inferior mesenteric nodes draining the gastrointestinal tract and adjacent organs such as the pancreas, spleen, and liver. The lateral aortic nodes are found on either side of the abdominal aorta anterior to the psoas major from the aortic hiatus of the diaphragm to the aortic bifurcation (Harisinghani, 2012). They receive lymph from the organs such as the suprarenal nodes, kidneys, ureters, and gonads. Lastly, the retroaortic nodes are concentrated at the third and fourth lumbar vertebrae. They drain the lymph from the posterior abdominal wall and feed directly into the cisterna chyli (Kenhub, 2019).

Celiac Nodes

The celiac nodes can be found around the origin of the celiac artery along the abdominal aorta. They drain the associated lymph nodes of the liver, gallbladder, spleen, pancreas, stomach, and upper gastrointestinal tract until the proximal duodenum. They then join the superior mesenteric and inferior mesenteric nodes to form the intestinal lymph trunk. The number of nodes in the bundle varies according to the source ranging from 3 to 15 cited (Harisinghani, 2012; Deaver, 1912).

Superior Mesenteric Nodes

The superior mesenteric nodes are located anterior to the abdominal aorta near the origin of the superior mesenteric artery. They receive lymph from the mesenteric, iliocolic, right colic, and middle colic nodes supplying the gastrointestinal tract from the distal duodenum to the proximal transverse colon. They then feed into the celiac nodes as well as the intestinal lymph trunk (Harisinghani, 2012).

Inferior Mesenteric Nodes

The inferior mesenteric nodes are a group of around 90 nodes situated near the inferior mesenteric artery, where it branches from the abdominal aorta. They receive drainage from peripheral nodes along the marginal artery and from the distal transverse colon, descending colon, sigmoid colon, and rectum above the pectinate line and feed into the superior mesenteric nodes (Harisinghani, 2012).

DRAINAGE

The superficial parietal vessels follow the path of adjacent blood vessels and drain the skin and subcutaneous tissue of the abdominal wall. The superficial vessels of the anterior abdominal wall drain into the axillary nodes above the umbilicus and the inguinal nodes below the umbilicus. Those of the lateral abdominal wall drain into the inguinal and lumbar nodes following the superficial circumflex iliac artery and the lumbar and iliolumbar arteries, respectively (Deaver, 1912).

The deep parietal vessels of the upper anterior abdominal wall drain into the internal thoracic nodes and eventually the anterior mediastinal, whereas those of the lower anterior abdominal wall terminate in the external iliac nodes. The upper vessels of the lateral wall also drain into the internal thoracic nodes, whereas the lower vessels end in the lumbar nodes. The visceral vessels drain the organs and follow their respective blood supply, eventually joining the cisterna chyli and thoracic duct (Fig. 15.2) (Richter and Feyerabend, 2012).

Drainage of the Liver and Gallbladder

The hepatic nodes consist of the hepatic, receiving lymph from the celiac nodes and located on the hepatic artery; the subpyloric, a group of four to five nodes at the bifurcation of the gastroduodenal artery; and the cystic nodes, on the neck of the gallbladder. These nodes feed into the celiac nodes.

The gallbladder contains two superior nodes, two intrahepatic nodes (medial and lateral), two extrahepatic nodes (medial and lateral), and two inferior nodes. The lymph of the gallbladder also drains into the cystic nodes eventually joining the hepatic lymph nodes (Richter and Feyerabend, 2012; Harisinghani, 2012).

Drainage of the Stomach

The nodes of the stomach consist of the left and right gastric nodes, which can be subdivided into superior and inferior categories. The superior nodes are located along the left gastric artery and contain the upper, lower, and paracardial nodes. The upper and lower nodes drain the lesser curvature of the stomach, situated between the two layers of the lesser omentum. The paracardial nodes are about five in number and drain the fundus and cardia of the stomach. These nodes drain into the left gastric nodes followed by the celiac nodes, whereas the upper and lower nodes drain directly into the celiac nodes (Harisinghani, 2012).

The inferior nodes of the stomach contain four to seven nodes and are also called the gastroomental nodes. They are located along the greater curvature of the stomach and drain into the pancreaticosplenic nodes on the left and the pyloric nodes on the right (Harisinghani, 2012).

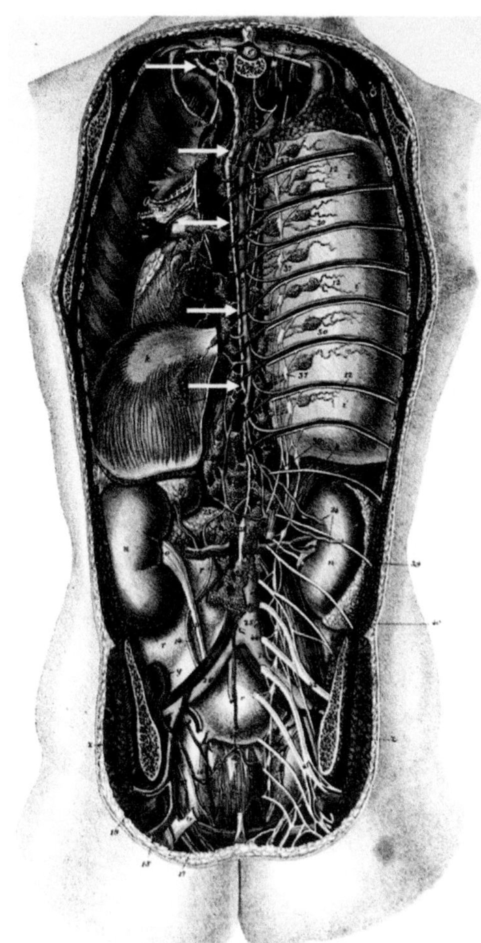

FIG. 15.2 Posterior view of the retropleural and retroperitoneal spaces from from Bourgery's 19th century. Traité complet de l'anatomie de l'homme comprenant la médecine operatoire.

Drainage of the Pancreas and Spleen

The pancreas has three main nodal groups containing the pyloric, pancreaticoduodenal, and the pancreaticosplenic lymph nodes. The pyloric nodes are six to eight in number, follow the gastroduodenal artery, and drain the head of the pancreas, the duodenum, and the right side of the greater curvature of the stomach. These nodes then end in the hepatic lymph nodes. The pancreaticoduodenal nodes are found along the pancreaticoduodenal arcade of vessels, drain the head of the pancreas and the duodenum, and drain to the pyloric nodes. Lastly, the pancreatic and splenic nodes are found along the splenic vessels draining the pancreas, spleen, and left side of the greater curvature of the stomach and feeding into the celiac nodes (Deaver, 1912; Harisinghani, 2012).

Drainage of the Intestines and Colon

The superior mesenteric parietal nodes receive lymph from three main groups of visceral nodes: the mesenteric, ileocolic, and mesocolic nodes. The mesenteric nodes range from 100 to 200 in number and are found between the layers of the mesentery along the vasa recta and branches of the superior mesenteric artery, draining the lymph of the small intestine. The ileocolic nodes are 10–20 in number and are situated in two groups along the ileocolic artery: one near the duodenum and the other around the lower trunk of the artery. Lastly, the mesocolic nodes are located between the transverse mesocolon around the right and left colic flexures, draining the colon (Harisinghani, 2012).

REFERENCES

Deaver, J.B., 1912. Surgical Anatomy: Abdomen, Pelvic Cavity, Lymphatics of Abdomen and Pelvis, Thorax, Lower Extremity. P. Blakiston's Son and Co, Philadelphia, pp. 392–396.

Harisinghani, M.G. (Ed.), 2012. Atlas of Lymph Node Anatomy. Springer, New York (Chapter 3).

Kenhub, 2019. Lymph Nodes of the Thorax and Abdomen https://www.kenhub.com/en/library/anatomy/lymph-nodes-of-the-thorax-and-abdomen/. https://doi.org/10.4103/0971-3026.195777.

Richter, E., Feyerabend, T., 2012. Normal Lymph Node Topography: CT Atlas. Springer, Berlin, pp. 81–95.

FURTHER READING

Arrivé, L., Azizi, L., Lewin, M., Hoeffel, C., Monnier-Cholley, L., Lacombe, C., Tubiana, J.M., 2007. MR lymphography of abdominal and retroperitoneal lymphatic vessels. Am. J. Roentgenol. 189 (5), 1051–1058.

Ohtani, O., Ohtani, Y., 2008. Lymph circulation in the liver. Anat. Rec. 291 (6), 643–652.

CHAPTER 16

Anatomical Variations Relevant to the Lateral Transpsoas Approach to the Lumbar Spine

JOE IWANAGA • R. SHANE TUBBS

INTRODUCTION

Variations along the pathways used for lateral transpsoas approaches to the lumbar spine should be appreciated by the spine surgeon. This chapter presents some of the common and uncommon anatomical variations that might be observed in patients undergoing such procedures. Some might be encountered on imaging and others, intraoperatively. Knowledge of such variations might help in better diagnosis of such patients and decrease operative complications.

Lumbar Vertebral Defects

Congenital block vertebra occurs as a result of a disturbance in segmentation of the somites during development of the vertebral column (Yochum, 1987). This results in fusion of adjacent vertebral bodies, with fusion of the apophyseal joint in approximately 50% of cases. While this variant is more typical of the cervical spine, it is also known to occur in the lumbar spine. In some cases, the two adjacent vertebrae fuse to form a solid block of bone. More often, a remnant of the intervertebral vertebral disc remains. A typical block vertebra has a decreased anterior/posterior diameter. As a result of the loss of the vertebral disc space, the vertebral foramina are frequently narrowed with congenital block vertebrae, but can be normally sized or enlarged.

Sagittal cleft vertebrae occur as a result of a failure of fusion of the two halves of the vertebral body. This is thought to be associated with the embryologic extension of the notochord longitudinally through the vertebral column during ossification (Hollinshead, 1982). Incomplete fusion of the two lateral chondral centers of the vertebral body results in a central sagittal constriction of the vertebral body. The sagittal cleft is created by the indentation of the endplate cortices (Yochum, 1987). From the frontal view, the body has the appearance of two triangular masses with opposing apices—hence the term butterfly vertebrae. The development of the ununited bodies is generally symmetrical (Yochum, 1987). Furthermore, the cleft results in an increase in the interpedicular distance (Yochum, 1987). The body may be cleft in the frontal plane. Enlarged fissures or Hahn's clefts may be seen. These are vascular channels within the vertebral body.

Lateral hemivertebrae (Figs. 16.1 and 16.2) appear as an absence of one lateral half of the vertebral body and develops when one of the two lateral ossification centers of the vertebral body fails to grow. The apex of the lateral hemivertebra is directed medially. Normal disk spaces are usually present above and below the affected level (Yochum, 1987). However, the endplates of the adjacent vertebrae are deformed, resulting in a trapezoid shape to those vertebrae. An isolated lateral hemivertebra will result in a scoliotic deformity, with the affected vertebra being located at the apex of the scoliotic curvature (Yochum, 1987). It has been hypothesized that hemivertebrae can result from a lack of vascularization to the defective side (Hollinshead, 1982).

Dorsal hemivertebrae appear as an absence of the anterior half of the vertebral body. The dorsal portion of the body tapers ventrally, and fibrous tissue replaces the absent ventral portion of the body. The adjacent vertebrae may demonstrate compensatory growth and come together in the defective area of the hemivertebra. Ventral hemivertebra is also a described anomaly. Dorsal and ventral hemivertebrae are much less frequent that lateral hemivertebrae (Taylor, 2000).

The limbus bone is a small, triangular bony ossicle often adjacent to the anterior superior aspect of the vertebral body (Jaeger, 1988). It is believed to result from a herniation of nuclear material through a

Surgical anatomy of the lateral transpsoas approach to the lumbar spine. https://doi.org/10.1016/B978-0-323-67376-1.00016-1

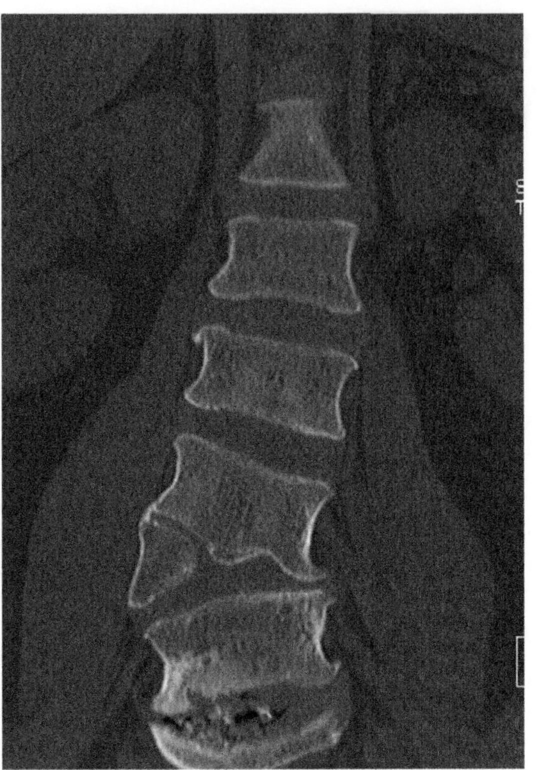

FIG. 16.1 Example of lumbar hemivertebra.

secondary ossification center for the corner of the vertebral body. This results in nonunion of the secondary ossification center, and thus the presence of a bony fragment (Yochum, 1987).

Nuclear impressions are invaginations in the vertebral endplates that result from notochordal remnants. They appear as broad curvilinear depressions of the endplate. They more commonly affect the inferior, rather than superior, endplate (Jaeger, 1988; Taylor, 2000). On a frontal view, the impressions create paramedian curvilinear indentations, creating the appearance of a double hump. This has been referred to as Cupid's bow contour (Taylor, 2000; Yochum, 1987).

Another vertebral disk variant, which can be confused with a nuclear impression, is a Schmorl's node. Vertical nucleus pulposus herniations, rather than notochordal remnants, are to blame for the endplate defects of Schmorl's nodes. Radiographically, a Schmorl's node appears as a squared off, rectangular rim of sclerosis protruding through the endplate. It can be centrally or peripherally located. This is different from the defect of nuclear impressions, in which there is a smooth, wavelike cortical surface irregularity involving nearly all of the endplate (Yochum, 1987).

Disruptions in arch formation can produce clefts in numerous parts of the vertebral arch. A retrosomatic cleft is found at the junction of the pedicle and vertebral body. It results as a failure of fusion between the

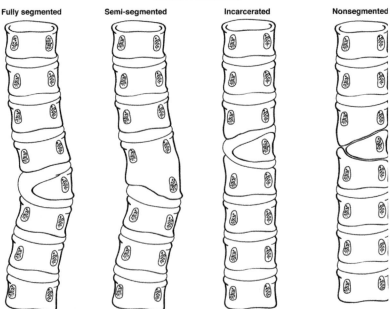

FIG. 16.2 Schematic drawing of several variations of hemivertebra.

ossifying neural arch and centrum. A cleft may also occur more posteriorly in the body of the pedicle itself. A retroisthmic cleft occurs on the lamina, behind the pars interarticularis.

One of the most recognized neural arch cleft defects is spina bifida. Spina bifida occulta, or rachischisis, is a defect in ossification at the spinous process or lamina (Hollinshead, 1982). The dorsal synchondrosis between the neural arches usually fuses during the first year of life. Failure of this fusion results in the formation of a dorsal cleft involving the spinous process or lamina. The size of cleft can vary from a small midline cleft to near absence of the vertebral arch. It is most commonly found in the lumbosacral region (Jaeger, 1988).

When a spina bifida occulta defect occurs at the first sacral vertebra with an elongated spinous process of the fifth lumbar vertebra, this is known as a knife clasp deformity. The long spinous process may result from a fusion of the L5 spinous process with the first sacral tubercle (Jaeger, 1988; Taylor, 2000). An anterior/posterior radiographic view will demonstrate with spina bifida defect at S1 with a vertical enlargement of the L5 spinous process. A lateral view will show distal enlargement of the spinous process. This entity is so named due to the pain it induces when the patient extends the lumbar spine (Yochum, 1987).

Spondylolysis is a vertebral arch cleft which occurs at the pars interarticularis (Fig. 16.3). This disruption of the pars can be either unilateral or bilateral. There is debate as to whether a congenital etiology exists for this entity. Spondylolisthesis is defined as an anterior displacement of a vertebral body relative to the body immediately inferior. Approximately, 90% of spondylolystheses involve the fifth lumbar vertebra (Yochum, 1987). There are multiple types of spondylolisthesis. Those of interest here are the types that would result from a congenital deformity, opposed to the acquired type. Dysplastic spondylolisthesis has a congenital implication with dysplasia in the neural arch of L5 or the sacrum, allowing anterior displacement of the former relative to the latter.

Split cord malformation is a congenital anomaly where a longitudinal diastasis divides the spinal cord or cauda equina, depending on a thoracic or lumbar location (Fig. 16.4). The division consists of either an osseous, cartilaginous, or fibrous band (Fig. 16.5). There is typically an increased interpediculate distance. Fifty percent of cases are associated with other vertebral anomalies, such as scoliosis, spina bifida occulta, and tethering of the spinal cord (Taylor, 2000; Yochum, 1987).

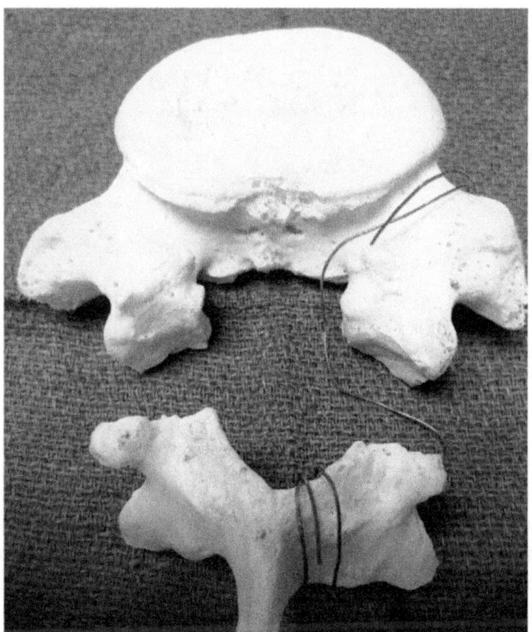

FIG. 16.3 Dry bone specimen of L5 spondylolysis.

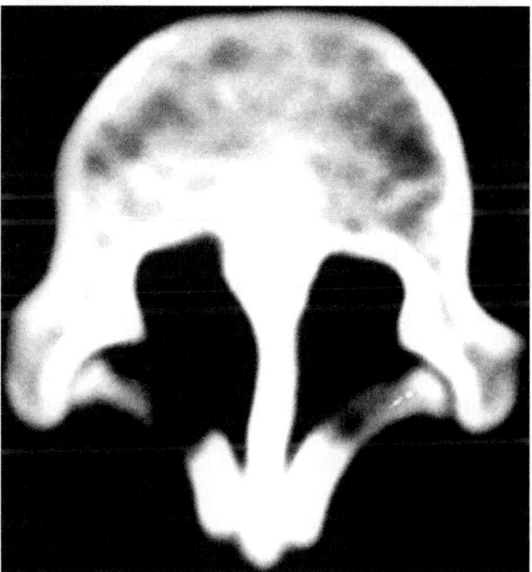

FIG. 16.4 CT of lumbar split cord malformation with bony partition.

Agenesis of a vertebral pedicle is more likely to occur in the cervical spine but has been documented in the lumbar region. Failure of development of the chondral center responsible for one side of the neural arch results in a unilaterally absent pedicle. The superior articular

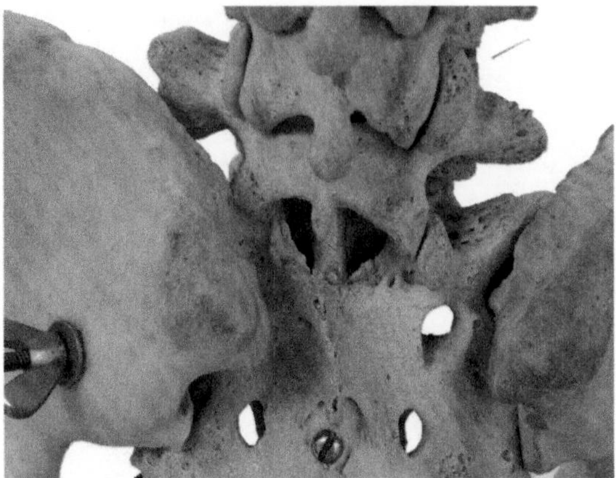

FIG. 16.5 Right lumbosacral tropism.

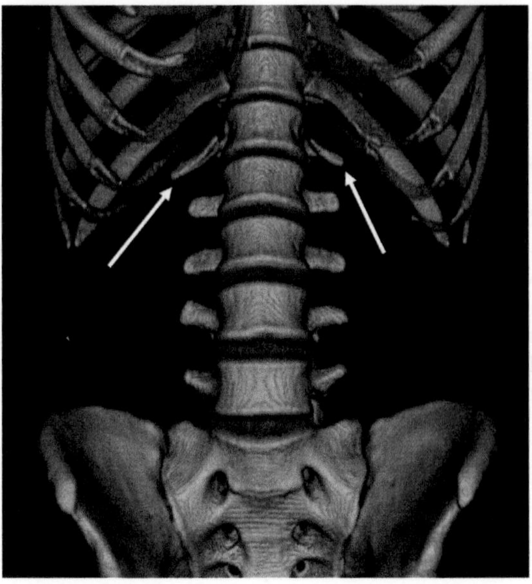

FIG. 16.6 Bilateral lumbar ribs (arrows).

process and transverse process at the affected level may be dysplastic. In addition, the contralateral pedicle is often hyperplastic, which occurs more frequently in the lumbar spine opposed to the cervical spine (Yochum, 1987).

Nonfusion of secondary centers of ossification is known to occur in the lumbar vertebrae. One common site is the apophysis of the transverse process of the first lumbar vertebra. Another nonfusion site, which typically occurs in the lumbar region, is the inferior articular process apophysis. Found here are joint surfaces covered with cartilage. These often occur around the third lumbar vertebra. A triangular bony ossicle is found at the tip of the inferior articular process, referred to as Oppenheimer's ossicle (Jaeger, 1988; Taylor, 2000). A similar entity in the superior articular process is much less common (Jaeger, 1988).

Variation in orientation of lumbosacral facet joints is known as tropism (Fig. 16.5). The L1-2 to L4-5 facet joints are oriented in the sagittal plane. L5-S1 facet joints are oriented in the coronal plane. Tropism occurs when this convention is broken for either the right or left apophyseal joint at a given level. This most commonly occurs at the L4-5 and L5-S1 levels. On frontal radiographic views, normal lumbar spine facet joints are visible as linear radiolucencies between the superior and inferior facet. Tropism presents as an absence of the radiolucency on the affected side (Taylor, 2000; Yochum, 1987).

The transverse processes in the lumbar spine are actually homologs of the ribs. Ribs of the lumbar vertebrae (Fig. 16.6) are actually more common than ribs of the cervical vertebrae (C7). The accessory process, a small tubercle projecting from the posterior surface of the transverse process medially, is the rudimentary true transverse process, in that it serves as an attachment for spinal muscles along with the mammillary process on the superior and lateral aspects of the superior articular facet (Jinkins, 2000). Rarely, an accessory process can be congenitally absent. This occurs more frequently in the fifth lumbar vertebra (Bergman et al., 1984; Hollinshead, 1982). In contrast to an absent accessory process, a styloid process is defined as an elongated accessory process, exceeding a length of 3–5 mm (Bergman et al., 1984). Occasionally, the mamillary and accessory processes are united by a bony bridge forming a foramen behind the transverse process.

Of all the vertebral transitional zones, the most commonly involved with anatomic variations is the lumbosacral. The typical human spine contains 24 presacral vertebrae. The 24th presacral vertebra, commonly identified as L5, may be partially or completely incorporated with the sacrum, either unilaterally or bilaterally. This is termed sacralization of L5 (Fig. 16.7). Conversely, the first sacral vertebra, S1, can take on characteristics of a lumbar vertebra, including articulation rather than fusion with the remainder of the sacrum, lumbar type facet joints, and a squared appearance in the sagittal plane. This is termed lumbarization of S1. Considered together, these variations are often referred to as a lumbosacral transitional vertebra (LSTV). The reported prevalence of LSTV ranges from 4% to 30% (Konin and Walz, 2010). There may be just four lumbar vertebrae in the absence of any fusion abnormalities.

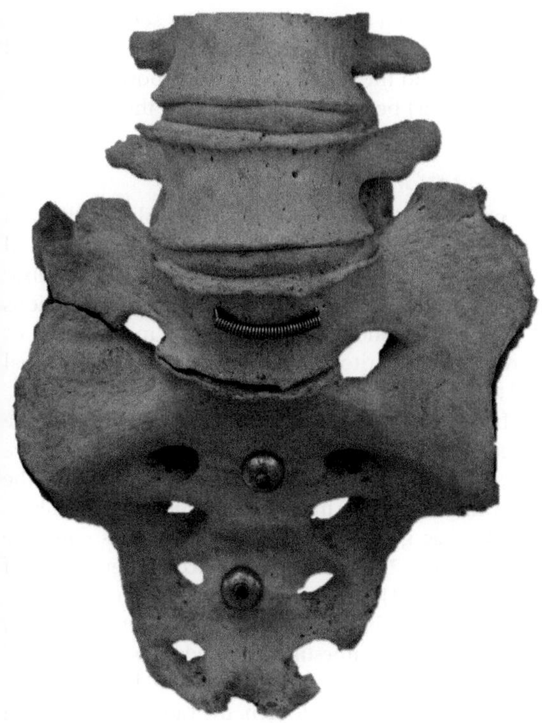

FIG. 16.7 Example of sacralization.

There are varying degrees of sacralization of the fifth lumbar vertebra (O'Connor, 1934). Castellvi et al. (1984) described a radiographic classification system identifying four types of LSTVs on the basis of morphologic characteristics.

Type I: Unilateral (Ia) or bilateral (Ib) dysplastic transverse process, measuring at least 19 mm in width in the craniocaudal dimension.

Type II: Incomplete unilateral (IIa) or bilateral (IIb) lumbarization/sacralization with an enlarged transverse process that has a diarthrodial joint between itself and the sacrum.

Type III: Unilateral (IIIa) or bilateral (IIIb) lumbarization/sacralization with complete osseous fusion of the transverse process to the sacrum.

Type IV: Unilateral type II transition with a type III on the contralateral side (Castellvi et al., 1984).

Other characteristics of LSTV include a decreased disc height between the lumbar transitional vertebra and the sacrum as compared to a normal L5-S1 disk. In fact, this space may be completely devoid of any disk material. Conversely, when a lumbarized S1 is present, the S1–S2 disc height is greater than the typical rudimentary disk present in a normal spine. In addition to the disk space, the vertebral body displays morphologic changes with LSTV. With sacralization of L 5, the lowest lumbar segment develops a wedged shaped. With lumbarization of S1, the highest sacral segment develops a squared appearance. Finally, the facet joints of the transition point must be considered. With a sacralized L5, the facet joints are typically hypoplastic, if not all together nonexistent with complete fusion of L5 to S1. With a lumbarized S1, S1-S2 facet joints can be identified, whereas a typical S1-S2 segment has osseous fusion (Konin and Walz, 2010).

MUSCULAR

Muscular variations are covered in the chapters dealing with the anterolateral and posterior abdominal wall chapters.

NERVES

Nerve variations are covered in the chapter devoted to the nerves.

OTHER RETROPERITONEAL STRUCTURES

Kidneys

Horseshoe kidneys (HSK) occur in approximately one in every 400 to 500 people (Fig. 16.8). An HSK is usually located lower than the normal kidney, so it is rarely injured by the upper part of a lumbar fixation. However, many HSKs have two to three accessory renal arteries of which the course is unpredictable. Not only the right and left parts of the HSK but also the isthmus between the right and left kidneys receive a plentiful blood supply from the abdominal aorta.

The incidence of kidney malrotation is approximately 1 in 1000 cases. Lateral malrotation is the least common type, and its true incidence is unknown. The laterally malrotated kidney could have a renal artery and vein that pass posterior to the kidney. The posteriorly malrotated kidney has a posterior renal hilum. Such malrotations result from a reverse or excessive rotation of the kidney during the fetal period. In these cases, the variant vessels are susceptible to injury during a lateral fusion procedure.

Ectopic kidneys occur in approximately 1 in 1000 in autopsy series, which is much higher than in clinical presentation (1 in 10,000) because only about 1 in 10 of these cases is ever diagnosed (Fig. 16.9). Crossed fused renal ectopia is a relatively uncommon congenital anomaly of the kidney. The autopsy incidence is approximately 1 in 2000.

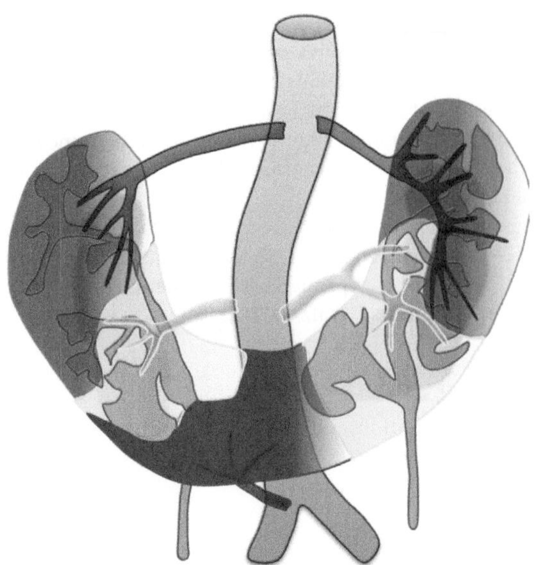

FIG. 16.8 Drawing of a horseshoe kidney and its vascular supply.

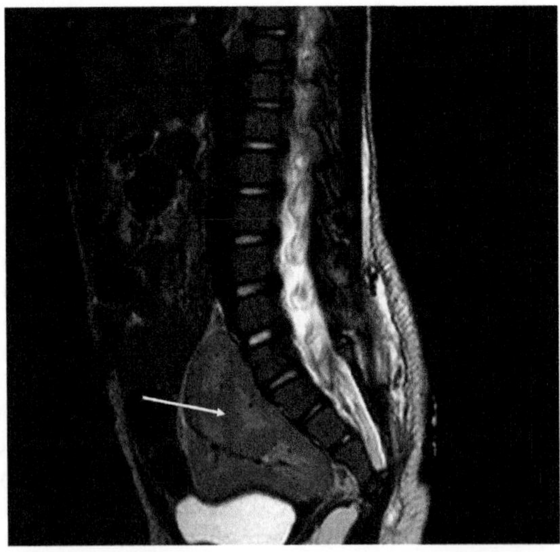

FIG. 16.9 MRI demonstrating a pelvic kidney at the arrow.

Ureters

The principal variation in the ureter is a more or less complete division into two. As a rule, the two ureters unite a little above the bladder, so that there is only one vesical orifice. When the division is complete there are two separate openings into the bladder. In rare cases, three or four ureters may be found. Several instances are recorded in which a supernumerary ureter, proceeding from the upper part of the kidney, opened directly into the urethra. Ureters have also been reported to open into the vagina, the seminal vesicle, or the prostatic urethra. The right ureter has been found passing behind the inferior vena cava (postcaval or retrocaval ureter) between that vessel and the aorta.

Left and Right Colon

The principal colonic variations probably result from irregular or defective development leading to mild embryologic abnormalities of bowel rotation and fixation. Examples are malrotation and abnormal fixations of the colon, shortened or absent mesocolon, or decreased retroperitoneal fat (Oyar et al., 2003; Unal et al., 2004).

The incidence of malrotation or nonrotation of the midgut is presumed to be approximately 1 in 500 live births. Two-thirds of cases are diagnosed during the newborn period. The male:female ratio is reportedly 2: 1 in this age group. However, male patients comprise approximately 20% of cases that occur after 1 year of age (Torres 1993). Nonrotation of the intestine is considered to occur in the second stage of midgut rotation. In nonrotation of the intestine, the midgut is only rotated to 90 degrees instead of the normal 270 degrees. As the midgut returns to the abdomen, the caudal limb (cecum and colon) enters the abdomen first and lies on the left side of the abdomen while the cecum localizes on the midline; the cranial limb (small intestine) then enters the abdomen and lies on the right. Nonrotation is the most common form of midgut malrotation. Most cases are symptomatic and diagnosed in infancy and childhood. However, adult cases have also been reported.

Mixed, partial, or incomplete rotation may result when rotation of the midgut stops in the second stage. The degrees of rotation vary from nonrotation (90 degrees) to normal (270 degrees); rotation usually stops at 180 degrees. As a result, the duodenum is usually fixed on the right, and the cecum is located in the left upper quadrant or close to the midline, just below the pylorus. The cecum, which can be duplicated, is fixed to the retroperitoneum by a peritoneal band called Ladd's ligament, which forms when the cecum and ascending colon attach to the abdominal wall during the third stage of midgut rotation. This band constrains the duodenum and frequently causes duodenal obstruction in infancy. The variety of the attachment of Ladd's band is considered to result from the degrees of midgut rotation.

Reverse rotation type of malrotation is extremely rare and comprises only 4% of all malrotation cases. Reverse rotation may be found in patients of any age from newborn to adult. Adult cases comprise approximately 75% of all cases; this differs from other types of malrotation, which are usually diagnosed in infancy. In this condition, the first 90-degree counterclockwise rotation of the midgut takes place; however, the subsequent 180-degree rotation occurs in the clockwise direction instead of in the normal counterclockwise direction.

Estrada (1962) classified reverse rotation of the midgut into two types according to the sequence of which limb, the cranial or caudal limb, reenters the abdominal cavity first. The type of reverse rotation in which the caudal limb reenters first is termed "retroarterial colon type"; the colon lies behind the superior mesenteric artery, and the small intestine is ventral to the colon and the artery. Another type of reverse rotation is termed "liver and entire colon ipsilateral type" and is extremely rare. In this type, the cranial limb reenters the abdomen first, the small intestine lies in front of the superior mesenteric artery and occupies the left side of the abdominal cavity, and the colon lies to the right with the cecum on the midline.

Reverse rotation has been classified into four types. Type 1 is the prearterial right-sided cecum type. This type involves very little actual reverse rotation with the exception of the first part of the jejunum. The rest of the midgut remains stationary. This type is very similar to nonrotation and is the type of reverse rotation most often mistaken for it. Type 2 is the prearterial left-sided cecum type. This type is characterized by a 180-degree reverse rotation of the distal midgut loop with mislocation of the splenic flexure. Type 3 is the retroarterial right-sided cecum type. In this type, it is considered that the caudal limb reenters the abdomen first, as in the retroarterial colon type and it is presumed that the caudal limb rotates and localizes normally but that the cranial limb rotates 90 degrees in a clockwise direction. Finally, type 4 is the retroarterial left-sided cecum type. In this type, the caudal limb reenters the abdomen first at a 180-degree clockwise rotation with mislocation of the splenic flexure, and the transverse colon and cecum are secondarily folded from their retroarterial position to a partial prearterial position.

The ascending colon does not usually have a mesentery, but is fused to the posterior wall of the abdomen, and its anterior surface is covered with peritoneum. However, there are various degrees of incomplete fixation of the ascending colon. Skandalakis and Gray (1994) described three types of attachment of the ascending colon to the abdominal wall: (A) normal retroperitoneal location of the colon; (B) paracolic gutter (deep paracolic groove but does not form a mesentery); and (C) mobile colonic mesentery. The frequency of a persistent right mesocolon is reported in up to about 35%. Absence of the mesocolon of the ascending colon is often associated with a mobile cecum. In one study, 55 of 87 cases demonstrated a mobile cecum alone, and 5 of 87 demonstrated a mobile cecum with the ascending colon (Skandalakis and Gray, 1994). A membrane termed Jackson's veil, which envelopes the ascending colon, is sometimes observed. This membrane was first reported by Jackson in 1911 and is also called the prececocolic fascia. This membrane may or may not be vascularized. It is most frequently observed in the ascending colon, and it may involve the cecum or hepatic flexure.

Gastrointestinal duplication is a rare anomaly and was observed in approximately 1 in 4500 cases in an autopsy study. Duplication of the colon constitutes approximately 15% of all alimentary tract duplications. The duplication is often located in the cecum and is associated with duplication of the vermiform appendix (i.e., type C). Both cystic and tubular types have been observed. In the tubular type, duplication extending throughout the entire colon has also been described. Such cases of entire colon duplication are known to be frequently associated with lower urinary tract and/or genital tract duplication.

A mobile splenic flexure is one of the more common colonic variations, occurring in 20% of cases (Saunders et al., 1995). Pancreaticogastric interposition of the splenic flexure and descending colon occurs in approximately 0.2% of cases (Unal et al., 2004). Anterolateral hepato-diaphragmatic interposition of the distal transverse colon and splenic flexure occurs in 1.3%–3% of individuals (Unal et al., 2004). Interposition of the colon between the spleen and diaphragm (cephalo-diaphragmatic or retrosplenic interposition) has been described in 0.03%–0.3% of cases. When this occurs the left colic flexure and distal part of transverse colon have been shown to be situated in the retroperitoneal space and sometimes between the kidney and psoas muscle (Oyar et al., 2003).

Although retroperitoneal, the descending colon, especially in the iliac fossa, has a short mesentery in approximately 33% of people (Moore and Dalley, 1999), which, however, is usually not long enough to cause volvulus of this part of the colon. A redundant loop of descending colon may occur which crosses the great vessels of abdomen to present itself, sometimes with the sigmoid colon on the right side of abdomen. In malrotation, an abnormal arrest in midgut rotation after the first 90 degrees of rotation occurs rendering the descending colon to lie anterior to the kidneys rather than lateral to them.

Interposition of the descending colon between psoas muscle and kidney (retrorenal position), which can be partial or complete, has been reported to occur in

0.7%–10% and tends to occur more frequently in young women and individuals with less intra-abdominal fat.

Inferior Vena Cava

Several variants of duplicated IVC exist; the most common of which is two distinct IVCs that arise from each iliac vein without a normal confluence. Duplication of the IVC results from persistence of both supracardinal veins. The prevalence is 0.2%–3%. The left IVC typically ends at the left renal vein, which crosses anterior to the aorta in the normal fashion to join the right IVC. This may be associated with retroaortic right renal vein, hemiazygos continuation of the IVC, significant asymmetry in the sizes of the left and right veins, and a communication between the right and left IVC in the position of the normal left common iliac vein. A left IVC results from regression of the right supracardinal vein with persistence of the left supracardinal vein. The prevalence is less than 0.5%.

The embryologic basis of double IVC with retroaortic right renal vein and hemiazygos continuation of the IVC is persistence of the left lumbar and thoracic supracardinal vein and the left suprasubcardinal anastomosis, together with failure of formation of the right subcardinal—hepatic anastomosis. In addition, the right renal vein and right IVC meet and cross posterior to the aorta to join the left IVC and continue cephalad as the hemiazygos vein. Thus, there is also persistence of the dorsal limb of the renal collar and regression of the ventral limb. The IVCs are noted to be continuous with their respective common iliac veins. Another variant complex is a double IVC with a retroaortic left renal vein and azygos continuation of the IVC. This results from persistence of the left supracardinal vein and the dorsal limb of the renal collar with regression of the ventral limb and failure of formation of the subcardinal-hepatic anastomosis.

Azygos continuation of the IVC has also been termed absence of the hepatic segment of the IVC with azygos continuation. The prevalence is approximately 0.5%. The embryonic event is theorized to be failure to form the right subcardinal-hepatic anastomosis, with resulting atrophy of the right subcardinal vein. Consequently, blood is shunted from the suprasubcardinal anastomosis through the retrocrural azygos vein, which is partially derived from the thoracic segment of the right supracardinal vein. The renal portion of the IVC receives blood return from both kidneys and passes posterior to the diaphragmatic crura to enter the thorax as the much enlarged azygos vein which joins the SVC at the normal location. The hepatic segment (often termed the posthepatic segment) is ordinarily not truly absent; rather, it drains directly into the right atrium. Since the postsubcardinal anastomosis does not contribute to formation of the IVC, each gonadal vein drains to the ipsilateral renal vein.

The absence of the IVC is one among infrequent subtypes of IVC abnormalities that are rarely seen in the general population, involving either that of entire IVC or that of its infrarenal segment. These two entities are relatively similar, but their etiopathogeneses are still controversial. The absence of the entire IVC is thought to be a result of an embryologic disorder, whereas perinatal thrombosis is hypothesized to lead to the development of an absent infrarenal IVC. With absence of the IVC, as in pathological obstruction, venous blood can return from the inferior part of the body through various pathways such as paraspinal, superficial abdominal collaterals, and the portal system. Absence of the entire posthepatic IVC suggests that all three paired venous systems failed to develop properly. Absence of the infrarenal IVC implies failure of development of the posterior cardinal and supracardinal veins. Since it is difficult to identify a single embryonic event that can lead to either of these scenarios, there is controversy as to whether these conditions are true embryonic anomalies or the result of perinatal IVC thrombosis. The external and internal iliac veins join to form enlarged ascending lumbar veins, which convey blood return from the lower extremities to the azygos and hemiazygos veins via anterior paravertebral veins. A normal suprarenal IVC is formed by confluence of the renal veins.

Renal Veins

The renal veins show less variation than do the renal arteries. One study found multiple renal veins to be rare on the left side (1%) and common on the right side (28%). In another study, the right renal vein was found to have one to three accessories (18% of 203 cases) and the left renal vein to have one or two accessories (9% of 203 cases). Poynter pointed out that the renal veins show a tendency to form two or more trunks as the arteries do, but in the veins the frequency is only about 7%. In about 2% of cases, the left renal vein may be retroaortic or even circumaortic(either single vessel or doubled with one limb anterior and the other posterior to the aorta reported frequency 1.5%–4.4% of all abdominal CT scans) or it may form a circumaortic renal venous collar (reported frequency 1.5%–8.7%). Dill et al. (2012), in an MRI study, found total left renal vein variations, retroaortic left renal vein, and circumaortic left renal veins in 71/2644 (2.68%), 44/2644

1.66%), and 27/2644 (1.02%), respectively. In cases vith a retroaortic left renal vein, the numbers of males and females with their corresponding percentages were 19/44 (43.2%) and 25/44 (56.8%), respectively. In cases with a circumaortic left renal vein, the numbers of males and females with their corresponding percentages were 13/27 (48.1%) and 14/27 (51.9%), espectively.

The right renal vein may be doubled, even though he left renal vein is usually single. The left renal may anastomose with the splenic vein and also receive lumbar veins. The renal and testicular veins show many irregularities when the left inferior vena cava persists.

Communication between the vena cava and accessory renal veins is not unusual nor is an anastomosis between the splenic and left renal veins. Lejars found the hemiazygos vein communicating with the left renal vein in 88% of subjects studied.

Aorta

The uppermost limit of the abdominal aorta is level vith the lower border of the T12 vertebra although his can be as high as T12 or low as L1. The aorta lies in the midline as it enters the abdomen, but it usually deviates very slightly to the left in its descent. Marked ortuosity of the aorta can also be found.

The most common point of the aortic bifurcation is opposite the lower part of L4, though the termination has been reported to vary from the upper third of L3 to the upper third of S1. A higher division is less common, though the aorta has been reported to divide as high as the second lumbar vertebra. The bifurcation of he aorta occurs just above or just below the highest part of the iliac crest.

Renal Arteries

tudies of the origins of right versus left renal arteries vith respect to vertebral levels have revealed the ollowing. In an angiographic study of 855 patients, Özkan et al. (2006) revealed that the right and left renal rteries originated between the upper margin of L1 and he lower margin of L2 in 98% and 97% of the patients, espectively. In the same study, they found that 23% of ight and 22% of left renal arteries originated at the ntervertebral disc between L1 and L2. Aubert and Koumare (1975) found that 14.49% (91/628) of right and 3.37% (87/632) of left renal arteries arose at the same evel, i.e., at the disk between L1 and L2. Renal angiographic studies by Edsman (1957) demonstrated that he right and left renal arteries originate at the disk between L1 and L2 in 31.5% (86/273) and 34.4% (86/50), respectively. The above findings establish that the vast majority of right and left renal arteries arise between the L1 and L2 vertebrae and generally at the level of the disk between them.

Çiçekcibaşi et al. (2005) found that the right and the left renal arteries originated between the upper margin of L1 and the upper one-third of L2 in 96% and 97.9%, respectively. Aubert and Koumare (1975) summarized the work of previous authors stating that the renal arteries originate from the abdominal aorta below the superior mesenteric artery at the level of L1. Angiographic studies by Edsman (1957) and Kincaid (1966) concluded that the renal artery arises from the aorta usually at the level of the lower third of L1 with a variation of one vertebral body cephalad or caudad. Renal arteries can be doubled, tripled, or quadrupled (Fig. 16.10).

Azygos Veins

The azygos vein originates in the thorax at the level of the 12th thoracic vertebra. It arises from lateral, intermediate, and/or medial roots or from any combination of the three. The lateral azygos root is found in 85% of bodies and arises by union of the ascending vein and subcostal vein. The intermediate root occurs in 34% of individuals. This root arises from the dorsal side of the vena cava near the level of the second lumbar segmental vein and often as a common trunk with the segmental, or right renal vein. The medial root occurs in 38% of subjects. They are small plexiform veins closely associated with the ventral side of the lumbar vertebral bodies dorsal to the aorta and its lumbar

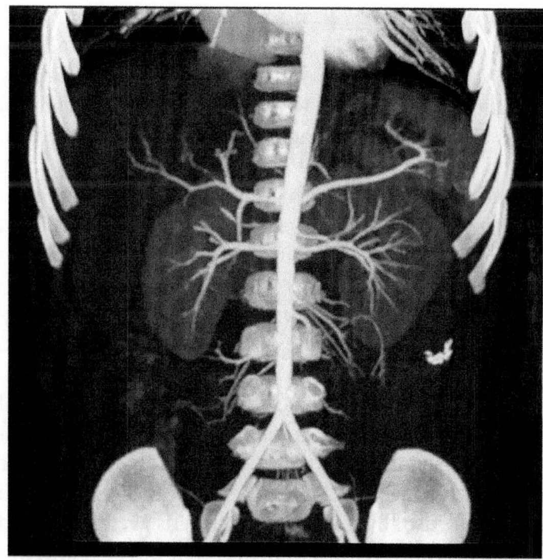

FIG. 16.10 CTA noting bilateral accessory renal arteries.

segmental branches. The azygos vein receives the hemiazygos vein, on its left margin, as a side or double branch at about the eighth and ninth vertebra. Slightly higher, at the sixth or seventh thoracic vertebra, it receives the accessory hemiazygos vein as a single trunk in 72% of individuals. The hemiazygos and accessory hemiazygos veins are incompletely formed in 15% of individuals. When this occurs the posterior intercostal veins on the left side of the thorax may drain into the azygos vein independently. In this case, the azygos vein lies on the midline. Rarely, the azygos vein passes through the aortic hiatus of the diaphragm. The azygos vein may be absent or doubled. The inferior vena cava has been seen continued into the azygos vein, which is then of course extremely large.

Iliolumbar Veins

The iliolumbar vein (ILV) travels laterally approximately 3–4 cm below the common iliac vein bifurcation and then tracks medially to laterally beside the body of the L5 vertebra. It then makes its way rostrally and posteriorly coursing between the lumbosacral trunk and obturator nerve. Reports of the ILV have described it as posterior to the obturator nerve located superficially and anterior to the lumbosacral trunk and drains the iliac fossa, iliacus, and psoas major muscle.

In an earlier study (Davis et al., 2019), we found the ILV on all but two sides (28/30; 93.3%). It arose as a common trunk from the common iliac vein on 14 sides (50%), as separate vessels (i.e., vertical and horizontal branches) from the common iliac vein on five sides (18%), as a single vertical branch on four sides (14%), and as more than two branches on three sides (11%). On two sides (7%), it arose from the very proximal external iliac vein. No specimen was found to have the ILV drain into the internal iliac vein or directly into the IVC. Left ILVs tended to have a more distal origin, but the overall length of the vessel to its vertical branch terminus was not significant when comparing left and right sides. ILVs had a mean length (origin of the vessel to the end of its vertical branch) of 3.7 cm (2.5–6.8 cm) and a mean width (at its origin) of 0.9 cm (0.5–1.5 cm). ILVs were significantly larger on right versus left sides, and although not statistically significant, the ILVs on the left tended to be longer. Left-sided ILVs tended to have more branches than right-sided veins. The majority of vertical branches of the ILV traveled anterior to the ventral rami of the lumbar spinal nerves, most commonly L4. However, some vertical branches traveled posterior to the ventral rami and again, usually L4. Two specimens were observed to have multiple vertical branches that traveled anterior and posterior to the L4 ventral ramus. The ILV and in particular, its vertical branches coursed next to the L4 and L5 vertebrae. For lateral transpsoas approaches, targeting the L4/L5 disk puts the ILV at most risk.

CONCLUSIONS

The spine surgeon performing lateral transpsoas approaches to the lumbar spine needs a good working knowledge of the potential anatomical variations along this pathway. Knowledge of such variants will decrease misdiagnosis and complications at operation.

REFERENCES

Aubert, J., Koumare, K., 1975. Variations of origin of the renal artery: a review covering 403 aortographies. Eur. Urol. 1, 182–188.

Bergman, R.A., Thompson, S.A., Afifi, A.K., 1984. Catalog of Human Variation. Urban & Schwarzenberg, Baltimore, p. 235.

Castellvi, A.E., Goldstein, L.A., Chan, D.P., 1984. Lumbosacral transitional vertebrae and their relationship with lumbar extradural defects. Spine 9, 493–495.

Çiçekcibaşi, A.E., Ziylan, T., Salbacak, A., Şeker, M., Büyükmumcu, M., Tuncer, I., 2005. An investigation of the origin, location and variations of the renal arteries in human fetuses and their clinical relevance. Ann. Anat. 187, 421–427.

Davis, M., Jenkins, S., Bordes, S., Iwanaga, J., Loukas, M., Uribe, J., Hynes, R.A., Tubbs, R.S., 2019. Iliolumbar vein: anatomy and surgical importance during lateral transpsoas and oblique approaches to lumbar spine. World Neurosurg.

Dill, A., Ayaz, U.Y., Karabacak, O.R., Tatar, I.G., Hekimoglu, B., 2012. Study of the left renal variations by means of magnetic resonance imaging. Surg. Radiol. Anat. 34L267-270.

Edsman, G., 1957. Angionephrography and suprarenal angiography; a roentgenologic study of the normal kidney, expansive renal and suprarenal lesions and renal aneurysms. Acta radiologica 1–141. Supplementum.

Hollinshead, W.H., 1982. Anatomy for Surgeons. Harper & Row, Philadelphia.

Jaeger, S.A., 1988. Atlas of Radiographic Positioning: Normal Anatomy and Developmental Variants. Appleton & Lange, Norwalk.

Kincaid, O.W., 1966. Normal Renal Angiogram: Renal Angiography. Year Book Medical Publishers, Chicago.

Konin, G.P., Walz, D.M., 2010. Lumbosacral transitional vertebrae: classification, imaging findings, and clinical relevance. Am. J. Neuroradiol. 31, 1778–1786.

Moore, K.L., Dalley, A.F., 1999. Abdomen. In: Moore, K.L., Dalley, A.F. (Eds.), Clinically Orientated Anatomy, fourth ed. Lippincott, Philadelphia, pp. 174–330.

Oyar, O., Yesildag, A., Malas, M., Gulsoy, U., 2003. Splenodiaphragmatic interposition of the descending colon. Surg. Radiol. Anat. 25, 434–438.

Özkan, U., Oğuzkurt, L., Tercan, F., Kızılkılıç, O., K, Z., KN, 2006. Renal artery origins and variations: angiographic evaluation of 855 consecutive patients. Diagn. Interv. Radiol. 183–186.

Saunders, B., Phillips, R., Williams, C., 1995. Intraoperative measurement of colonic anatomy and attachments with relevance to colonoscopy. Br. J. Surg. 82, 1491–1493.

Skandalakis, J.E., Gray, S.T. (Eds.), 1994. The Peritoneum. Embryology for Surgeons: The Embryological Basis for the Treatment of Congenital Anomalies, second ed. Williams & Wilkins, Baltimore, p. 1101.

Taylor, J.A.M., 2000. Skeletal Imaging: Atlas of the Spine and Extremities. Saunders, Philadelphia.

Unal, B., Kara, S., Aktaş, A., Bilgili, Y., 2004. Anatomic variations of the colon detected on abdominal CT scans. Tani. Girisim. Radyol. 10, 304–308.

Yochum, T.R., 1987. Essentials of Skeletal Radiology. Williams & Wilkins, Baltimore.

FURTHER READING

Atar, M., Hatipoglu, N.K., Soylemez, H., Pendegul, N., Bozkurt, Y., Gumus, H., Sancaktutar, A.A., Kuday, S., Bodakci, M.N., 2013. Relationship between colon and kidney: a critical point for percutaneous procedures. Scand. J. Urol. 47, 122–125.

Bhatnagar, B., Sharma, C., Gupta, S., Mathur, M., Reddy, D., 2004. Study on the anatomical dimensions of the human sigmoid colon. Clin. Anat. 17, 236–243.

Faure, J.P., Richer, J.P., Chansigaud, J.P., Scepi, M., Irani, J., Ferrie, J.C., Kamina, P., 2001. A prospective radiological anatomical study of the variations of the position of the colon in the left pararenal space. Surg. Radiol. Anat. 23, 335–339.

Indrajit, G., Sudeshna, M., Subhra, M., 2012. A redundant loop of descending colon and right sided sigmoid colon. Int. J. Anat. Var. 5, 11–13.

Pinto, A., Brunese, L., Noviello, D., Catalano, O., 1996. Colonic interposition between kidney and psoas muscle: anatomical variation studied with CT. Radiol. Med. 94, 58–60.

Poynter, C.W.M., 1922. Congenital Anomalies in the Arteries and Veins of Man with Bibliography, vol. 22. The University Studies of the University of Nebraska, pp. 1–106.

Prassopoulos, P., Gourtsoyiannis, N., Cavouras, D., Pantelidis, N., 1994. Interposition of the colon between the kidney and the psoas muscle: a normal anatomic variation studied by CT. Abdom. Imaging 19, 446–448.

Ramachandran, I., Rodgers, P., Elabassy, M., Sinha, R., 2009. Multidetector computed tomography of the mesocolon: review of anatomy and pathology. Curr. Probl. Diagn. Radiol. 38, 84–90.

CHAPTER 17

Technique: Lateral Transpsoas Approaches to the Lumbar Spine

ALEXANDER VON GLINSKI • DIA R. HALALMEH • SEONG-JIN MOON • MARC D. MOISI • ROD J. OSKOUIAN

INTRODUCTION

Ever since Dandy described the first surgical treatment for lumbar disc disease in 1929, surgeons have continued to develop new minimally invasive approaches. Love was the first to report his technique of lumbar discectomy through a minimally invasive interlaminar approach without laminectomy in 1939, and it inspired modern microdiscectomy (Love, 1939). With the rise of endoscopic procedures during the 1990s, spine surgeons also adopted endoscopes. Mayer and Brock (1993) described a lumbar discectomy procedure using an endoscope in 1993. Smith and Foley (1998) developed a microendoscopic discectomy system that used tubular retractors to perform disc removal, laminectomy, facetectomy, etc. with direct visualization under an endoscope (Smith and Foley, 1998). Not until the 1970s was a lateral approach described to remove thoracic discs (Maiman et al., 1984). Currently, open approaches are still more commonly used in spine surgeries. Minimally invasive procedures provide the advantages of less trauma to the tissue, less postoperative pain, and faster wound healing. As the field of minimally invasive spine surgery evolves, surgeons continue to develop new surgical approaches. Among these, Ozgur et al. (2006) first described the technique of extreme lateral interbody fusion to approach the lumbar spine.

Patient Selection

Initially, Ozgur et al. included patients who presented with axial low back pain without severe central canal stenosis after having undergone at least 6 months of conservative, traditional nonoperative management. Contraindications included significant central canal stenosis, significant rotatory scoliosis, and moderate to severe spondylolisthesis (Ozgur et al., 2006). At our institution, we use the lateral transpsoas approach for single- or multilevel approaches to intervertebral degenerative spinal disease, for adult degenerative scoliosis (especially in the coronal plane), and for any case where indirect decompression is required. It can be used for corpectomies, intrabody fusions, and anterior column resection. Patients with BMI >30 are especially well-suited candidates. Furthermore, its minimally invasive character particularly benefits patients who are older and often multimorbid.

Patient Positioning

Prior to positioning the patient, the left- or the right-sided approach should be chosen with consideration of the following factors:

1. Previous retroperitoneal surgery
2. Position of iliac crest in relation to the target level. In doubt, preoperative standing bending radiographs are useful
3. Collapsed or open disc space, presence of lateral listhesis
4. Vascular variations that could preclude the approach

In general, we typically choose a left-sided access approach (Fig. 17.1) when all other variables have been accounted for to establish a routine for the operating room staff. A key aspect of successful lateral lumbar interbody fusion (LLIF) surgery is proper initial positioning of the patient, required to maintain safety and provide comfortable access. This is also essential to minimize the number of incisions, to avert injury to neural elements, vascular, visceral, and reproductive tissues, and to optimize cage placement. Implementation of the following strategies will most likely improve patient outcomes. With general endotracheal anesthesia achieved and intravenous lines started, the patient is placed on a radiolucent surgical table in a true 90 degrees right lateral decubitus position with the left side elevated and taped in this position. A cross-table

Surgical anatomy of the lateral transpsoas approach to the lumbar spine. https://doi.org/10.1016/B978-0-323-67376-1.00017-3

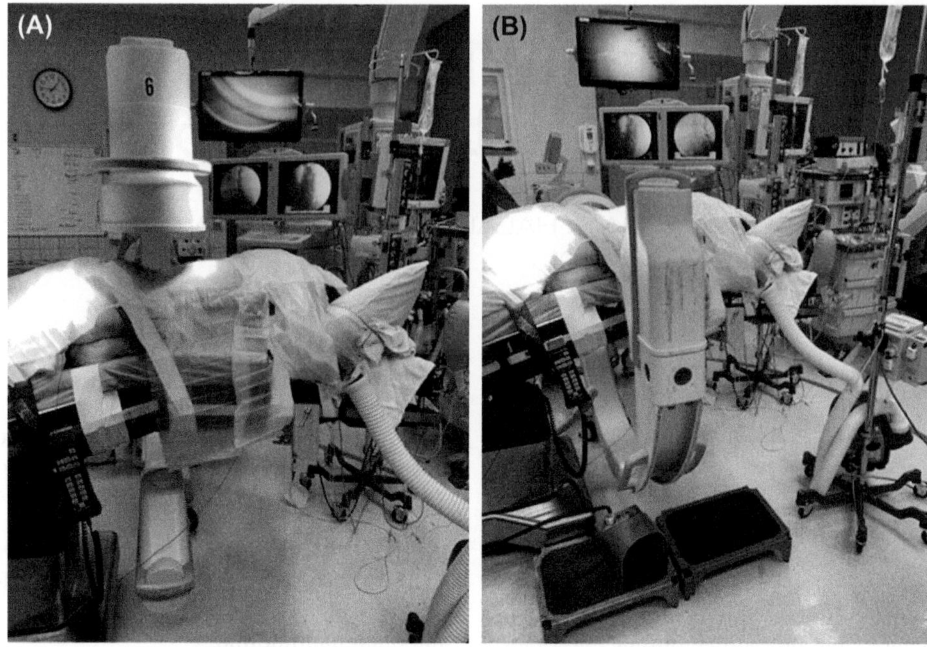

FIG. 17.1 Preoperative C-arm positioning for lateral **(A)** and anteroposterior **(B)** views.

anteroposterior (AP) image helps to confirm the true 90 degrees position.

The lumbar spine should be flexed (Fig. 17.2) so as to increase the distance between the iliac crest and the rib cage, which is especially useful at upper lumbar levels and at L4–L5. Therefore, while the patient is placed in the lateral decubitus position, his or her greater trochanter is placed over or slightly inferior to the table break after electrodes are installed for EMG neuromonitoring. The patient is positioned with at least 20–30 degrees bendable break at its midportion, serving to increase the distance between the iliac crest and inferior costal margin and open intercostal spaces. At times, it is helpful to place a bump/roll under the contralateral flank. Lateral flexion of the lower lumbar levels is then accomplished by slightly breaking the table to 20–30 degrees to achieve easier access to the L1–L5 levels. Additionally, the psoas muscle is relaxed by modestly flexing the hips and the knees (20–30 degrees). Note that overbreaking of the table should be avoided so as not to stretch the lumbar plexus within the psoas muscle. Adhesive tape over the thoracic, subaxillary, and pelvic regions is essential to secure the patient in place and ensure safety. Moreover, an axillary roll should be placed to avert brachial plexus compression, and bony prominences are padded to prevent pressure sores. Arm boards (Fig. 17.2) are also used to suspend the patient's arm securely in the neutral position and to minimize pressure points, with the shoulders and elbows typically flexed to 90 degrees. Once the patient is fixed securely to the operating room table, a fluoroscope (C-arm) is placed anteriorly with the surgeon at the surgical working site posterior to the patient. The iliac crest should be marked. EMG electrodes are placed, and the patient is secured in place using adhesive tape.

The table is rotated as necessary, especially in multilevel cases, to obtain true AP and lateral images of the target disc spaces. The characteristics of true AP images include midline spinous process, symmetrical pedicles that are equidistant from the spinous process, and linear superior endplate (Fig. 17.3). On the lateral view, distinct and linear superior endplates should be seen (Fig. 17.3). The patient must be perpendicular to the plane of the floor, and the C-arm beam should be matched with the lumbar lordosis to ensure good quality of lateral and AP views. The lateral view is obtained when the C-arm is horizontal; the AP view is obtained when the C-arm is vertical. For multilevel cases, subsequent table repositioning and obtaining new AP and lateral orientations for each level are advised owing to variations of anatomy.

The AP and lateral views should be examined meticulously to identify anatomical abnormalities that could impede access to the target disc. For instance, long 11th and 12th ribs could overlie the operative portal, making access to upper lumbar levels very difficult. In this setting, rib segments can be sacrificed, or an intercostal approach is advisable. Nevertheless, a rib-sparing technique has been described, resulting in improved patient outcomes, less postoperative surgical site pain, and earlier discharge (Moisi et al., 2016). Similarly, a high

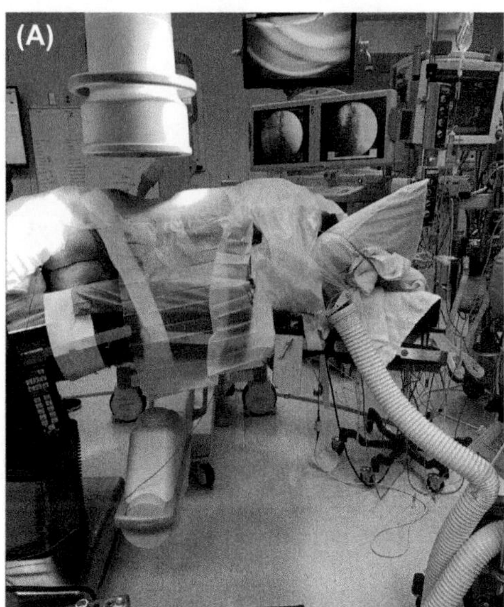

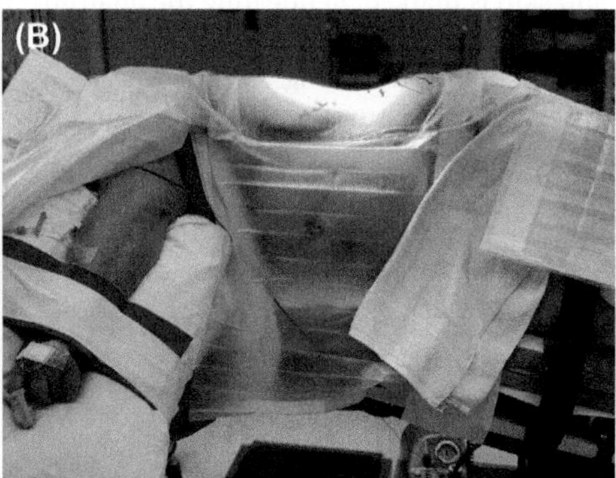

FIG. 17.2 **(A)** The patient is supported and secured in the lateral decubitus position. The pressure points are padded, and the C-arm is positioned anteriorly for the lateral view. Proper positioning of the patient prior to taping and "breaking" the table. The patient is then secured to the table at the following locations: just below the iliac crest and over the thoracic region. **(B)** Patient's arm is suspended using the arm board. Shoulder is elevated 90 degrees, and elbow is extended almost 180 degrees. Pads should be placed especially in the axilla to avoid plexus brachialis injury. Tape should be used to secure the position.

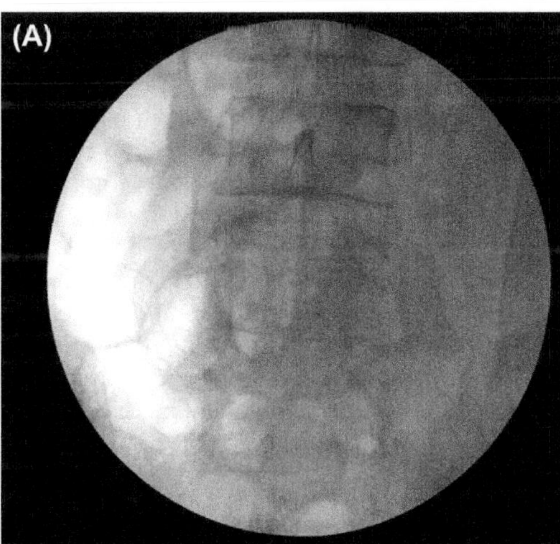

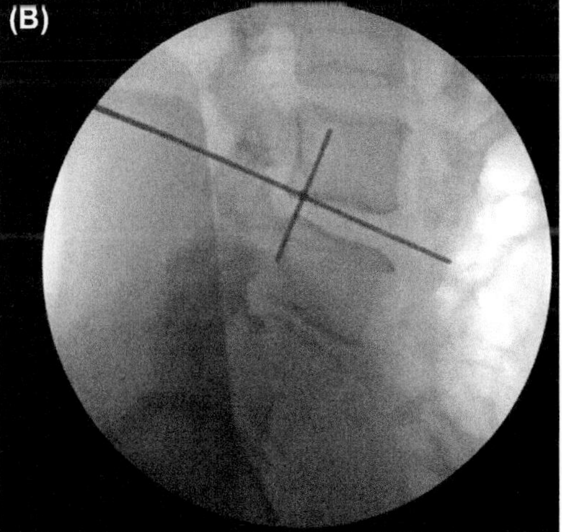

FIG. 17.3 **(A)** Intraoperative anteroposterior (AP) fluoroscopic view. Anterior fluoroscopy should be obtained to ensure the true lateral position of the patient. True AP shows a spinous process that is midway between the two pedicles. Distinguishable superior and inferior endplates should be seen. Notice no "double endplate" shadow. **(B)** Intraoperative lateral fluoroscopic view. Notice no "double pedicle" shadows are seen. The disc space of interest is marked on AP and lateral views.

iliac crest at the L4 or L5 level can obstruct access to lower lumbar disc spaces. In these circumstances, a standing AP image with lateral flexion is highly recommended to establish accessibility to the discs of interest. On the basis of this information, the surgeon determines which side of the patient should be approached. In addition, L4–L5 level can be accessed using an angled retractor into the disc space, avoiding the iliac crest (Fig. 17.4).

Planning and Localization

Under lateral imaging guidance, the target segment is confirmed, and skin is marked, delineating the anatomical orientation of the target disc (anterior and posterior border of the vertebral body, along with its location). Following confirmation of true AP and lateral views, the surgical site is prepared, and the skin is draped in the usual manner. The retractor arm should be mounted posteriorly at the same level as the patient's scapula (Fig. 17.5). Before the incision is made, the number of the levels treated should be taken into account depending on how many levels are to be operated upon.

Opening and Disc Exposure

The incision is typically made from the posterior border toward the anterior border, just past the approximate halfway point. It is essential to maintain the surgical working plane perpendicular to the sagittal plane of the target discs to avoid vascular or neural injury. Two principal incisions determine the technique of the lateral approach: the lateral incision and the posterolateral incision. The latter is typically used for retroperitoneal access, and it is posterior to the direct lateral incision just over the lateral border of the erector spinae muscle. Two techniques, single-incision and two-incision, have been described for gaining access to the psoas muscle. The posterolateral incision is part of the two-incision technique, and it facilitates safe access of the initial dilator to the lateral border of the psoas muscle.

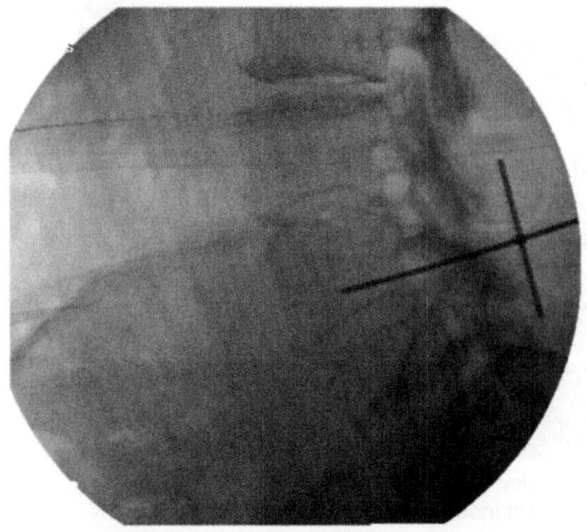

FIG. 17.4 Intraoperative lateral fluoroscopic view. The iliac crest is seen here blocking the view of the L4/L5 disc space.

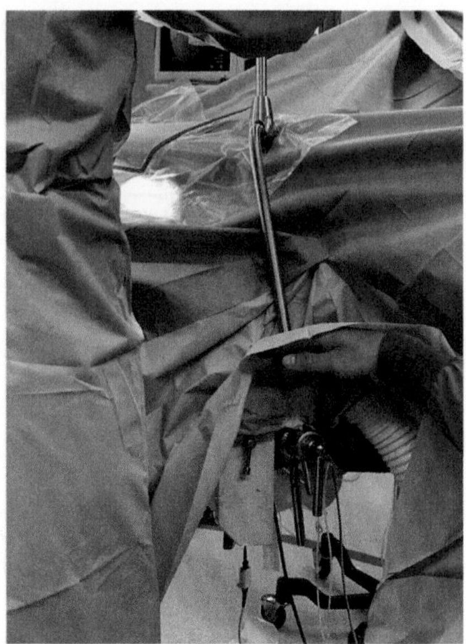

FIG. 17.5 Posterior retractor arm placement.

Two-Incision Technique

Retroperitoneal access can be achieved using the two-incision technique. This involves a posterolateral incision through which the surgeon's index finger guides the initial dilator through the retroperitoneal space to the psoas muscle, taking care not to injure the abdominal contents. While the retroperitoneal content is palpated through the posterolateral incision and before the initial dilator is docked, a gentle sweeping motion of the intraabdominal organs anteriorly and dissection of any remaining fat from the psoas muscle are used to create a safe path for subsequent placement of the dilators and retractor system. The tip of the index finger is then turned upward toward the direct lateral incision to meet the initial dilator and guide its passage down to the lateral surface of the psoas muscle.

One-Incision Technique

Once the skin is marked, a direct lateral incision is sharply made in a fashion parallel to the muscle fibers of the abdominal wall. The incision is carried down through subcutaneous fat layers to the abdominal musculature until the superficial fascia of the external oblique muscle is exposed (Fig. 17.6). At this point, electrocautery should be avoided in the initial incision to preclude injury to the sensitive superficial sensory nerves within the skin. A small self-retaining retractor can be used to facilitate the initial blunt dissection.

The external oblique is then sharply incised, and a Peon clamp is subsequently used to dissect bluntly through fibers of the external oblique, internal oblique, and transversus abdominus muscles (Fig. 17.7). The retroperitoneal fat is exposed after bluntly passing through the transversalis fascia, taking care not to enter the peritoneal cavity.

Index finger palpation is then used to help identify the lateral border of the psoas and quadratus muscles. The surgeon gently sweeps the retroperitoneal fat forward, along with the peritoneal content, by advancing the finger. This allows the peritoneal content to fall forward away from the operative portal. Extreme caution is needed during the single-incision technique when the retroperitoneal space is initially approached. At our institution, we use the single-incision technique.

Neuromonitoring

Comprehension of EMG neuromonitoring enables the surgeon to identify a safe trajectory to the target disc more easily, thereby facilitating a safe passage through the psoas muscle and minimizing the risk to the lumbar plexus (Figs. 17.8 and 17.9). The lumbar plexus is located between the superficial and deep layers of the psoas muscle, the bulk of it lying mostly within the posterior third of the psoas muscle (Ebraheim et al., 1997). Therefore, timely EMG monitoring of the neural elements is essential as the surgeon traverses this muscle.

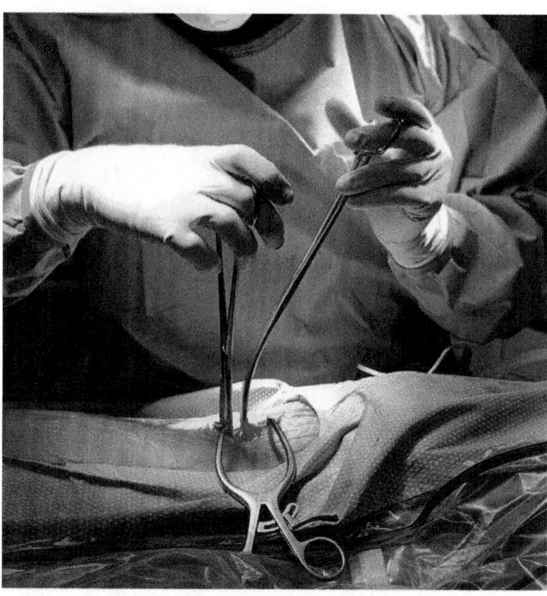

FIG. 17.7 Peon clamps can be used to help the blunt dissection.

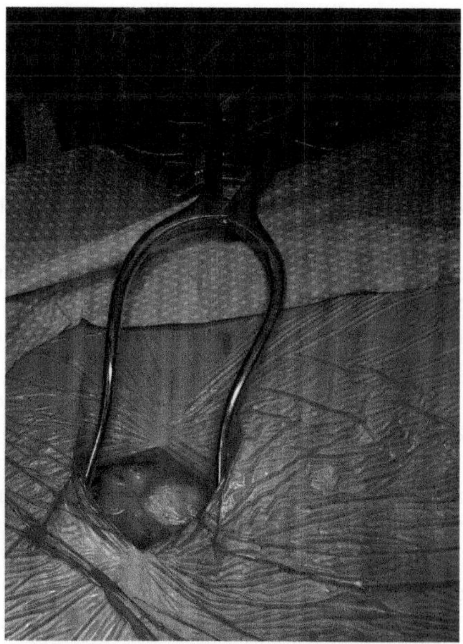

FIG. 17.6 Skin retractor placement after skin incision.

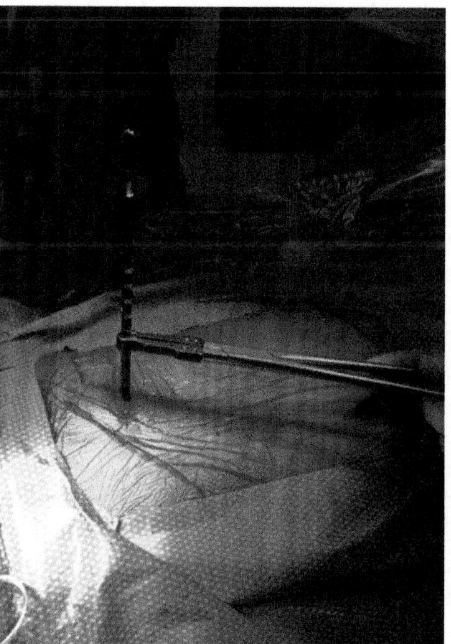

FIG. 17.8 Intraoperative neuromonitoring.

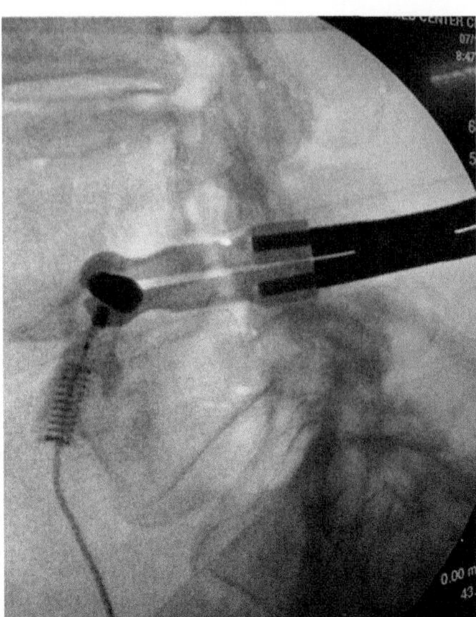

FIG. 17.9 Lateral fluoroscopic image demonstrating the use of neuromonitoring probes to map the lumbar plexus.

The EMG probe should be targeted toward the anterior third of the psoas muscle away from the lumbar plexus, and care should be taken to avoid injuring the vascular structures anteriorly.

Intraoperative "train of four" (TOF) testing is typically performed to ensure that muscle relaxants are not interfering with the EMG monitoring. During TOF testing, four consecutive stimulations with four corresponding responses are observed. The fourth response should be 75% or more of the initial response. Peripheral stimulation is then used to identify nerves within the substance of psoas muscle in relation to the surgical field. The lower the threshold for evoking an action potential, the closer the probe is to a nerve. Subsequent advancement of the EMG probe tip along the psoas muscle down to the disc space is confirmed by fluoroscopy (Berends et al., 2016).

Dilators and Retractor Placement

Three sequential dilators are typically placed, and triggered EMG neuromonitoring is used to ensure adequate distance from the lumbar plexus and a safe plane of dissection (Fig. 17.10). The dilators have stimulating electrodes on their distal ends, providing real-time EMG monitoring during placement through the psoas muscle.

Correct placement of the dilators on the lateral surface of the psoas muscle should be verified by lateral fluoroscopy. Blunt dissection is then carried down along the psoas muscle with real-time EMG neuromonitoring provided by the stimulating electrodes at the tips of the dilators. The trajectory of the dilators should

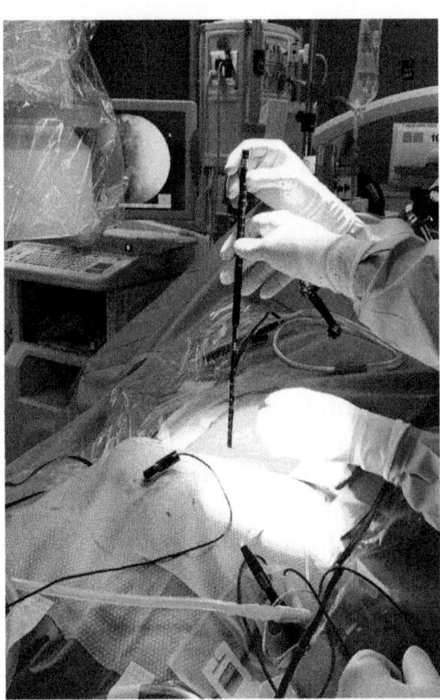

FIG. 17.10 Placing the dilator while continuously monitoring is crucial for preventing approach-related plexus injuries.

target the anterior and, to a lesser extent, the middle third of the psoas muscle to minimize the risk to the lumbar plexus. Again, lateral fluoroscopy is used to ensure optimal placement of the dilators over the junction of middle to posterior thirds of the target disc space. Once proper positioning of the initial dilator is confirmed, a K-wire is inserted under fluoroscopic guidance through the initial dilator and to halfway across the disc space. With the initial dilator resting on the annulus of the disc, a proper blade length of the retractor system can be chosen using the depth marks on the initial dilator at the skin edge (Fig. 17.11).

To allow adequate time for assembling the retractor system, the surgeon should communicate the desired blade length to the scrub technician/nurse while performing sequential dilation. After the last dilator is placed, a table-mounted retractor is docked over the dilators on the junction of the middle and posterior thirds of the target disc, taking care not to expand the blades past the midpoint of the vertebral body to avoid segmental vessel injury. Slow rotating motion is used to advance the retractor through the surgical corridor. The retractor handle should be parallel to the disc space to visualize the monopolar probe and ensure alignment with the C-arm. The retractor is then secured to the operating table, and lateral fluoroscopy is once again used to confirm the correct trajectory and disc space and to ensure proper placement of the retractor over the target disc (Fig. 17.12).

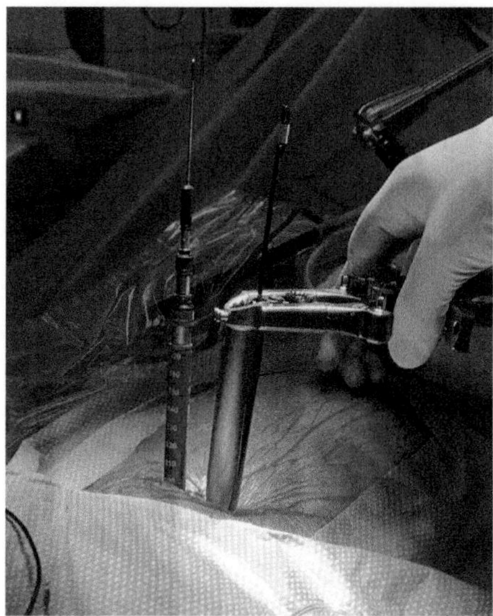

FIG. 17.11 Retractor placement. Retractor length is determined using the last dilator tube as guide. In this case, a 100-mm retractor was chosen.

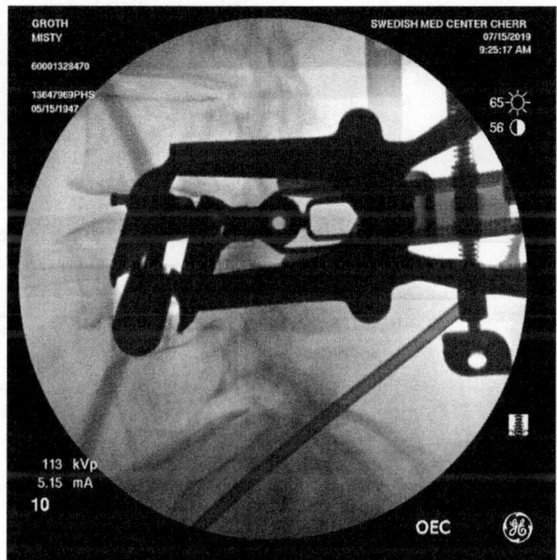

FIG. 17.12 Retractor placement using fluoroscopy. Positioning of the retractor depends on the procedure.

Once the retractor is adjusted to the desired position, the dilators are removed, leaving the K-wire in place. A small amount of soft tissue typically remains at the base of the retractor; therefore, the stimulating probe can be used to check for proximity to neural elements (Fig. 17.13).

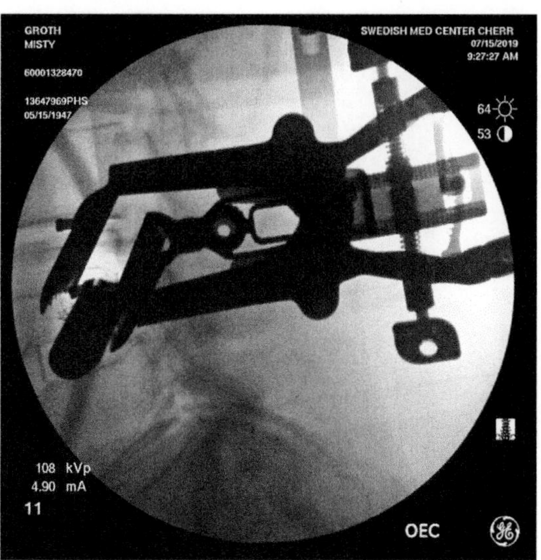

FIG. 17.13 Lateral fluoroscopy showing placement of the retractor over the junction of the middle and posterior thirds of the disc. The retractor blades should not be expanded too far into the posterior third of the disc (where descending nerve roots are at risk) or too far into the anterior border of the vertebral body (where vascular structures are at risk).

When the retractor is in final position, the shim should be placed to keep the posterior blade and retractor from moving (Fig. 17.14). Should it be necessary, bipolar electrocautery must be used cautiously to minimize the risk to nearby nerves. Next, the monopolar EMG probe can secure its position. It should be inserted into the groove of the posterior blade to ensure adequate distance from nearby nerve roots. Once the posterior blade is situated a safe distance from nerve roots, the shim can be deployed, and shim impactors can be inserted until they are flush with the tips of the blades. Posterior intradiscal shim insertion helps to prevent retractor displacement prior to fixing the desired position of the retractor. Shim location is verified using AP fluoroscopy (DiGiorgio et al., 2017) (Fig. 17.14). The authors prefer to use live fluoroscopy along with EMG monitoring to guide appropriate placement of the probes, dilators, and retractors, thereby facilitating quick and accurate docking of the instruments (Fig. 17.15). Consequently, there is less overall radiation exposure than when multiple shots are obtained while advancing cautiously toward the target disc.

Discectomy

Once the anterior border of the disc space is identified, a lateral annulotomy is performed using a bayoneted annulotomy knife (Fig. 17.16). Care must be taken to

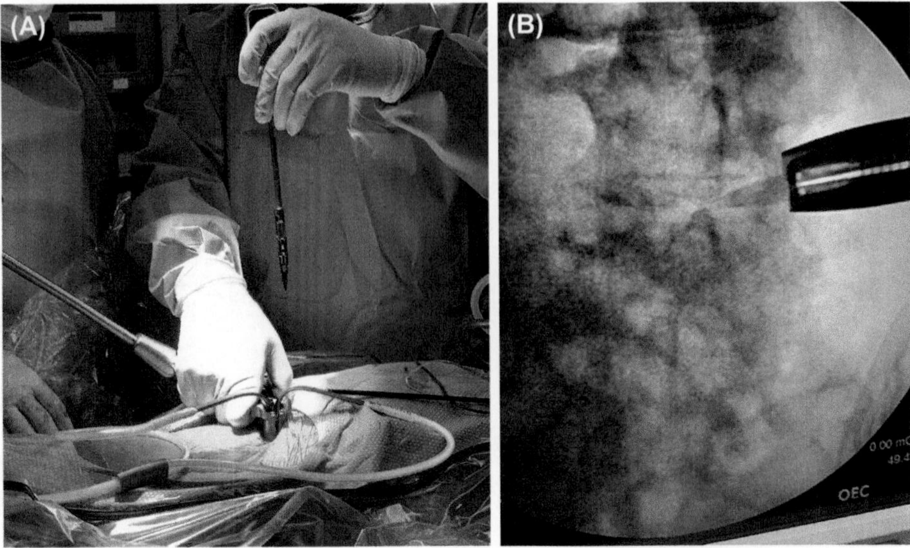

FIG. 17.14 Shim **(A)** and placement under fluoroscopy **(B)**.

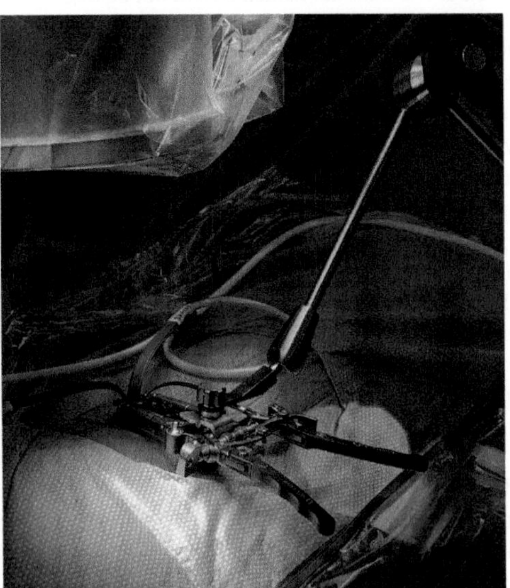
FIG. 17.15 Intraoperative retractor placement.

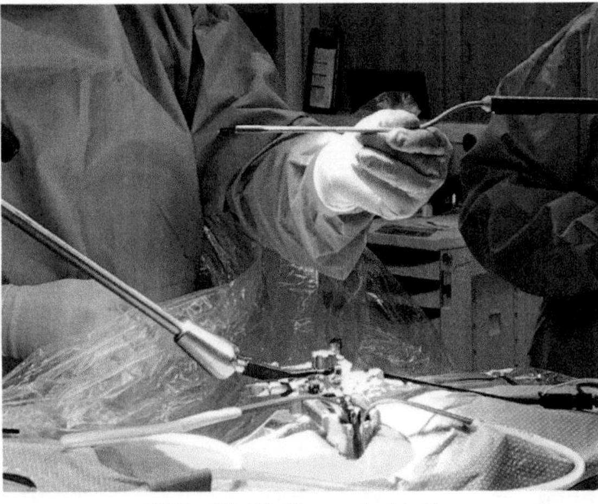
FIG. 17.16 Bayoneted knife.

avoid traversing the anterior longitudinal ligament (ALL) and anteriorly situated vessels and nerves. The annulotomy incision should roughly match the width of the desired implant. Complete discectomy is accomplished using pituitary rongeurs, curettes, and a boxcutter. A blunt intradiscal device (Figs. 17.17 and 17.18) is then used to release the contralateral annulus and disrupt the disc from both endplates. A boxcutter can be used to remove the remaining parts of the disc (Figs. 17.19 and 17.20).

Preservation of the cortical endplates with complete removal of the cartilaginous disc is required for proper and stable implant placement. Therefore, overresection of the endplate should be avoided to minimize the risk of subsidence. However, adequate discectomy and endplate decortication are necessary to restore disc height and reduce the risk of cage subsidence. Each step is performed under fluoroscopic guidance. It is crucial not to shift the patient's position during the procedure unless necessary. Accidental displacement of the patient can lead to nonorthogonal insertion of the instruments and consequent vessel and nerve injury (Berjano et al.,

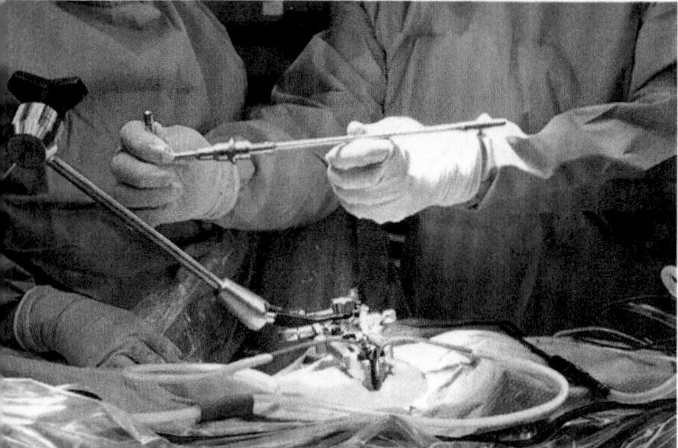

FIG. 17.17 Blunt intradiscal device.

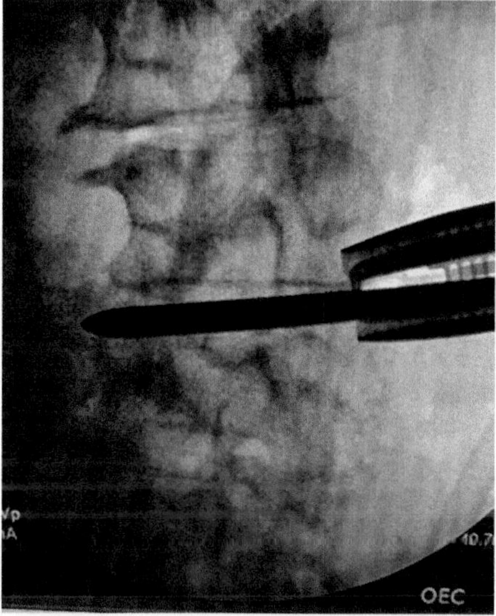

FIG. 17.18 Blunt intradiscal device.

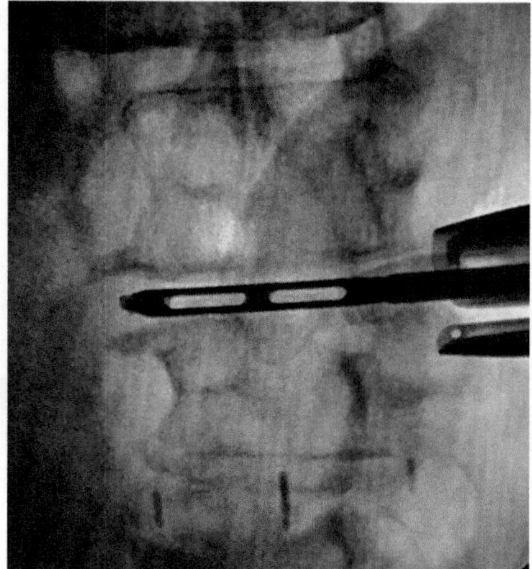

FIG. 17.19 Boxcutter

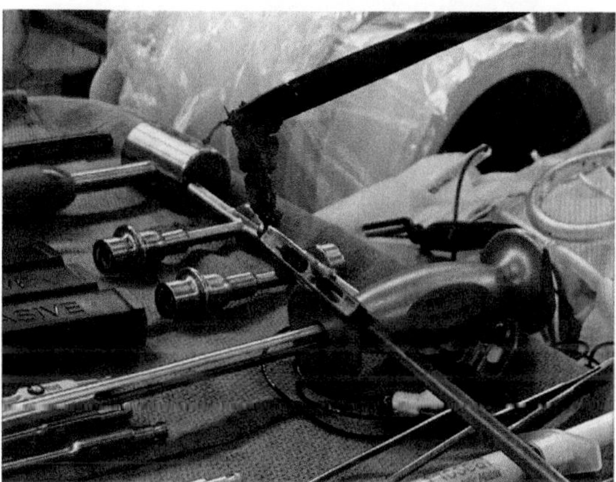

FIG. 17.20 Boxcutter

2015). To prevent intensive bleeding from the endplate, we use Fluroseal, which can be further used to prepare the cage (Fig. 17.21).

Graft Placement

After the disc is completely removed, adequate disc height and foraminal size are restored with trial positioning, and the appropriate size of the interbody implant is determined. Correct placement of the trial is confirmed using biplanar fluoroscopy (Fig. 17.22). Care must be taken not to injure the endplate by oversizing the height of the trial. A slap hammer is then used to assist with removal of trials. Once the proper size of the implant has been identified, the implant is packed with autograft and/or allograft or other synthetic materials, taking care not to overpack it.

The interbody cage is typically porous, so the bone graft can grow through it and fuse with the adjacent vertebral bodies (Figs. 17.23 and 17.24). The implant is attached to the inserter and impacted into the center of the disc space under fluoroscopic guidance and the endplates protected (Figs. 17.25 and 17.26). The interbody spacer can be inserted using grafting slides, which are important for graft containment and protection of the endplates upon graft impaction.

The implant should be always large enough to span the apophyseal ring, which ensures anatomical stability of the implant, solid fusion, and reduced risk of subsidence (Berjano et al., 2015). In addition, the instrument trajectory should always remain perpendicular to the disc space during placement of the implant to avoid

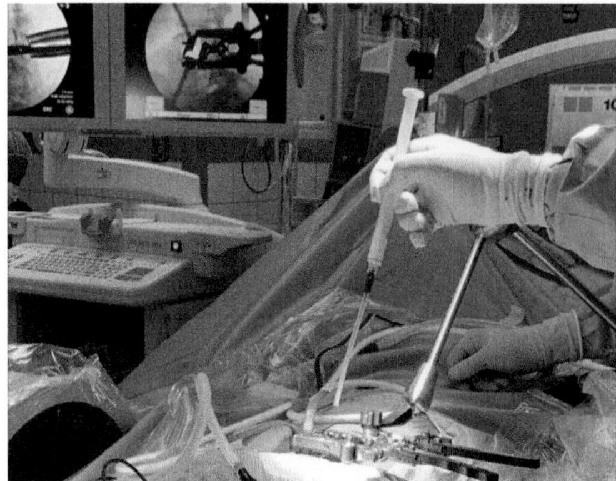

FIG. 17.21 Use of fluroseal.

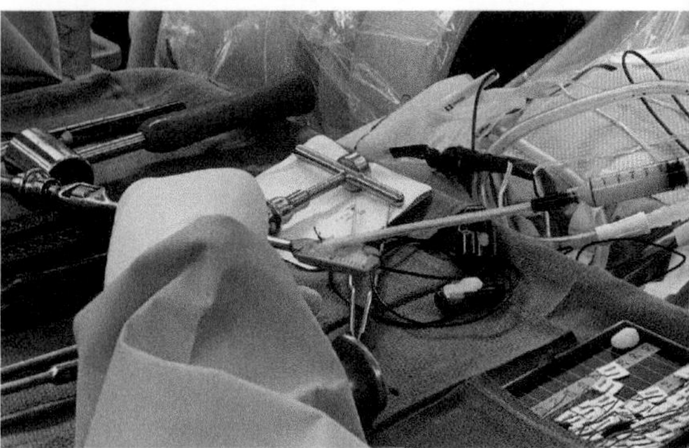

FIG. 17.23 Cage prepped with fluroseal

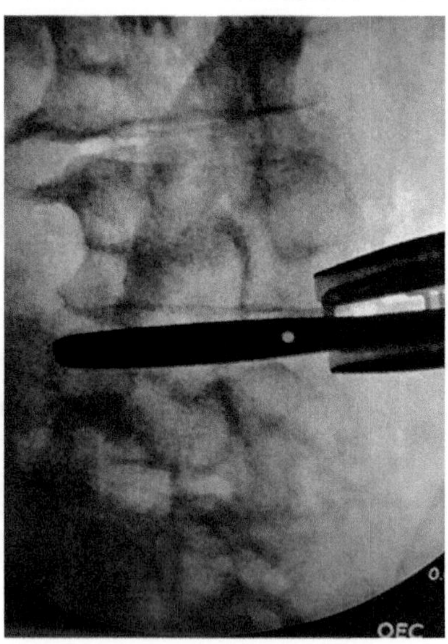

FIG. 17.22 Trial seen on fluoroscopy

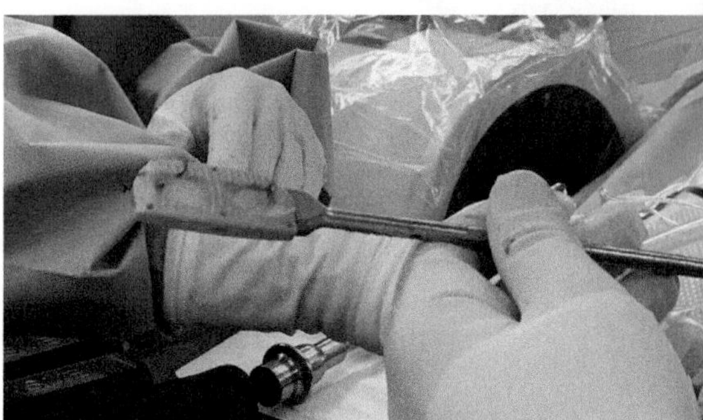

FIG. 17.24 Cage prepped with fluroseal

injury to nearby neurovascular elements and ensure proper placement of the implant. This can be confirmed by an observer with continuous feedback on the surgeon's position and the trajectory plane.

Anterior Longitudinal Ligament Release

In cases where the anterior column needs to be lengthened, the ALL can be released without the need for an open approach, minimizing tissue disruption and morbidity. In terms of a recently published anatomical realignment classification, a stand-alone lateral approach with an ALL would be considered an anterior column realignment (ACR) + Schwab grad 1. A 20

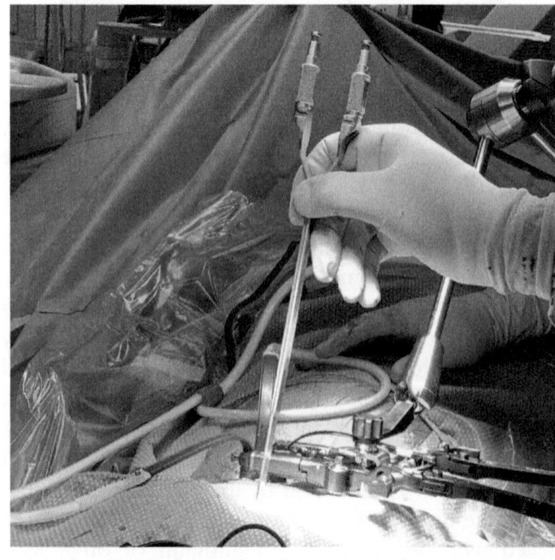

FIG. 17.25 Protecting the endplate from fracture.

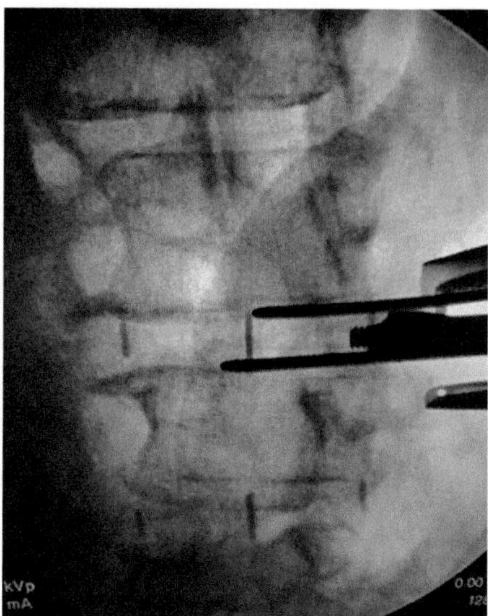
FIG. 17.26 Fluoroscopy

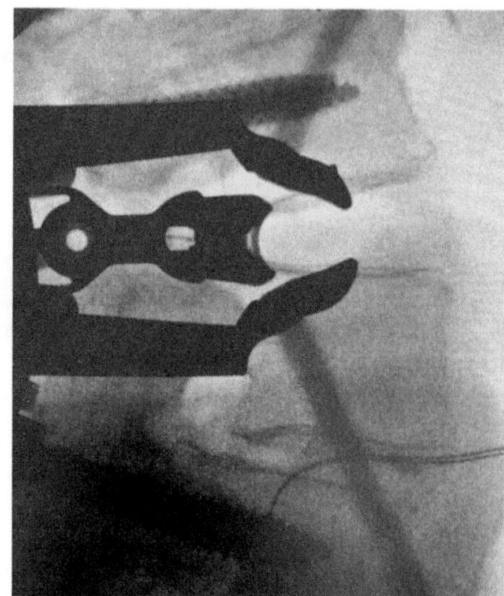
FIG. 17.27 Lateral fluoroscopy with retractor in place.

degrees or 30 degrees hyperlordotic cage is used depending on the amount of segmental lordosis restoration desired and the accessibility of the disc space. Approximately 7.8 degrees of segmental lordosis, with a range of 1–14 degrees, can be gained with a 30 degrees cage (Uribe et al., 2018). This avoids complications that would otherwise occur with spinal osteotomies such as greater decrease in foraminal height and subsequent neural compression and epidural bleeding [9]. In the surgical treatment of kyphotic deformities, discectomies should be performed along with ALL release to ensure anterior release of the spine and correction of the sagittal Cobb angle (Birnbaum et al., 2001). In scoliotic cases, LLIF with posterior percutaneous pedicle screw instrumentation modestly increases the lordosis and provides significant (40%–75%) correction of the coronal curve (Berjano and Lamartina, 2013). When the retractor is placed, the shim blade anchors it into the posterior disc space (Fig. 17.27).

Before the ALL is released, an annulotomy and extensive discectomy should performed, with the surgeon paying careful attention to endplate preparation and preservation. The ALL itself should be sectioned sequentially using a dilator that is brought into the disc space. Complete ALL release can be confirmed by mobilization of the adjacent vertebral body endplates with minimal resistance and further radiological observation of an obvious "fish-mouth" opening of the ventral disc space. After the endplates are prepared (Figs. 17.28 and 17.29), different sizes and angulations can now

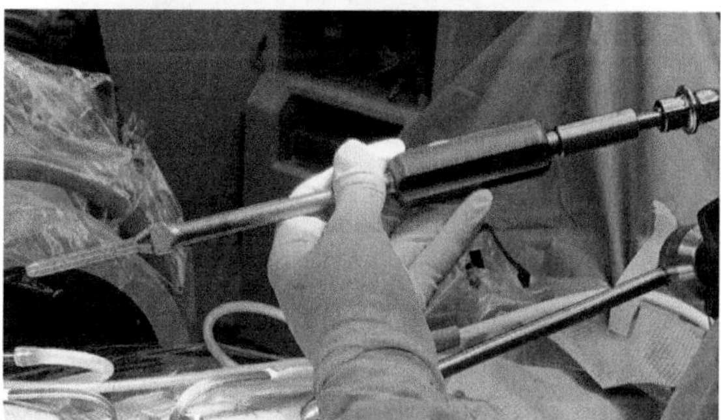
FIG. 17.28 Anterior inderdiscal distractor closed.

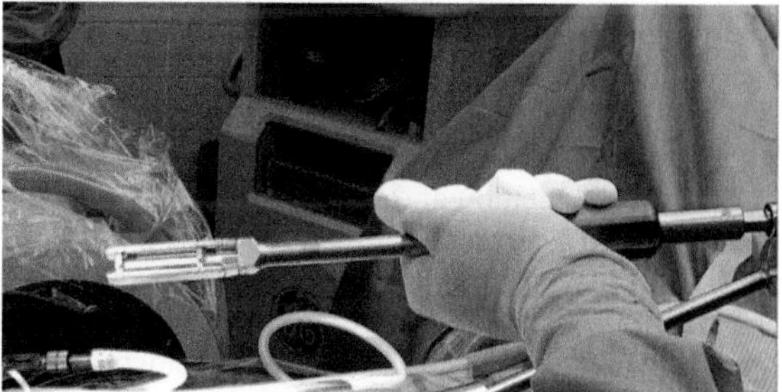
FIG. 17.29 Anterior inderdiscal distractor opened.

be put into the disc space to determine the right size and degree of angulation (Fig. 17.30).

Once selected, an appropriately sized lordotic PEEK (polyetheretherketone) cage with integrated screw fixation can be implanted (Fig. 17.31). If ALL release and fusion with lordotic cages are performed, LLIF should

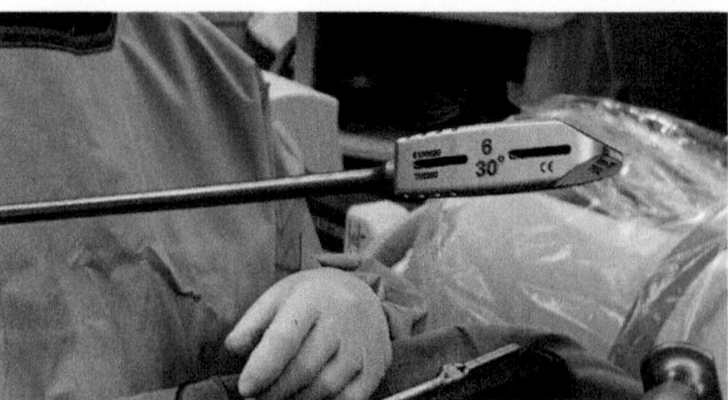

FIG. 17.30 Trial.

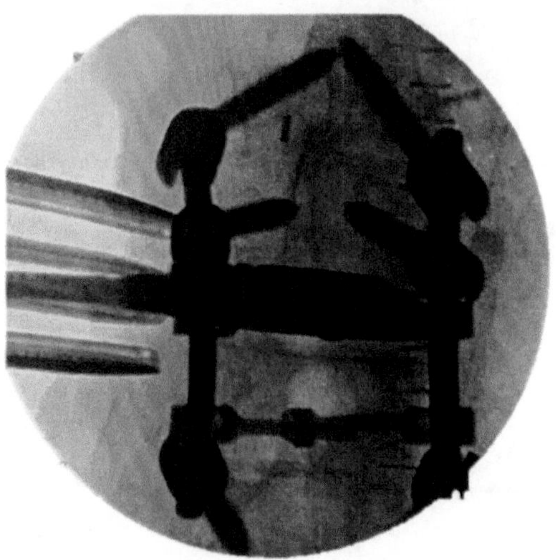

FIG. 17.31 Cage and screw set placement.

be supplemented with pedicle screw fixation to eliminate potential complications such as implant subsidence and to provide significant stability.

Closure

After cage implantation and fluoroscopic confirmation, the shims and light guides are removed. The retractor system is detached, and the blades are removed slowly, watching for any excessive bleeding. Final AP and lateral images are obtained to ensure proper placement of the cage. Hemostasis is achieved via bipolar cautery, and the surgical site is irrigated. The table is unbent, returning the patient to the neutral position. Finally, the fascia over the external oblique is sutured using single Vicryl sutures, followed by closure of the skin and subcutaneous layers.

REFERENCES

Berends, H.I., Journée, H.L., Rácz, I., van Loon, J., Härtl, R., Spruit, M., 2016. Multimodality intraoperative neuromonitoring in extreme lateral interbody fusion. Transcranial electrical stimulation as indispensable rearview. Eur. Spine J. 25 (5), 1581–1586.

Berjano, P., Lamartina, C., 2013. Far lateral approaches (XLIF) in adult scoliosis. Eur. Spine J. 22 (Suppl. 2), S242–S253.

Berjano, P., Damilano, M., Ismael, M., Longo, A., Bruno, A., Lamartina, C., 2015. Anterior column realignment (ACR) technique for correction of sagittal imbalance. Eur. Spine J. 24 (Suppl. 3), 451–453.

Birnbaum, K., Siebert, C.H., Hinkelmann, J., Prescher, A., Niethard, F.U., 2001. Correction of kyphotic deformity before and after transection of the anterior longitudinal ligament–a cadaver study. Arch. Orthop. Trauma Surg. 121 (3), 142–147.

DiGiorgio, A.M., Edwards, C.S., Virk, M.S., Mummaneni, P.V., Chou, D., 2017. Stereotactic navigation for the prepsoas oblique lateral lumbar interbody fusion: technical note and case series. Neurosurg. Focus 43 (2), E14.

Ebraheim, N.A., Xu, R., Huntoon, M., Yeasting, R.A., 1997. Location of the extraforaminal lumbar nerve roots. An anatomic study. Clin. Orthop. Relat. Res. (340), 230–235.

Love, J.G., 1939. Protruded intervertebral disks: with a note regarding hypertrophy of ligamenta flava. Jama 113 (23), 2029–2035.

Maiman, D.J., Larson, S.J., Luck, E., El-Ghatit, A., 1984. Lateral extracavitary approach to the spine for thoracic disc herniation: report of 23 cases. Neurosurgery 14 (2), 178–182.

Mayer, H.M., Brock, M., 1993. Percutaneous endoscopic discectomy: surgical technique and preliminary results compared to microsurgical discectomy. J. Neurosurg. 78 (2), 216–225.

Moisi, M., Fisahn, C., Tubbs, R.S., Page, J., Rice, R., Paulson, D., et al., 2016. Lateral thoracic osteoplastic rib-sparing technique used for lateral spine surgery: technical note. Cureus 8 (7), e668.

Ozgur, B.M., Aryan, H.E., Pimenta, L., Taylor, W.R., 2006. Extreme Lateral Interbody Fusion (XLIF): a novel surgical technique for anterior lumbar interbody fusion. Spine J. 6 (4), 435–443.

Smith, M.M., Foley, K.T., 1998. Micro endoscopic discectomy (MED): the first 100 cases. Neurosurgery 43 (3), 701.

Uribe, J.S., Schwab, F., Mundis, G.M., Xu, D.S., Januszewski, J., Kanter, A.S., et al., 2018. The comprehensive anatomical spinal osteotomy and anterior column realignment classification. J. Neurosurg. Spine 29 (5), 565–575.

FURTHER READING

Dandy, W.E., 1989. Loose cartilage from intervertebral disk simulating tumor of the spinal cord. By Walter E. Dandy, 1929. Clin. Orthop. Relat. Res. (238), 4–8.

CHAPTER 18

Autonomics of the Abdomen

GRAHAM DUPONT • R. SHANE TUBBS

INTRODUCTION

The autonomic nervous system is divided into two parts, the sympathetic and parasympathetic, both of which are governed by upper motor neurons that are derived from the hypothalamus. Upper motor neurons from the anterior hypothalamus govern lower parasympathetic fibers, and neurons from the posterior hypothalamus, sympathetic fibers. These fibers then descend into the brainstem and spinal cord as hypothalamospinal tracts.

In the sympathetic nervous system, the hypothalamospinal tracts travel in the white matter posterolateral to the dorsal horn of the spinal cord to end on neuronal cell bodies within the intermediolateral horns between the first thoracic and first or second lumbar segments. Axons from these spinal cord nuclei travel laterally through the ventral rootlets and enter the sympathetic trunk by way of a white ramus communicans. After entering the sympathetic trunk, they can synapse in a sympathetic ganglion either at their respective spinal level or superior or inferior to that level. After the synapse, postganglionic (postsynaptic) fibers can leave the sympathetic trunk and travel to their visceral target primarily along blood vessels within the body cavities or into the head. Some postganglionic fibers are not distributed to the viscera but instead reenter a spinal nerve segment via a gray ramus communicans to be distributed to smooth muscle (arrector pili), blood vessels, and glands in the skin of the extremities and walls of the body cavities. As the source neurons for the sympathetic system lie primarily within the thoracic spinal cord, it is only here that one finds white rami communicans (T1-L2). In contrast, gray rami communicantes are found at all spinal levels, so postganglionic fibers distributed to the somatic body superior or inferior to the thoracic spinal cord must ascend or descend within the sympathetic trunk. Topographically, the white rami communicans are found slightly lateral to the gray ramus communicans; also, they are generally larger owing to the density of myelinated fibers. Furthermore, white ramus communicantes carry visceral afferent fibers from the body cavities. In the upper lumbar region, the white rami usually ascend obliquely from a given ganglion since they typically arise from a nerve from the next more superior level (Hollinshead, 1956). Gray rami tend to run horizontally or travel only slightly inferiorly from a ganglion to their corresponding nerve segment.

Sympathetic Trunk Ganglia

The sympathetic trunk (Fig. 18.1) can be traced from the skull base to the lowest part of the vertebral column. Its lowest unpaired ganglion, the ganglion impar (ganglion of Walther), joins the two trunks anterior to the coccyx. In the neck, the sympathetic trunks travel posterior to the carotid sheath in a paravertebral location in the thorax just anterior to the costovertebral junction. In the abdomen, after passing posterior to the medial arcuate ligament, these trunks take a more anterior route along the anterolateral aspect of the bodies of the lumbar vertebrae and anterior sacrum, where they are found posterior to the common iliac vessels. There are commonly 3 cervical, 11 thoracic, 4 lumbar, and 4 to 5 sacral ganglia. These ganglia range in size from 6 mm to 6 cm (Hollinshead, 1956). The most constant and usually the largest of them is located on the second lumbar vertebra. The lumbar segments of the sympathetic trunks pass between the psoas major and inferior vena cava on the right side and between the psoas major and aorta on the left (Fig. 18.2). The sacral segment of the sympathetic trunk conveys two or three branches (sacral splanchnics) to the inferior hypogastric plexus, which will be discussed later. Other branches of the lumbosacral sympathetic trunk include vascular, osseous, and articular twigs (Woodburne and Burkel, 1988).

Sympathetic Splanchnic Nerves

To reach the abdomen, preganglionic splanchnic nerves from the thoracic sympathetic trunks descend through

Surgical anatomy of the lateral transpsoas approach to the lumbar spine. https://doi.org/10.1016/B978-0-323-67376-1.00018-5

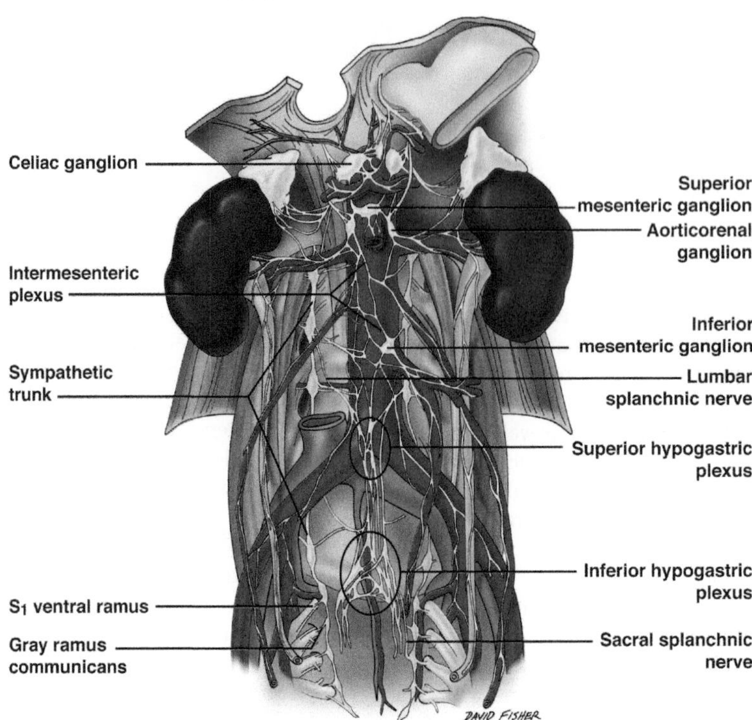

FIG. 18.1 Schematic drawing of the autonomic nerves of the retroperitoneum. Note the sympathetic splanchnic nerves (not labeled) and posterior trunk of the vagus nerve (not labeled) entering into the celiac ganglia.

the diaphragm to synapse in preaortic (prevertebral) ganglia. The greater splanchnic nerve, arising from segments T5 to T9, terminates on the celiac ganglia; the lesser splanchnic nerve, arising from segments T10–T11, terminates on the celiac or aorticorenal ganglia; and the least (lowest) splanchnic (if present) derived from T12 terminates on the aorticorenal ganglia. There is a fourth, or accessory, splanchnic nerve in 4% of cases with a course and termination similar to the least splanchnic nerve (Hollinshead, 1956). The preaortic plexus formed by the aforementioned ganglia and nerves (derived from both sympathetic and vagal fibers and both visceral sensory and visceral motor neurons) progresses inferiorly and anterior to the descending abdominal aorta. Preganglionic branches of the sympathetic trunk that exit directly without synapsing are known as lumbar and sacral splanchnics. These branches contribute to the formation of the intermesenteric plexus, inferior mesenteric plexus, and superior hypogastric plexus, which are the distal prolongation of the preaortic plexus inferior to the bifurcation of the descending abdominal aorta. Some authors have found that the S2 ganglion provides most of the sacral splanchnic branches (Baader and Herrmann, 2003). Some of the lumbar splanchnics, especially the more inferior branches, tend to travel posterior to the common iliac arteries. It should be emphasized that the term splanchnic (referring to the viscera) does not indicate whether a nerve is pre- or postganglionic. Although the sympathetic splanchnics of the abdomen and pelvis are indeed preganglionic, the splanchnics superior to T5 that travel primarily to the heart and lungs are postganglionic.

Parasympathetic Pathways—Vagus Nerve

As indicated by the term "craniosacral outflow," the central neuronal cell bodies of the parasympathetic nervous system are found in the brainstem and sacral spinal cord. Four cranial nerves have brainstem nuclei that participate in the parasympathetic system; only the vagus nerve will be considered in this review as it is the only participating parasympathetic nerve that travels to the abdomen. Generally, it provides parasympathetic fibers to the entire abdomen, stretching to a

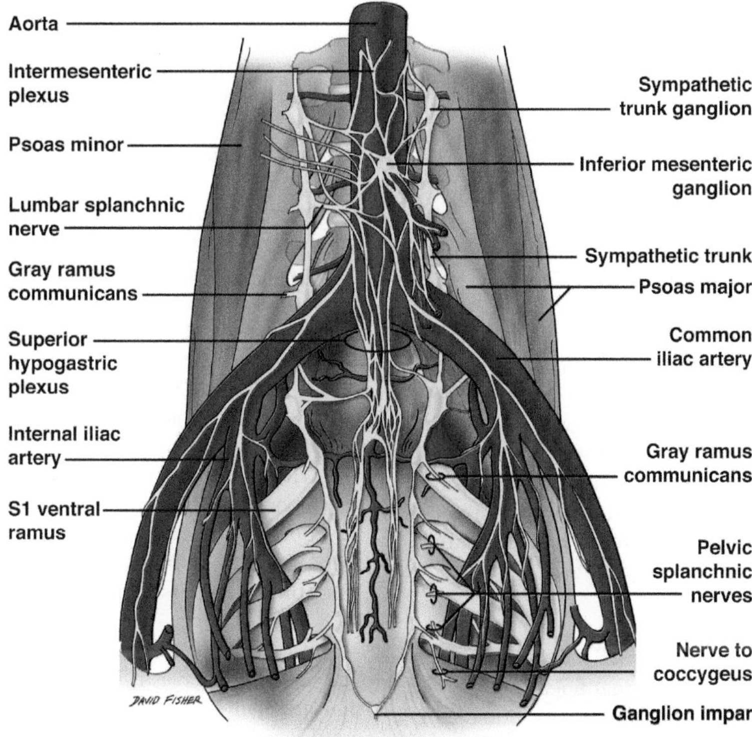

FIG. 18.2 Lower aspect of the abdominopelvic cavity noting the autonomic nerves in this area and their relationship to the aorta and common iliac arteries.

point approximated by the splenic flexure of the colon. These fibers arise from the brainstem, specifically the dorsal motor nucleus of the medulla oblongata. Interestingly, most vagus nerve fibers are sensory not motor. The vagus nerve descends within the neck as a component of the carotid sheath and after entering the thorax traverses the mediastinum posterior to the hila of the lungs. The left vagus nerve forms a plexus anterior to the esophagus while the right portion forms a plexus posterior to it. The vagus nerves are then reconstructed near the diaphragm as the anterior and posterior vagal trunks. These two vagal trunks traverse the esophageal hiatus together with the esophagus and intermingle with sympathetic ganglia in this region such as the celiac ganglion. Subsequent to the emergence of the trunks within the abdomen, the vagal and sympathetic fibers become indistinguishably variegated. The anterior trunk travels primarily to the hepatic plexus that serves the liver, its associated ducts, and the stomach. The posterior trunk (Fig. 18.1) sends a large branch into the celiac plexus with distal branches to the gastrointestinal tract proximal to the splenic flexure and to the pancreas, spleen, and kidneys. There is no synapsing of vagal nerve fibers within the abovementioned sympathetic ganglia because the vagus nerve synapses with enteric ganglia (submucosal or Meissner's plexus, and intramuscular or Auerbach's plexus) near or on its target organs. Visceral afferent fibers of the vagus nerve have their origin cells in the nodose ganglion near the skull base and terminate in the solitary nucleus (Crosby et al., 1962).

Parasympathetic Pathways—Pelvic Splanchnic Nerves

The sacral portion of the parasympathetic nervous system is found within segments S2-S4 of the spinal cord. These neuronal cell bodies are found in a location comparable to the intermediolateral horn of the thoracic and upper lumbar spinal cord. Postganglionic fibers of these neurons supply the pelvis and abdomen approximately distal to the splenic flexure. These nerves, also known as the pelvic splanchnics (Fig. 18.2) or nervi erigentes (erotic), are seen soon after their emergence from the anterior sacral foramina (S2—S4) and give rise to 3—10 branches. It is important to note that most of these fibers are located in the S3 spinal nerve.

AUTONOMIC PLEXUSES OF THE ABDOMINOPELVIC REGION

Phrenic Plexus

This collection of nerves, derived from branches of the celiac ganglia and vagus nerves, travels with the inferior phrenic arteries and is disseminated alongside those vessels to the diaphragm, parietal peritoneum, suprarenal gland, inferior vena cava, esophagus, and gastroesophageal junction (Hollinshead, 1956). The right phrenic plexus communicates at the foramen of the vena cava with the right phrenic nerve and there is a small (phrenic) ganglion at this location (Woodburne and Burkel, 1988). Fibers from the left side communicate with the esophagus, and on both sides, fibers from the celiac ganglion communicate with the phrenic nerve. In addition to supplying the aforementioned structures, branches are also sent to the suprarenal plexus. The branches of the phrenic plexus destined for the suprarenal gland are preganglionic.

Celiac Plexus

This plexus is formed by fibers derived from thoracic sympathetic splanchnic nerves, vagal fibers, and the celiac ganglia (Fig. 18.1). Subsidiaries of it include the hepatic, left gastric, gastroduodenal, and splenic plexuses. It should be noted that this plexus is not simply the nerve fibers associated with the celiac artery but rather the plexus in the region of the celiac, superior mesenteric, and renal arteries. Thus, this collection of fibers lies anterior and lateral to the aorta and anterior to the crura of the diaphragm. The celiac ganglia are typically covered anteriorly on the right by the inferior vena cava. The celiac plexus is distributed primarily to foregut derivatives such as the liver, spleen, and stomach.

Superior Mesenteric Plexus

The superior mesenteric plexus is the largest offshoot of the celiac plexus and is a continuation of its inferior part. This mesh of sympathetic and vagal fibers lies on the anterior surface of the aorta at the level of the superior mesenteric artery. Its ganglia (Fig. 18.1) can be fused to the celiac ganglia so that the two cannot be distinguished. This plexus becomes less dense as it follows the superior mesenteric artery to the derivatives of the midgut such as the small intestine, cecum, appendix, and ascending and transverse colon.

Suprarenal Plexus

Branches of the celiac plexus and ganglion, phrenic and greater splanchnic nerves donate to the suprarenal plexus, which in turn sends its fibers principally to the medullary portion of the suprarenal gland. These branches are described as much larger than others relative to the size of the organ that is supplied.

Renal Plexus

This plexus is a lateral prolongation of the celiac plexus and derives most of its fibers from the aorticorenal ganglia and least splanchnic nerves. Postganglionic fibers are derived from the celiac ganglion, and most preganglionic fibers are derived from T11 to T12 (L1). This plexus interdigitates with the plexuses of the suprarenal glands and ovaries. The aorticorenal ganglia are found near this region at the junction of the left and right renal arteries with the aorta. Small renal ganglia are often found along the posterosuperior aspect of the renal artery. There are communications between the renal and suprarenal plexuses and also with the ureteric plexus (see below). Parasympathetic fibers to the renal plexus are derived from the vagus nerve, and they reach the renal plexus by passing through the celiac plexus.

Ureteric Plexus

This plexus of nerves is derived from both the abdominal and pelvic regions. Fibers to its upper segments are derived from the renal, intermesenteric, and superior hypogastric plexuses. The nerve supply to its lower segments is from the inferior hypogastric plexus and is associated with innervation of the urinary bladder. Segmentally, sympathetic fibers to the ureteric plexus are derived from the T11 to L2 levels of the spinal cord. Preganglionic vagal fibers reach the ureteric plexus via the celiac plexus and, in at least its inferior one-third, synapse on ganglia in the wall of the ureter.

Ovarian Plexus

The ovarian plexus is closely associated with the ureteric plexus and receives branches from many of the same sources. This collection of nerves travels with the ovarian vessels. The parasympathetic input to it is from the vagus nerve; however, fibers can also be derived from the inferior hypogastric plexus (Crosby et al., 1962). Sympathetic fibers reach the ovary from the T10 to T11 spinal levels. Postganglionic fibers arise either from cells in the ovarian ganglion at the origin of the ovarian artery or from neurons in the celiac and renal plexuses (Crosby et al., 1962). The ovarian plexus is distributed to the ovary, broad ligament, and oviduct and communicates with the uterine plexus. The fibers along the oviduct are termed the plexus of Jacques. Intraovarian ganglion cells (ganglion of Elis) can be scattered along the ovarian plexus. Winterhalter (1896) described a sympathetic ganglion of the ovary.

Intermesenteric Plexus

These fibers (Fig. 18.1) are found on the aorta between the superior and inferior mesenteric plexuses and are directly continuous with more proximal preaortic nerve fibers, the nerve plexuses along the renal and ovarian arteries and the nerve plexus along the proximal ureter. Each of these plexuses contains small ganglia (Baljet and Drukker, 1981).

Inferior Mesenteric Plexus

This plexus consists of nerve strands and minute ganglia. Its distal prolongation, reinforced by lumbar splanchnic nerves, becomes the superior hypogastric plexus inferior to the aortic bifurcation. Some authors believe that pelvic splanchnic fibers (parasympathetic) travel backward from the inferior hypogastric plexus to the inferior mesenteric plexus to be distributed to the hindgut (i.e., descending colon, sigmoid colon, and rectum). The superior rectal plexus is a continuation of the inferior mesenteric plexus along the superior rectal artery. These fibers supply the lower portion of the sigmoid colon and rectum.

Superior Hypogastric Plexus

The superior hypogastric plexus (presacral nerve or plexus of Hovelacque) (Figs. 18.2 and 18.3) is a retroperitoneal structure, fixated anterior to the aortic bifurcation, bounded by left common iliac vein, median sacral vessels, fifth lumbar vertebrae, sacral promontory, and common iliac arteries. Authors and texts have referred to this plexus as the presacral nerve; however, not only is it usually not a single nerve, having complicated meshwork in the pelvis, it is also prelumbar. The superior hypogastric plexus is found within the extraperitoneal connective tissue along the midline, and slightly leftward. It is formed from branches of the aortic plexus (sympathetic and parasympathetic), and lumbar splanchnic (sympathetic) nerves, and pelvic splanchnic (parasympathetic) nerves that project upward from the inferior hypogastric plexus via the hypogastric nerves. Visceral afferent nerves also traverse the superior hypogastric plexus. The intermediate portion of the ureteric plexus is formed from contributions of the superior hypogastric plexus and hypogastric nerve, usually penetrating the muscular coat of the uterus or accompany blood vessels to the adventitia. The superior hypogastric plexus supplies innervation to the pelvic wall of the rectum and internal anal sphincter, by way of following the inferior mesenteric and superior rectal arteries. The plexus also supplies parts of the perineum. This parasympathetic supply inhibits the rectal muscles and facilitatory to internal anal sphincter tone, thus providing resistance to defecation.

The superior hypogastric plexus is most often plexiform in appearance, though there are deviations from plexiform appearance. The plexus may be formed

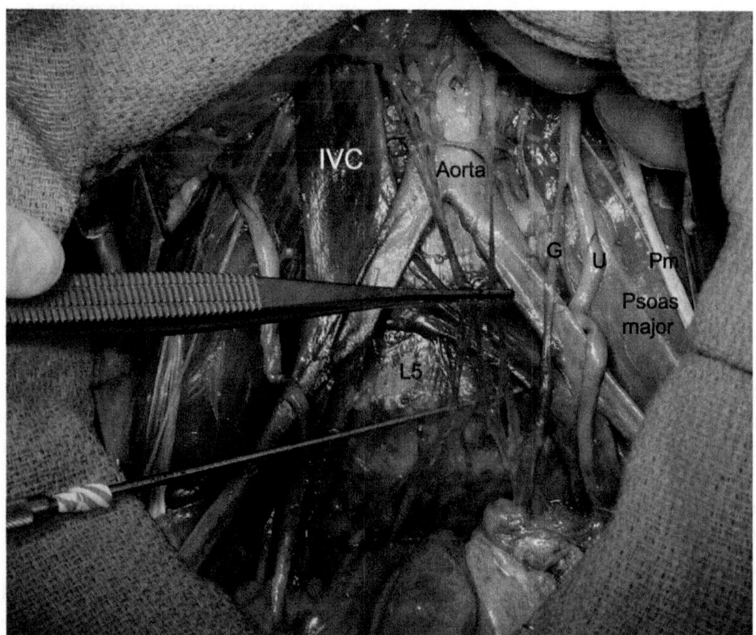

FIG. 18.3 Cadaveric dissection of the superior hypogastric plexus (held with forceps and running over probe. Note the inferior vena cava (IVC) and fifth lumbar vertebra (L5). On the left side, the gonadal vein (G), ureter (U), and psoas minor (Pm) are seen.

from a singly thin, rounded nerve; a wide plexiform morphology; a broad, bandlike trunk with scattered nerve bundles; and two distinct nerves in close proximity to one another.

Type I

This variation (17.14%) appears as a single, thin rounded, nerve. Paraskevas et al. (2008) refer to this nerve in their study as the *presacral* nerve; however, in the current text its contemporary denomination, the *prelumbar* nerve, will be used. The prelumbar nerve forms below the abdominal aortic bifurcation, traverses the left side of the body, anterior to left common iliac vein, and subsequently bifurcates into respective two hypogastric nerves. This nerve maintains close proximity to the superior rectal artery and peritoneum along its course.

Type II

This variation (28.57%) appears in the classical plexiform arrangement covering the area between the common iliac arteries.

Type III

This variation (22.85%) is a broader, quadrated, thicker trunk with nerve bundles intermingled with connective tissue. This trunk usually extends from the abdominal aorta bifurcation to the sacral promontory.

Type IV

This variation (31.44%) appears as two nerves that run alongside one another before separating. These two nerves run medially at the level of the fifth lumbar vertebrae and separate laterally at the first sacral vertebrae and then separate.

Though the superior hypogastric plexus is said to be bounded by the sacral promontory, a significant number of specimen (37.14%; $n = 35$) had the plexus extend up to 12.3 mm beyond the sacral promontory. The plexus may be situated as close as 6.1 mm to the right of the midline, be as wide as 41.2 mm, and as long as 98 mm (Paraskevas et al., 2008). Delmas (1928) examined the configuration of the superior hypogastric plexus and found that the superior hypogastric plexus consistently received branches from the third and fourth sympathetic ganglion. The plexus is derived from three roots, two lateral and one intermediate, the former being from the pelvic visceral nerves, the latter being a continuation of the abdominal aorta plexus. Argentino (1934) describes one type of superior hypogastric plexus in which there were three distinct roots covered by a fibrous connective sheath. Savas (1958) dissected 126 cadavers, male and female, and found a common nerve trunk in 63.5% of specimen; thin striplike trunk in 23.8%; and a wide plexiform configuration in 12.7%. Furthermore, Savas (1958) was one of the first to assert that firstly that the presacral nerve was prelumbar and that it does not in fact exist and is simply a part of the superior hypogastric plexus. Paraskevas (2008) also located sympathetic fibers stemming not only from the lumbar region but also from thoracic sympathetics through the celiac plexus.

EJACULATORY DISORDERS FROM LUMBAR INTERBODY FUSIONS

Male sexual function is governed by the superior hypogastric plexus, allowing for normal sperm transit through innervation of the smooth muscle of the ductus deferens and seminal vesicle. Sympathetic innervation of the male structures from the plexus allows for contraction of the smooth muscle of the genital tract resulting in the emission of semen. Reflux of semen into the bladder is prevented by simultaneous sympathetic stimulation of urethral proximal muscles and sphincteric closure of the neck of the bladder (Paraskevas et al., 2008). Approaches to the spine for lumbar interbody fusion surgery result in noticeable incidence of retrograde ejaculation. Lindley et al. (2012) notes that while anterior lumbar interbody fusion (ALIF) has gained popularity, retrograde ejaculation occurred in 7.4% of patients undergoing ALIF, and 9.8% undergoing artificial disc replacement. Sasso et al. (2003) reported an incidence of retrograde ejaculation following ALIF ranging between 0.42% and 5.9%. The incidence of retrograde ejaculation may be lowered by using retroperitoneal exposure of the L4-L5 and L5-S1 disk spaces, as opposed to the transperitoneal approach which was reported to result in a 10 times higher incidence of retrograde ejaculation (Sasso et al., 2003). Accessing the disk space and vertebral bodies through the retroperitoneal tissue requires avoidance of the great vessels, lumbosacral plexus, while also paying close attention to avoiding the superior hypogastric plexus. Cutting through tissue without careful blunt dissection may sever the connections between the superior hypogastric plexus and the seminal vesicles, ductus deferens, and other pelvic ejaculatory structures, and subsequently result in ejaculatory disorders.

Inferior Hypogastric Plexus

The inferior hypogastric plexus (Fig. 18.1) is formed from the fusion of the superior hypogastric plexus, pelvic splanchnics, and sacral splanchnics incorporated with visceral afferent fibers. It is located at the level of the ductus deferens and terminal pelvic ureter. It subsequently follows the posterolateral aspect and passage of the seminal vesicle (Drizenko et al., 2003). Some authors have reported a contribution of S1-S5 spinal nerves to the inferior hypogastric plexus. However, Baljet and Drukker (1981) found that most nerve fibers entering this plexus from the sacral nerves arise from the S3 ventral rami. In women, transection of the uterosacral ligaments can result in disruption of most of the hypogastric fibers (Maas et al., 2005). Most of this plexus is found at the level of the inferior vesical vessels, so it does not reach inferiorly to the pelvic floor (Fritsch, 1989). Frankenhäuser (1866) described a ganglion at the lateral side of the cervix within the inferior hypogastric plexus, and Lee (1841) had probably referred to the same structure over two decades earlier. The sympathetic fibers in the inferior hypogastric plexus are vasomotor, motor to smooth muscle sphincters, and inhibitory to peristalsis. In men, the inferior hypogastric plexus is described by Röthlisberger et al. (2018) as spreading in a fanlike pattern; dorsally, these nerves carry parasympathetics toward the sacral plexus via the splanchnic nerves; dorsomedially, branches are sent to the rectum; ventrally, there are branches to the bladder, seminal vesicles, prostate, and urethra. The inferior hypogastric plexus also provides a pelvic nerve branch to the rhabdosphincter. Most afferent pain fibers from the pelvis return to the CNS along sympathetic pathways. The cervix, vagina, trigone of the bladder, and rectum are exceptions to this rule; pain fibers from those areas travel along parasympathetic pathways (S2–S4). Moszkowicz et al. (2011) found that the intersection of the ureter with the posterior wall of the uterine artery precisely located the junction of the hypogastric nerve and inferior hypogastric plexus and that anteroinferior branches to the sexual organs originated from the anteroinferior angle of the inferior hypogastric plexus and were concentrated in the posterolateral wall of the vagina.

Subdivisions of the Inferior Hypogastric Plexus

The subdivisions of the inferior hypogastric plexus can be named according to either the organs they supply or the vessels that accompany them. These divisions intercommunicate freely so their names are arbitrary.

Uterovaginal plexus

This extension of the inferior hypogastric plexus is located against the supravaginal portion of the cervix on either side of the uterus. The autonomic fibers within this plexus are primarily vasomotor and are referred to as the lateral nerves of Latarjet and Rochet (1922). As stated previously, the uterine part of this plexus communicates with the ovarian plexus. The uterovaginal plexus is found just lateral to the uterosacral ligaments as they attach to the uterus.

Some of its fibers travel with the uterine vessels and not through the uterosacral ligaments. There are many of these fibers in the cardinal ligament medial to the uterine artery. The inferior branches of this plexus (e.g., cavernous nerves) are distributed to the vaginal wall, erectile tissue of the vestibular bulbs, the greater vestibular glands, and the erectile tissue of the clitoris and are therefore important in the female's sexual response. Preganglionic sympathetic fibers arise from the T10 to L2 levels of the spinal cord. The fimbria, ampulla, and ovary receive their nerve supply from the ovarian plexus (T10 to T11). The nerve supplies to the remainder of the oviduct and uterus are derived from levels L1 and L2. The vagina receives its sympathetic innervation by way of the uterovaginal plexus, but its afferent pain fibers travel with parasympathetic fibers from the pelvic splanchnic nerves (S2-S4). The lowest part of the vagina receives somatic afferent innervation from branches of the pudendal nerve. Pelvic splanchnic fibers to the vagina synapse in the cervical ganglion. Potentially, afferent fibers from the uterus reach the spinal cord by way of the 10th through 12th thoracic nerves and first lumbar nerve.

Vesicoureteric plexus

The urinary bladder receives direct branches from the inferior hypogastric plexus and indirect fibers traveling along the ureter and inferior vesical artery (Baader and Herrmann, 2003). The uterovaginal and vesicoureteric plexuses intermingle to varying degrees. The vesicoureteric plexus to the urinary bladder travels via the vesical blood vessels and contains small ganglia (Baljet and Drukker, 1981), which have been excised in patients with hypersensitive bladder disorders such as interstitial cystitis (Gillespie, 1994). The parasympathetic innervation of the urinary bladder results in contraction of the detrusor muscle, thereby serving the emptying reflex. The sympathetic nervous system supplies the smooth muscle of the trigone and the regional blood vessels. Sensory information is conducted along both the sympathetic and parasympathetic nerves, but pain due to overdistension is carried primarily by the sympathetic system (Woodburne and Burkel, 1988). Once the bladder is full (sensed by the visceral afferent fibers within this plexus), the smooth muscle in its dome (detrusor) contracts, thereby increasing intravesical pressure. Next, the somatic innervation of the pelvic diaphragm and external urethral sphincter by the pudendal nerve (perineal branch) enable this muscle to be relaxed so that urine can be expelled through the urethra.

Middle rectal plexus

This offshoot of the posterior part of the inferior hypogastric plexus is formed from four to eight nerves, often along the middle rectal artery to the rectum, and provides the rectum with sympathetic and parasympathetic innervation. The inferior hypogastric plexus also sends direct branches to this plexus. Some authors have stated that the rectum only receives motor innervation from parasympathetic fibers. Afferent pain fibers from the rectum travel with parasympathetic fibers (S2-S4).

Cavernous plexus

These are extensions of the inferior hypogastric plexus out to the erectile tissue of the female and pelvic floor and prostate of the male. Some authors have stated that the cavernous nerves are derived entirely from the vaginal plexus. However, the cavernous nerves in the female are derived not from the vaginal plexus but rather from the most inferior fibers of the inferior hypogastric plexus (Baader and Herrmann, 2003). These fibers innervate the corpora cavernosa by penetrating the urogenital diaphragm (Lepor et al., 1985). Stimulation of these fibers results in clitoral engorgement, vaginal lengthening, and increased vaginal flow (Crosby et al., 1962). In males, the cavernous nerves arise from the anteroinferior border of the inferior hypogastric plexus and travel tangentially to the posterolateral aspect of the prostate. These fibers then cross the pelvic floor in front of the prostatic apex and superior surface of the cavernous body (Drizenko et al., 2003).

Visceral pain pathways of the abdominopelvic region

Visceral afferents (slow conducting fibers) tend to predominate in parasympathetic nerves, but there are fewer of them in sympathetic nerves. For example, 90% of the fibers in the vagus nerve are sensory compared with 20% in the greater splanchnic nerve. However, pelvic visceral pain returns to the spinal cord primarily via the sympathetic nervous system (e.g., sacral splanchnics, superior hypogastric plexus, ureteric plexus, and ovarian plexus). This is the mechanism underlying the success of presacral neurectomy for the relief of dysmenorrhea. Intraperitoneal structures are said to reside above the "pelvic pain line," and afferent pain fibers from these structures travel along sympathetic nerves. Subperitoneal structures are said to lie below the "pelvic pain line," and afferent pain fibers from this region travel along parasympathetic nerves (S2–S4). For example, pain from the cervix, vagina, vesical trigone, and rectum returns to the cord via the pelvic splanchnics. Visceral pain that utilizes the pelvic splanchnic nerves (S2–S4) is known not to enter via the dorsal roots of these spinal nerves but rather through ventral roots (Hardy and Naftel, 2002). By entering through the ventral roots, these visceral pain fibers have less contact with somatic afferent fibers so there is less referred pain. Some authors have also stated that pain fibers from the ovary, distal oviduct, and uterus can travel with the ureteric plexus, which includes vagal nerve fibers. However, others have argued that the vagus nerve within the abdominopelvic region does not convey pain information because its brainstem relay center (solitary nucleus) does not convey information to the thalamus and cortex, so its information does not reach the level of consciousness (Hardy and Naftel, 2002). Evidence for pain fibers that are conveyed by the vagus is found in some women who continue to have menstrual cramping following spinal cord transection (Crosby et al., 1962). Further evidence for this pathway lies in the ability of women to experience orgasm following complete spinal cord transection. Visceral pain fibers terminate primarily on the lateral edge of the gray matter of the spinal cord close to the intermediolateral cell column. This is in contrast to somatic afferents, which terminate primarily in the medial parts of the dorsal gray matter (Hardy and Naftel, 2002). In general, sympathetic afferent fibers from the liver, spleen, pancreas, and stomach travel to cord segments T6 through T9; from the ileum and jejunum to segments T8 to T12; from the suprarenal gland to segments T6 to L2; from the kidneys to segments T10 to L1; and from the colon to segments T8 to S2. The upper portion of the proximal vagina is said to be almost insensitive (Crosby et al., 1962).

REFERENCES

Argentino, A., 1934. Riceche morfologiche sul cosideto "nervo presacrale". Anat Bericht 28, 7.

Baader, B., Herrmann, M., 2003. Topography of the pelvic autonomic nervous system and its potential impact on surgical intervention in the pelvis. Clin. Anat. 16, 119–130.

Baljet, B., Drukker, J., 1981. Some aspects of the innervation of the abdominal and pelvic organs in the human female fetus. Acta Anat. 111, 222–230.

Crosby, E.C., Humphrey, T., Lauer, E.W., 1962. Correlative Anatomy of the Nervous System. The Macmillan Company, New York.

Delmas, J., Laux, G, 1928. Constitution, forme et rapports du nerf prèsacrè. Anat Bericht 12 (1928), 420.

Drizenko, A., Goullet, E., Mauroy, B., Demondion, X., Bonnal, J.-L., Biserte, J., Abbou, C., 2003. The inferior hypogastric plexus (pelvic plexus): its importance in neural preservation techniques. Surg. Radiol. Anat. 25 (1), 6–15.

Frankenhäuser, I., 1866. Nerven der weiblichenGeschlechtorgane. Jena Ztschr.

Fritsch, H., 1989. Topography of the pelvic autonomic nerves in human fetuses between 21–29 weeks of gestation. Anat. Embryol. 180, 57–64.

Gillespie, L., 1994. Destruction of the vesicoureteric plexus for the treatment of hypersensitive bladder disorders. Br. J. Urol. 74, 40–43.

Hardy, G.P., Naftel, J.P., 2002. Viscerosensory pathways. In: Haines, D.E. (Ed.), Fundamental Neuroscience. Churchill Livingstone, New York, pp. 293–302.

Hollinshead, W.H., 1956. Anatomy for Surgeons: The Thorax, Abdomen, and Pelvis, vol. 2. Hoeber Harper, New York.

Latarjet, A., Rochet, P., 1922. Le plexus hypogastrique chez la femme. Gyn. Obs. 6, 225–243.

Lee, C., 1841. The anatomy of the nerves of the uterus. Philos. Trans. 14, 34–54.

Lepor, H., Gregerman, M., Crosby, R., Mostofi, F.K., Walsh, P.C., 1985. Precise localization of the autonomic nerves from the pelvic plexus to the corpora cavernosa: a detailed anatomical study of the adult male pelvis. J. Urol. 133, 207–212.

Lindley, E.M., McBeth, Z., Henry, S.E., Burger, E.L., Cain, C.M., Patel, V.V., 2012. Retrograde ejaculation following anterior lumbar spine surgery. The Spine Journal 12 (9), S135.

Maas, C.P., Kenter, G.G., Trimbos, J.B., Deruiter, M.C., 2005. Anatomical basis for nerve-sparing radical hysterectomy: immunohisto- chemical study of the pelvic autonomic nerves. Acta Obstet. Gynecol. Scand. 84, 868–874.

Moszkowicz, D., Alsaid, B., Bessede, T., Penna, C., Benoit, G., Peschaud, F., 2011. Female pelvic autonomic neuroanatomy based on conventional macroscopic and computer-assisted anatomic dissections. Surg. Radiol. Anat. 33, 397–404.

Paraskevas, G., Tsitsopoulos, P., Papaziogas, B., Natsis, K., Martoglou, S., Stoltidou, A., Kitsoulis, P., 2008. Variability in superior hypogastric plexus morphology and its clinical applications: A cadaveric study. Sur. Radio. Anat. 30 (6), 481–488.

Röthlisberger, R., Aurore, V., Boemke, S., Bangerter, H., Bergmann, M., Thalmann, G.N., Djonov, V., 2018. The anatomy of the male inferior hypogastric plexus: what should we know for nerve sparing surgery. Clin. Anat. 31 (6).

Savas, A., 1958. Contribution in presacral nerve study. In: Proceedings of the Aristotle University of Thessaloniki, vol 2, pp. 283–297. Greece.

Sasso, R.C., Burkus, J.K., LeHuec, J.C., 2003. Retrograde ejaculation after anterior lumbar interbody fusion: Transperitoneal versus retroperitoneal exposure. Spine 28 (10), 1023–1026.

Winterhalter, E., 1896. Ein sympathisches ganglion immenschlichen ovarium. Arch. Gynak 51, 1–49.

Woodburne, R.T., Burkel, W.E., 1988. Essentials of Human Anatomy, eighth ed. Oxford University Press, New York.

FURTHER READING

Carter, J.E., 1998. Surgical treatment for chronic pelvic pain. J. Soc. Laparoendosc. Surg. 2, 129–139.

Perry, C.P., 2000. Peripheral neuropathies causing chronic pelvic pain. J. Am. Assoc. Gynecol. Laparoscopists 7, 281–287.

Pollitt, C.I., Salota, V., Leschinskiy, D., 2011. Chemical neurolysis of the superior hypogastric plexus for chronic noncancer pelvic pain. Int. J. Gynaecol. Obstet. 114, 160–161.

CHAPTER 19

The Abdominal Aorta

MISHAN LISTMANN • R. SHANE TUBBS

INTRODUCTION

The abdominal part of the aorta (Fig. 19.1) begins at the diaphragm's aortic hiatus anterior to the 12th thoracic vertebra. The abdominal aorta has anterior, lateral, and posterior branches. The bifurcation level is at the fourth lumbar vertebra or the intervertebral disc between the fourth and fifth lumbar vertebrae, slightly to the left of the midline (Mirjalili et al., 2012), and the angle of bifurcation varies (Moussallem et al., 2012) (Fig. 19.2). The results of computed tomography have revealed that the mean adult diameter of the aorta inferior to the renal arteries' origin is 16–18 mm in females and 19–21 mm in males (Rogers et al., 2013;

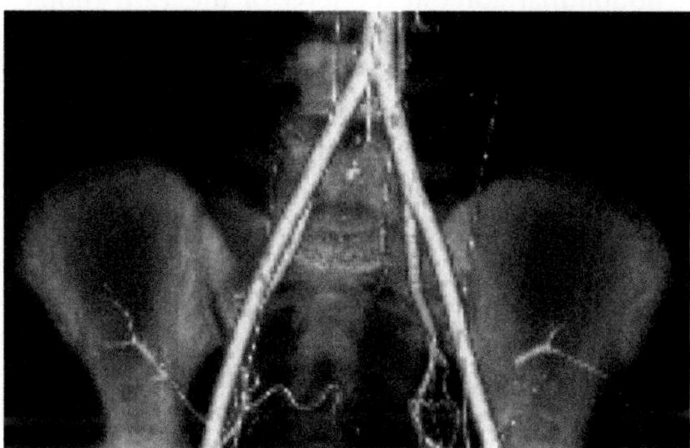

FIG. 19.2 CT angiography noting the aortic bifurcation.

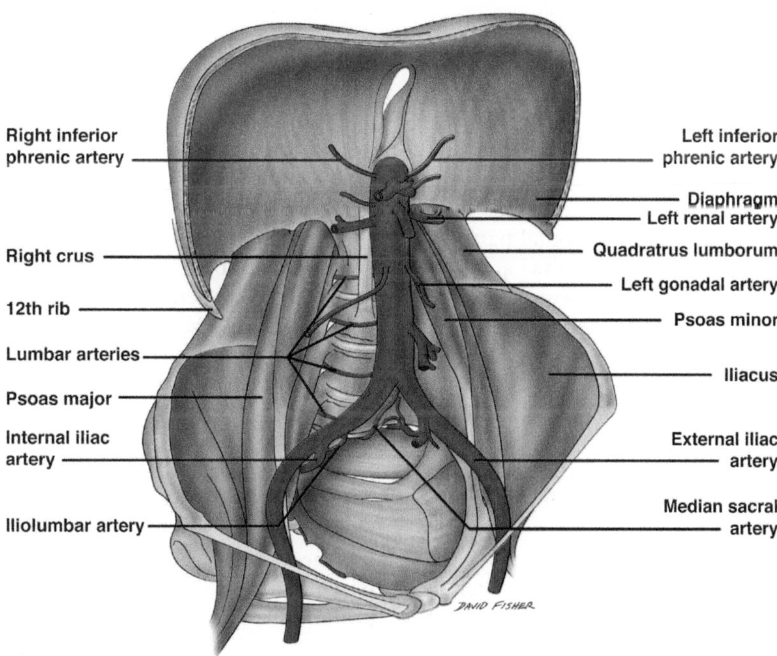

FIG. 19.1 Schematic view of the abdominal part of the aorta and its branches. The three midline visceral arteries are not labeled, but from top-down are the celiac trunk, superior mesenteric artery, and inferior mesenteric artery.

Surgical anatomy of the lateral transpsoas approach to the lumbar spine. https://doi.org/10.1016/B978-0-323-67376-1.00019-7

Jasper et al., 2014). The mean caliber declines slightly from distal to proximal. Frequently, the abdominal aorta becomes ectatic and tortuous in the elderly.

This chapter is meant as a review of the basic anatomy of the abdominal part of the aorta and its branches. Such anatomical knowledge is important for the lateral transpsoas spine surgeon.

Celiac Trunk

The celiac trunk (Fig. 19.1) arises most commonly from the abdominal aorta at the level of the 12th thoracic vertebra just inferior to the aortic hiatus and supplies the foregut's structures. It is 1–3 cm long and passes nearly horizontally anterior and slightly to the right superior to the splenic vein's body and the pancreas. Usually, it trifurcates into the left gastric, common hepatic, and splenic arteries. Several variations can occur: the celiac trunk can give rise to the superior mesenteric artery or one or both of the inferior phrenic arteries. Furthermore, the abdominal aorta can give rise to the left gastric artery, which normally is a branch of the celiac trunk (Panagouli et al., 2013) to which the omental bursa lies anterior. The celiac plexus surrounds the celiac trunk, and in rare cases, the median arcuate ligament (Dunbar syndrome) can compress the celiac trunk (Ho et al., 2017).

Superior Mesenteric Artery

The superior mesenteric artery (Fig. 19.1) originates approximately 3 cm distal to the celiac trunk at the level of the body of the first lumbar vertebra (Mirjalili et al., 2012). This artery supplies midgut structures and courses caudally and anteriorly over the pancreas' uncinate process and the duodenum's horizontal part. The left renal vein separates it from the aorta, and it is located posterior to the pancreas' body. Several anatomical variations have been described (Tubbs et al., 2016).

Inferior Mesenteric Artery

The inferior mesenteric artery (Fig. 19.1), which has a smaller diameter compared with the superior mesenteric, originates at the third lumbar vertebra approximately 3–4 cm proximal to the aorta's bifurcation.

Suprarenal Arteries

The two middle suprarenal arteries proceed laterally over the diaphragm's crua to the suprarenal gland, where it anastomoses with the ipsilateral inferior phrenic and renal arteries' suprarenal branches (Toni et al., 1988). The right middle suprarenal artery travels posterior to the inferior vena cava near the right celiac ganglion, and the left middle suprarenal artery travels near the left celiac ganglion, the pancreas' superior border, and the splenic artery.

Renal Arteries

The renal arteries (Fig. 19.1) arise perpendicularly from the aorta just inferior to the superior mesenteric artery's origin from the aorta at approximately the level of the first lumbar vertebra (Mirjalili et al., 2012). The right renal artery is the longer of the two and runs posterior to the inferior vena cava, right renal vein, the pancreas' head, and the duodenum's descending part. In contrast, the left renal artery courses behind the left renal vein, the pancreas' body, and the splenic vein. The renal arteries vary frequently in their origin, course, and branching patterns.

Gonadal Arteries

The gonadal arteries (Fig. 19.1) are two long, slender vessels that arise from the aorta slightly inferior to the renal arteries and travel distally in close proximity to the ureter and genitofemoral nerve to supply the ovaries and testicles.

Inferior Phrenic Arteries

Normally, the inferior phrenic arteries (Fig. 19.1) branch from the aorta just superior to the celiac trunk at the level of the 12th thoracic vertebra or originate from the celiac trunk directly. Occasionally, they can originate from the renal arteries (Loukas et al., 2005; Gwon et al., 2007), and they supply the diaphragm's inferior surface. Before they divide into ascending and descending branches, each artery ascends laterally, anterior to the diaphragm's crus near the ipsilateral suprarenal gland's medial border. The left ascending branch passes posterior to the esophagus and bifurcates anteriorly on the esophageal hiatus' left side. One of the branches courses anteriorly to the diaphragm's central tendon and forms an anastomosis with its counterpart, whereas the other branch helps supply the thoracic wall together with the musculophrenic and pericardiacophrenic arteries. The right ascending branch courses posterior to the inferior vena cava before it bifurcates;

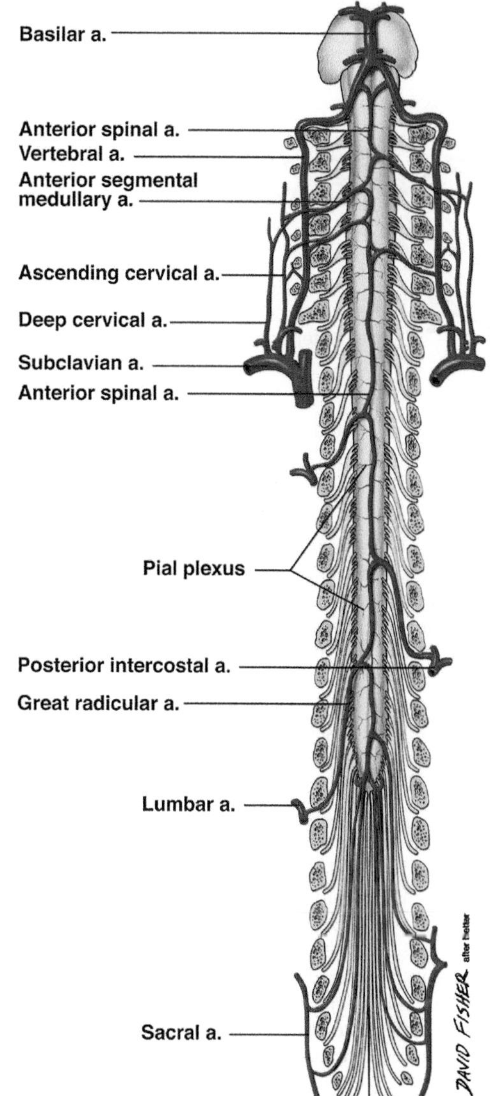

FIG. 19.3 Schematic drawing of the arterial blood supply to the spinal cord and indicated the great radicular artery.

one branch runs on the diaphragm's inferior aspect, whereas the other anastomoses with its counterpart anterior to the diaphragm's central tendon. Two or three small superior suprarenal arteries arise from the inferior phrenic artery.

Lumbar Arteries

In series with the posterior intercostal arteries, the aorta gives rise usually to four lumbar arteries from its dorsal surface on each side (Fig. 19.1). Occasionally, a fifth, smaller pair of lumbar arteries emerges from the median sacral artery, but the iliolumbar arteries provide these frequently. The lumbar arteries pass posterior to the sympathetic trunk and tendinous arches; the psoas major's attachments to the vertebral bodies form posterolateral from the first to the fourth lumbar vertebral bodies. The right lumbar arteries travel posterior to the inferior vena cava. The first left lumbar artery and the superior two right lumbar arteries rest behind the diaphragm's corresponding crus. Just beyond the intervertebral foramina, each lumbar artery divides into a medial branch that gives off ganglionic and spinal branches: a middle branch, from which anastomotic and dorsal branches arise, and a lateral branch, which provides blood to the abdominal wall (Arslan et al., 2011).

The spinal branch referred to as the great radicular artery (of Adamkiewicz) originates frequently from an upper lumbar artery, particularly on the left side (Biglioli et al., 2004), and its injury can lead to spinal cord infarction with resultant neurological compromise (Figs. 19.3 and 19.4).

The lumbar arteries' lateral branches course between the internal abdominal oblique and transversus abdominis by passing posterior to the psoas major and anterior to the quadratus lumborum to supply the posterior abdominal wall's muscles and skin. The lumbar arteries join the lower posterior intercostal, subcostal, iliolumbar, deep circumflex iliac, and inferior epigastric arteries to form an anastomosis that supplies the back muscles, vertebrae and their joints, and the skin of the back.

Median Sacral Artery

Most commonly, the median sacral artery (Fig. 19.1) arises from the aorta's posterior aspect slightly above its bifurcation and descends near the midline toward the coccyx. As mentioned above, it can give rise to the fifth lumbar artery.

CONCLUSIONS

The anatomy of the aorta in the abdomen and its major branches is very important to the retroperitoneal spine surgeon.

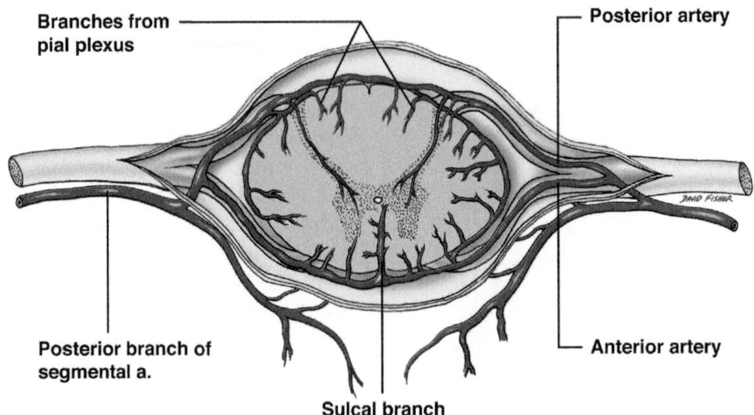

FIG. 19.4 Axial section of the spinal cord noting the arterial blood supply to the internal aspect of the spinal cord. Compare with Fig. 19.3.

REFERENCES

Arslan, M., et al., 2011. Surgical view of the lumbar arteries and their branches: an anatomical study. Neurosurgery 68, 16–22.

Biglioli, P., et al., 2004. Upper and lower spinal cord blood supply: the continuity of the anterior spinal artery and the relevance of the lumbar arteries. J. Thorac. Cardiovasc. Surg. 127, 1188–1192.

Gwon, D.I., et al., 2007. Inferior phrenic artery: anatomy, variations, pathologic conditions, and interventional management. RadioGraphics 27, 687–705.

Ho, K.K.F., et al., 2017. Outcome predictors in median arcuate ligament syndrome. J. Vasc. Surg. 65, 1745–1752.

Jasper, A., et al., 2014. Evaluation of normal abdominal aortic diameters in the Indian population using computed tomography. J. Postgrad. Med. 60, 57–60.

Loukas, M., Hullett, J., Wagner, T., 2005. Clinical anatomy of the inferior phrenic artery. Clin. Anat. 18, 357–365.

Mirjalili, S.A., et al., 2012. A reappraisal of adult thoracic surface anatomy. Clin. Anat. 25, 827–834.

Moussallem, C.D., et al., 2012. Relationship of the lumbar lordosis angle to the abdominal aortic bifurcation and inferior vena cava confluence levels. Clin. Anat. 25, 866–871.

Panagouli, E., et al., 2013. Variations in the anatomy of the celiac trunk: a systematic review and clinical implications. Ann. Anat. 195, 501–511.

Rogers, I.S., et al., 2013. Distribution, determinants, and normal reference values of thoracic and abdominal aortic diameters by computed tomography (from the Framingham Heart Study). Am. J. Cardiol. 111, 1510–1516.

Toni, R., et al., 1988. Clinical anatomy of the suprarenal arteries: a quantitative approach by aortography. Surg. Radiol. Anat. 10, 297–302.

Tubbs, R.S., Shoja, M., Loukas, M., 2016. Bergman's Comprehensive Encyclopedia of Human Anatomic Variation. Wiley Blackwell, New Jersey.

FURTHER READING

Fleischmann, D., et al., 2001. Quantitative determination of age-related geometric changes in the normal abdominal aorta. J. Vasc. Surg. 33, 97–105.

Goldberg, B.B., McGahan, J., 2006. Atlas of Ultrasound Measurements, second ed. Elsevier Mosby, Boston.

Groeneveld, M.E., et al., 2018. Systematic review of circulating, biomechanical, and genetic markers for the prediction of abdominal aortic aneurysm growth and rupture. J Am. Heart Assoc. 7.

Kiil, B.J., et al., 2009. The lumbar artery perforators: a cadaveric and clinical anatomical study. Plast. Reconstr. Surg. 123, 1229–1238.

Winston, C.B., et al., 2007. CT angiography for delineation of celiac and superior mesenteric artery variants in patients undergoing hepatobiliary and pancreatic surgery. AJR Am. J. Roentgenol. 189, 13–19.

CHAPTER 20

The Inferior Vena Cava and Its Branches and Connections in the Abdomen

MISHAN LISTMANN • R. SHANE TUBBS

INTRODUCTION

The inferior vena cava (Figs. 20.1–20.4) drains blood from almost all structures inferior to the diaphragm. Most of its course is within the abdomen, but a small segment extends into the pericardium in the thoracic cavity. It begins at the level of the fifth lumbar vertebra, approximately 1 cm to the right of the midline, at the junction of the left and right common iliac veins (Standring, 2016). Then, it follows the anterior surface of the vertebral column as it travels superiorly to the right of the aorta. Next, it passes through a deep indentation on the liver's posterior surface, where it is enveloped completely in hepatic tissue at times before it exits the abdominal cavity.

Because of its proximity to the lumbar spine, lateral transpsoas surgery, particularly on the right side, can encounter branches of the inferior vena cava. Furthermore, other important veins in the retroperitoneum include the ascending lumbar and its tributaries. Therefore, spine surgeons performing such procedures require a thorough knowledge of this anatomy.

Anatomical Associations Within the Abdominal Cavity

The inferior vena cava is located behind the dorsal parietal peritoneum and, at its origin, is immediately posterior to the right common iliac artery. As it ascends through the abdominal cavity, it passes behind the root of the small intestine's mesentery, the right gonadal artery, and the duodenum's horizontal part. It continues superiorly along the head of the pancreas' posterior surface and the duodenum's first part, separated from these structures by the bile duct and hepatic portal vein. Superior to the duodenum, the inferior vena cava and its overlaying layer of parietal peritoneum constitute the omental foramen's posterior wall.

The vertebral bodies of L3–L5 and their intervertebral discs, the anterior longitudinal ligament, the right sympathetic trunk, and the right third and fourth lumbar arteries are posterior to the inferior vena cava in the abdominal cavity's inferior region, and the right psoas major is situated posterolateral to it. In the abdominal cavity's superior aspect, the inferior vena cava overlays the right renal and middle suprarenal arteries, the right suprarenal gland's medial border, the right inferior phrenic arteries, and the right celiac ganglion.

The right lobe, duodenum's descending part, right kidney's medial margin, and the right ureter lay to the right of the inferior vena cava (Standring, 2016), whereas the liver's caudate lobe, the diaphragm's right crus, and the abdominal aorta are on its left.

The adult inferior vena cava can measure up to 30 mm in diameter, and its cross-sectional shape fluctuates between round and flat depending upon venous load. The inferior vena cava's complex embryogenesis gives rise to many anatomical variants documented well. Common variants include azygos extension, a double inferior vena cava in which the left vessel drains usually into the left renal vein, or a left-sided inferior vena cava (Ang et al., 2013; Spentzouris et al., 2014).

Tributaries

The inferior vena cava drains the common iliac veins at its origin over the fifth lumbar vertebral body. From inferior to superior, it is joined by the lumbar, right gonadal, renal, right suprarenal, hepatic, and inferior phrenic veins.

Lumbar Veins

Four pairs of lumbar veins drain blood from the regions of the posterior, lateral, and anterior abdominal walls and travel with the corresponding lumbar arteries (Figs. 20.7 and 20.8). The lumbar veins anastomose with the azygos and hemiazygos veins' tributaries (Fig. 20.5) posteriorly, and the epigastric, circumflex iliac, and lateral thoracic veins' tributaries anteriorly.

Surgical anatomy of the lateral transpsoas approach to the lumbar spine. https://doi.org/10.1016/B978-0-323-67376-1.00020-3

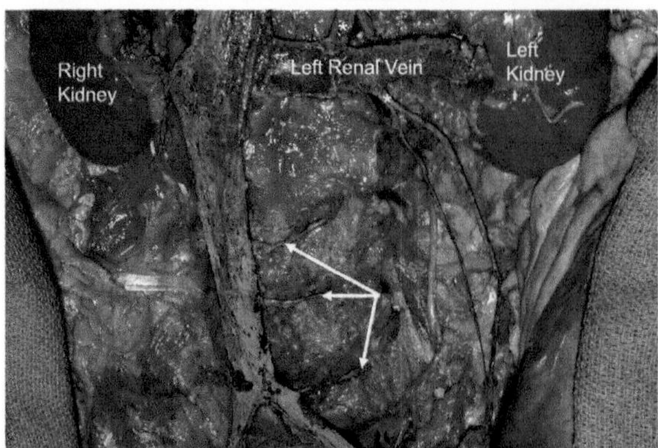

FIG. 20.1 Cadaveric view of the inferior vena cava, colored in blue. Note the lumbar veins (arrows) with the lowest vein here arising from the iliolumbar vein and the left suprarenal vein (upper asterisk) and left gonadal vein (lower asterisk). The right gonadal vein (not marked) is seen coursing over the right renal vein (not marked) and draining into the inferior vena cava.

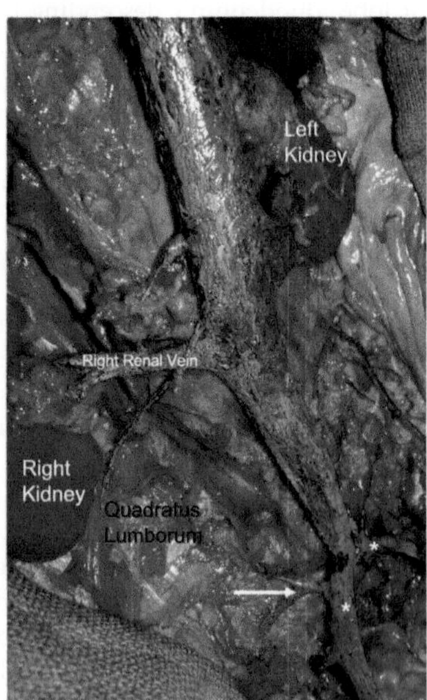

FIG. 20.2 Note the left and right common iliac veins (asterisks) and right iliolumbar vein (arrow).

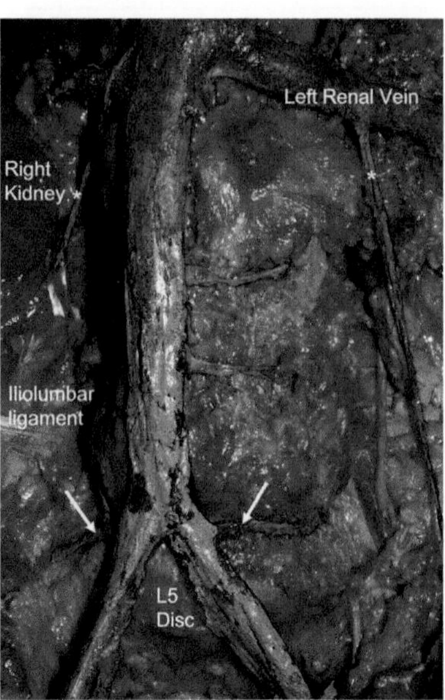

FIG. 20.3 The left and right gonadal veins are marked with asterisks, and the left and right iliolumbar veins with arrows. For orientation of level, note the iliolumbar ligament and L5's intervertebral disc.

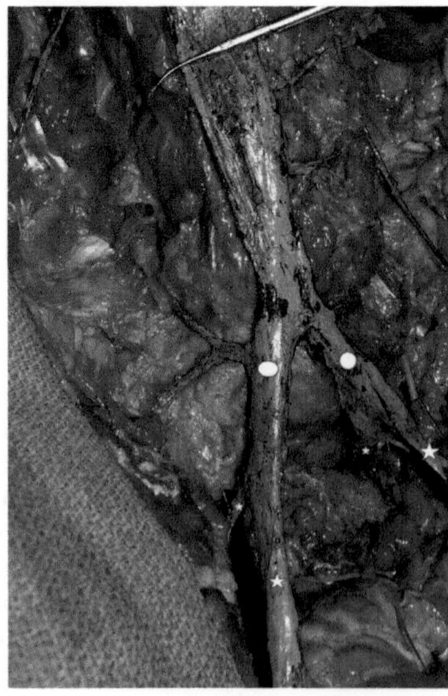

FIG. 20.4 Here, the common iliac veins are marked with white circles, the external iliac veins with stars, and the internal iliac veins with asterisks.

Should the inferior vena cava become compressed, these communications can serve as collateral routes of venous drainage from the pelvis and lower limbs. Although they are smaller vessels, the internal and external vertebral venous plexuses (Fig. 20.6) also may provide alternative drainage routes via the lumbar veins.

Typically, the third and fourth lumbar veins wrap around their corresponding vertebral bodies to join the inferior vena cava at its posterior wall. The left lumbar veins must cross the midline to reach the right-sided inferior vena cava and, therefore, are longer. The first and second lumbar veins demonstrate much more variability

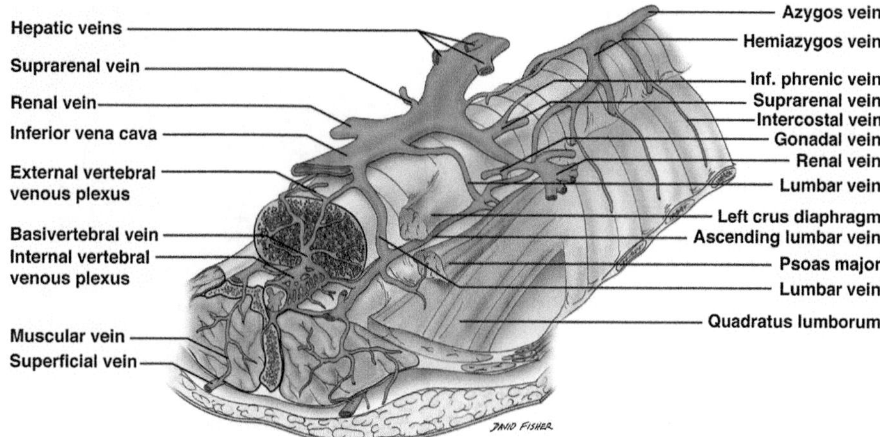

FIG. 20.5 Schematic drawing of the inferior vena cava and its connections to the azygos and vertebral venous systems.

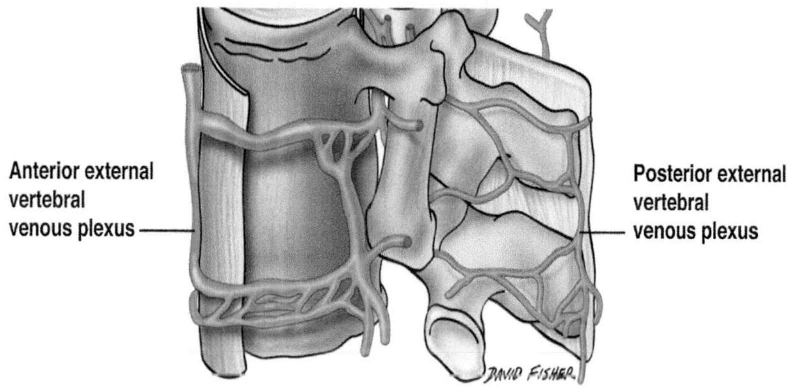

FIG. 20.6 Lateral view of parts of the vertebral venous plexus (Batson's plexus).

than do the third and fourth, and either may empty into the inferior vena cava, the ascending lumbar (Fig. 20.5), the lumbar azygos, or the renal veins (on the left: Standring, 2016). Often, they anastomose, and often, the first lumbar vein passes inferiorly to merge with the second, while occasionally, it may drain directly into the ascending lumbar vein or pass anteriorly across L1's body to join the lumbar azygos vein. The second lumbar vein may join the inferior vena cava at or near its junction with the renal veins or, occasionally, join the third lumbar or ascending lumbar vein.

Ascending Lumbar Veins

The paired ascending lumbar veins (Fig. 20.5) course medial to the psoas major and connect the common iliac veins with the iliolumbar and individual ipsilateral lumbar veins. They run parallel and lateral to the vertebral column from the base of the spine to the thoracolumbar junction. The ascending lumbar vein's course and connections are highly variable, and in rare cases, it may be absent entirely or in part on one side. Often, it merges with the subcostal vein to form the azygos vein on the right and the hemiazygos on the left (Standring, 2016). The azygos and hemiazygos veins track along the body of T12's anterior surface and then pass into the thoracic cavity deep to, or through, the diaphragm's crura.

Gonadal Veins

The right gonadal vein drains directly into the inferior vena cava approximately 2 cm inferior to the left renal vein in adults (Standring, 2016), although, occasionally, it may drain into the right renal vein (Tubbs et al., 2016). The left gonadal vein (Fig. 20.3) drains into the left renal vein. The gonadal veins may be found in duplicate for all or part of their length.

Renal Veins

The renal veins usually travel anterior to the renal arteries. The left renal vein (Fig. 20.1) is three times longer than the right, and typically, they measure approximately 7.5 and 2.5 cm, respectively. The left renal vein courses along the posterior abdominal wall, deep into the pancreas and splenic vein, and passes between the proximal superior mesenteric artery and the abdominal aorta before it empties into the inferior vena cava. The right renal vein (Fig. 20.2) travels posterior to the duodenum's descending part, or in some cases, the head of the pancreas' lateral part.

Suprarenal Veins

In most cases, the suprarenal gland drains only into one vein. The shorter right vein empties directly into the inferior vena cava at the T12 level, whereas the longer left suprarenal vein (Fig. 20.5) empties typically into the left renal vein and, occasionally, merges with the left inferior phrenic vein. Several anatomical variations of this vein have been documented (Cesmebasi et al., 2014).

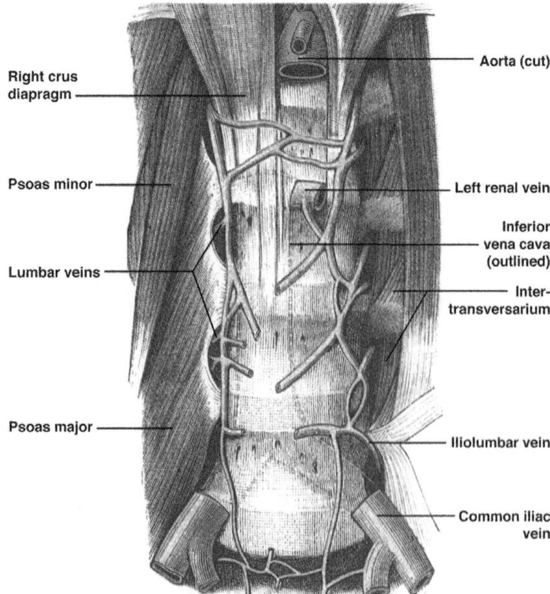

FIG. 20.7 Drawing of many of the inferior vena cavas' tributaries, which has been removed, but its position outlined. Note the lumbar veins and their relation with the vertebral bodies and the psoas major's tendinous slips (after Testut).

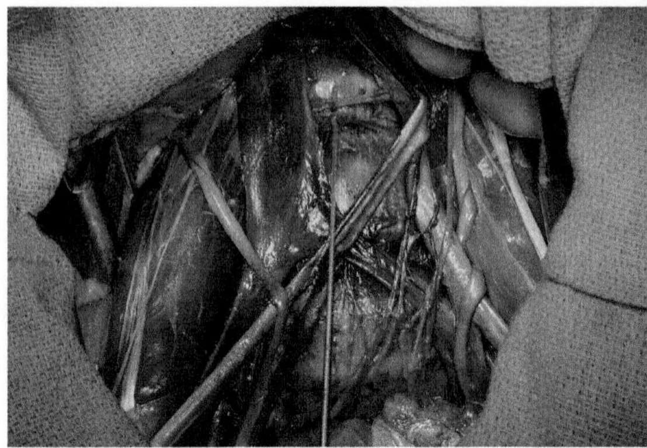

FIG. 20.8 Cadaveric dissection of the proximal inferior vena cava. The aortic bifurcation is retracted to the left with forceps to illustrate a lumbar vein (over the tip of the pointer) draining into the posterolateral aspect of the inferior vena cava. Note the left common iliac vein's relation to the iliac arteries.

Inferior Phrenic Veins

Typically, the inferior phrenic veins originate in the thoracic cavity on the diaphragm's superior surface but run along its inferior surface for most of their length and join the vena cava on its posterolateral side. Both inferior phrenic veins receive multiple tributaries from the diaphragm. The right vein courses to the right of the caval foramen, whereas the left runs to the left of the esophageal hiatus. The left inferior phrenic vein communicates often with the left gastric vein, and in cases of portal hypertension, it may become dilated (Standring, 2016). Both inferior phrenic veins empty typically into the inferior vena cava as it enters the abdominal cavity and, occasionally, merge anteriorly into a short common trunk. The right inferior phrenic vein drains occasionally into the right hepatic vein or inferior vena cava superior to the diaphragm, whereas the left drains frequently into the left suprarenal, left hepatic, or left renal veins.

REFERENCES

Ang, W.C., Doyle, T., Stringer, M.D., 2013. Left-sided and duplicate inferior vena cava: a case series and review. Clin. Anat. 26, 990–1001.

Cesmebasi, A., et al., 2014. A review of the anatomy and clinical significance of adrenal veins. Clin. Anat. 27, 1253–1263.

Spentzouris, G., et al., 2014. The clinical anatomy of the inferior vena cava: a review of common congenital anomalies and considerations for clinicians. Clin. Anat. 27, 1234–1243.

Standring, S., 2016. Gray's Anatomy. Elsevier, Philadelphia.

Tubbs, R.S., Shoja, M., Loukas, M., 2016. Bergman's Comprehensive Encyclopedia of Human Anatomic Variation. Wiley Blackwell, New Jersey.

FURTHER READING

Lolis, E., Panagouli, E., Venieratos, D., 2011. Study of the ascending lumbar and iliolumbar veins: surgical anatomy, clinical implications and review of the literature. Ann. Anat. 193, 516–529.

Loukas, M., et al., 2005. An anatomical classification of the variations of the inferior phrenic vein. Surg. Radiol. Anat. 27, 566–574.

Moeller, T.B., 2000. Normal Findings in CT and MRI. Thieme, New York.

Morita, S., et al., 2007. Flow direction of ascending lumbar veins on magnetic resonance angiography and venography: would "descending lumbar veins" be a more precise name physiologically? Abdom. Imag. 32, 749–753.

CHAPTER 21

Lateral Approaches to the Thoracolumbar Junction—Anatomical Considerations

ZANE TYMCHACK • ANDREW JACK • ALEXANDER VON GLINSKI • ROD J. OSKOUIAN • R. SHANE TUBBS

INTRODUCTION

Lateral approaches to the spine present particular anatomical challenges and considerations for the spine surgeon. Perhaps most challenging, the thoracolumbar junction represents an especially complex region with its convergence of the retroperitoneal space, the thoracic cavity, the diaphragm, and the thoracolumbar spine. The lower rib cage and the diaphragm present an especial dilemma for the spine surgeon (Uribe et al., 2011).

The thoracolumbar spine is generally thought of as comprising the T11-L2 motion segments and is a natural transition zone in the spine (1). It represents a transition zone between the relatively rigid, rib-bearing, thoracic spine and the more mobile lumbar spine (Figs. 21.1–21.4) (2). It represents a neutral zone between the natural kyphosis of the thoracic spine and the lordotic lumbar spine (3). It encompasses a transition zone of the neural elements from spinal cord level to conus level to nerve root level. Because of these features, the thoracolumbar spine is a common location for certain spinal pathologies, particularly traumatic lesions (Vaccaro et al., 2004). However, it is not spared nontraumatic pathologies (Uribe et al., 2010). Therefore, it is essential that the spine surgeon have a thorough knowledge of the anatomical considerations and challenges of this region.

Given the morbidity associated with anterior approaches, lateral surgery has gained popularity by providing a lateral view of the spinal canal and avoiding morbidities associated with entry into the chest (Uribe et al., 2011). Furthermore, the surgeon is better able to visualize the pathology and the thecal sac than in more ventral approaches, which require resection of the pathological area in order to visualize the thecal sac (Uribe et al., 2011; Dakwar et al., 2012). The lateral approach to this region, especially a minimally invasive approach, allows unparalleled access for safe neural decompression, endplate preparation for fusion, and placement of implants for restoration of normal alignment (Mirbaha, 1973; Moskovich et al., 1993; McCormick, 1995).

REGIONAL ANATOMY OF THE THORACOLUMBAR JUNCTION

Chest/Lateral Abdominal Wall

At the level of the thoracolumbar spine, the chest and lateral abdominal wall muscles of significance are the latissimus dorsi, the external and internal intercostals, the transversus abdominis, and the external and internal oblique abdominis muscles. The fibers of these muscles can be split bluntly to allow access to the retroperitoneal/retropleural compartments. Depending on the level(s) being accessed during surgery, the rib cage can pose an obstacle. Typically, the 11th and 12th ribs are floating ribs in that they do not have an attachment to the sternum or to the costal cartilage of the 7th rib. Ribs 8–10 do not directly attach to the sternum but have cartilaginous connections with the costal cartilage of the seventh rib. Exposure at the thoracolumbar junction (T11–L1) differs from higher levels owing to a more caudal orientation of the ribs (Angevin and McCormick, 2001). Therefore, the rib incision is two levels above the involved segment (a T-10 incision is made for a T-12 resection), and both incision and rib resection are extended anteriorly by 2–4 cm (Angevin and McCormick, 2001). Otherwise, if the rib at the involved segment is resected, the upper ribs will cover the surgically treated level (Angevin and McCormick, 2001). An intercostal (between ribs) or transcostal

Surgical anatomy of the lateral transpsoas approach to the lumbar spine. https://doi.org/10.1016/B978-0-323-67376-1.00021-5

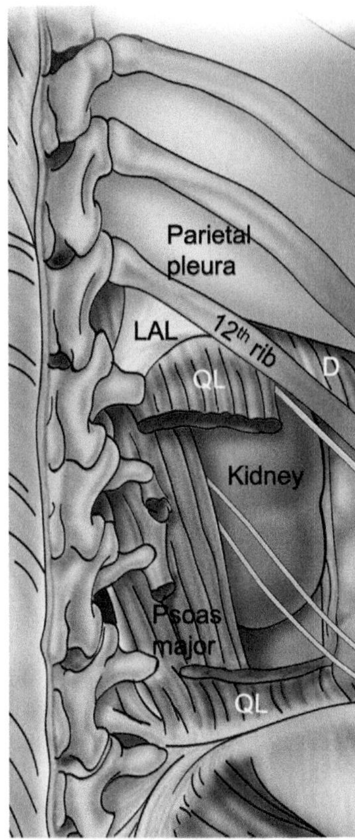

FIG. 21.1 Schematic drawing of the thoracolumbar junction from a posterior view. Diaphragm (D), Quadratus lumborum muscle (QL) and lumbocostal ligament (LAL).

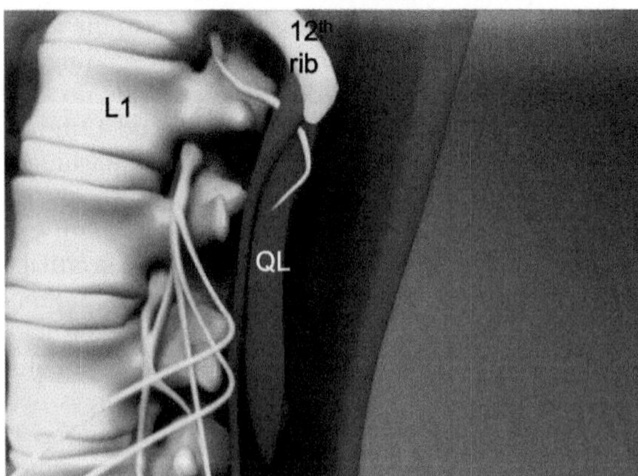

FIG. 21.2 Schematic view of the thoracolumbar junction from a lateral view.

(resection of a portion of rib) approach can be used to access the lateral thoracolumbar spine with no real consequence so long as the visceral pleura remains intact (Resnick and Benzel, 1998). The neurovascular bundle lies deep to the inferior border of the rib and can be preserved during lateral approaches to the spine requiring an intercostal or transcostal approach. Sacrificing the neurovascular bundle does not usually result in any significant morbidity, apart from leaving the patient with a patch of chest wall anesthesia that is usually temporary. Furthermore, it is critical to avoid ensnaring the intercostal nerves that run inferior to each rib to prevent postthoracotomy neuralgia (Angevin and McCormick, 2001).

Retroperitoneal Space

The retroperitoneal space is entered when the lumbar spine is accessed during lateral access spine surgery. It is separated from the peritoneal cavity by the peritoneum. The peritoneum is a serous membrane that has both visceral and parietal layers; the visceral layer covers the abdominal organs, while the parietal layer attaches to the abdominal wall. The retroperitoneal space contains structures related to the urogenital tract (kidneys and ureters), the gastrointestinal tract (duodenum, ascending/descending colon and portions of the pancreas), the vascular system (aorta, inferior vena cava), and musculoskeletal tissue (iliopsoas muscle).

The retropleural space is accessed when the lateral thoracolumbar spine is approached above the level of the diaphragm. It is a potential space between the pleura and the chest wall. The pleura, like the peritoneum, is a serous membrane with two layers, visceral and parietal. The visceral layer covers the lungs, while the parietal layer attaches to the chest wall. The surgeon should attempt to preserve both the visceral and parietal pleura during dissection to avoid complications such as hemopneumothorax (Resnick and Benzel, 1998). Typically, the parietal pleura can be violated with no significant morbidity. Even when the parietal pleura is inadvertently violated, we seldom leave a tube thoracostomy. However, violation of the visceral pleura can result in the feared complication of tension pneumothorax, and the surgeon should give strong consideration to tube thoracostomy in the immediate postoperative period.

Diaphragm

Much of the complexity of lateral approaches to the thoracolumbar junction arises from the anatomical challenges presented by the diaphragm. The diaphragm is a musculotendinous structure that divides the thoracic and abdominal compartments. Superiorly, it is covered by the parietal pleura and pericardium. Inferiorly, it is covered by an extension of the transversalis fascia and the peritoneum. It has surgically relevant

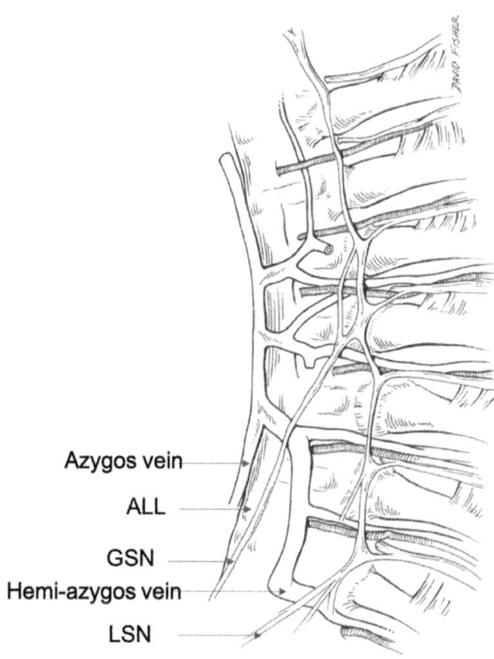

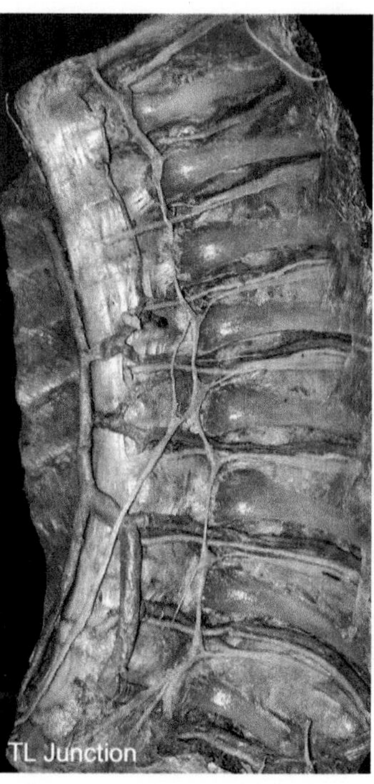

FIG. 21.3 Anterior view of the thoracolumbar junction in a cadaveric dissection (right). Note the neurovascular structures in this location as indicated on the line drawing (left). Anterior longitudinal ligament (ALL), greater splanchnic nerve (GSN) and lesser splanchnic nerve (LSN).

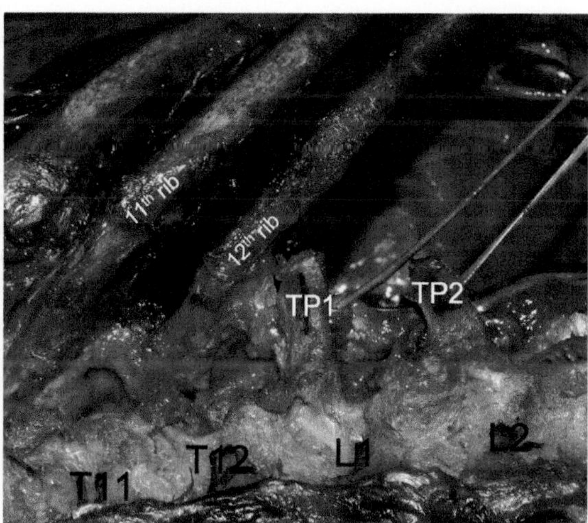

FIG. 21.4 Right cadaveric dissection of the thoracolumbar junction noting the relationship between the 12th rib, L1 transverse process (TP1), and body of T12. Note the transverse process of L2 (TP2) and the subcostal nerve (left) and iliohypogastric nerve (right).

attachments laterally to the medial portion of the 7th and 8th ribs anteriorly, the 9th and 10th ribs laterally, and the 11th and 12th ribs posterolaterally. Posteriorly, the diaphragmatic attachments are made up of the attachments of the lateral and medial arcuate ligaments. The lateral arcuate ligament spans the quadratus lumborum muscle and attaches laterally to the 12th rib, and medially to the transverse process of L1. The medial arcuate ligament spans the psoas muscle and attaches laterally to the transverse process of L1 and medially to the diaphragmatic crura (Dakwar et al., 2012). The right and left crura are tendinous structures that extend from the inferior diaphragm to the anterior lumbar vertebral bodies. The medal fibers of the crura meet to form the aortic hiatus. There is some variation between the right and left crura. The right extends more caudally, inserting on to L1-3, whereas the left extends to insert on to L1-2. These attachments become surgically relevant when a true retroperitoneal/retropleural approach is taken to the lateral thoracolumbar spine. The diaphragm can be mobilized anteriorly by releasing its lateral and posterior attachments, thereby avoiding having to repair it during a trans-diaphragmatic approach (Uribe et al., 2011; Dakwar et al., 2012). The lateral attachments can be detached using subperiosteal dissection during approach with a Cobb or Alexander dissector. However, the posterior attachments should be incised sharply for adequate mobilization of the diaphragm anteriorly. With such adequate mobilization, access to the retroperitoneal/retropleural compartments allows the surgeon to approach from both the left and right sides with relative safety. A thorough review of the patient's individual anatomy, paying close attention to vascular, genitourinary, and gastrointestinal structures, is still important for avoiding complications. Many surgeons choose a left-sided approach, preferring a relative working proximity to the aorta rather than the inferior vena cava as injuries to arterial structures tend to be easier to repair than those to veins.

CONCLUSIONS

Lateral approaches to the thoracolumbar junction provide the spine surgeon with unparalleled access for reconstruction of the anterior column between T11 and L2. This can now be done in a relatively minimally invasive fashion with good results. However, a thorough understanding of the retroperitoneal and retropleural spaces, and the diaphragm's relationship to each, is vital for avoiding complications.

REFERENCES

Angevin, P.D., McCormick, P.C., 2001. Retropleural thoracotomy. Technical note. Neurosurg. Focus 10 (1).

Dakwar, E., Ahmadian, A., Uribe, J.S., 2012. The anatomical relationship of the diaphragm to the thoracolumbar junction during the minimally invasive lateral extracoelomic (retropleural/retroperitoneal) approach. J. Neurosurg. Spine 16 (4), 359–364.

McCormick, P.C., 1995. Retropleural approach to the thoracic and thoracolumbar spine. Neurosurgery 37 (5), 908–914.

Mirbaha, M.M., 1973. Anterior approach to the thoracolumbar junction of the spine by a retroperitoneal-extrapleural technic. Clin. Orthop. Relat. Res. 91, 41–47.

Moskovich, R., Benson, D., Zhang, Z.H., Kabins, M., 1993. Extracoelomic approach to the spine. J. Bone Joint Surg. Br. 75 (6), 886–893.

Resnick, D.K., Benzel, E.C., 1998. Lateral extracavitary approach for thoracic and thoracolumbar spine trauma: operative complications. Neurosurgery 43 (4), 796–802 discussion 802-793.

Uribe, J.S., Dakwar, E., Cardona, R.F., Vale, F.L., 2011. Minimally invasive lateral retropleural thoracolumbar approach: cadaveric feasibility study and report of 4 clinical cases. Neurosurgery 68 (1 Suppl. Operative), 32–39 discussion 39.

Uribe, J.S., Dakwar, E., Le, T.V., Christian, G., Serrano, S., Smith, W.D., 2010. Minimally invasive surgery treatment for thoracic spine tumor removal: a mini-open, lateral approach. Spine 35 (26 Suppl. l), S347–S354.

Vaccaro, A.R., Kim, D.H., Brodke, D.S., Harris, M., Chapman, J.R., Schildhauer, T., Routt, M.L., Sasso, R.C., 2004. Diagnosis and management of thoracolumbar spine fractures. Instr. Course Lect. 53, 359–373.

CHAPTER 22

Lateral Approaches to the Thoracic Spine

MAXWELL T. LAWS • ALEXANDER VON GLINSKI • DIA R. HALALMEH • MARC D. MOISI • ROD J. OSKOUIAN

INTRODUCTION

Most historical surgical approaches to the spine were developed to treat spinal tuberculosis, as the disease commonly invades the vertebral end plate and intervertebral discs. Percival Pott reported on the debridement of paravertebral tuberculous abscesses and subsequent washout with antiseptic solutions in 1788 (Flamm, 1992). The first documented anterior attempt via a posterior approach to the thoracic spine for treating Pott's disease was performed by Menard in 1895. He performed a costotransversectomy in patients with paraplegia resulting from tuberculous spondylitis, allowing for abscess drainage and subsequent decompression of the vertebral canal (Menard, 1895). Unfortunately, these approaches could not provide adequate exposure to the ventral segments of the spinal cord: as a result, they could not completely address pathology in those areas. The chest cavity poses significant anatomical challenges due to proximity of vital structures (e.g., aorta, heart, lungs, and esophagus); viable anterior approaches to the ventral thoracic spine were not possible until the mid-20th century. During that time, a transthoracic anterior approach was developed, often credited to Hodgson and Stock. They popularized this approach through the publication of an extensive series on treatment outcomes for patients with Pott's disease treated in Hong Kong using their anterior approach, paired with radical debridement and an autologous bone graft (Hodgson and Stock, 2006). Their work established the model for the transthoracic approach and has been widely adopted and modified since.

The transthoracic approach has been the standard for anterior spine procedures since its inception, allowing for the treatment of a variety of thoracic pathologies including infections (e.g., tuberculosis, osteomyelitis, and parasitic infections), trauma (e.g., fracture dislocation and compression fracture), tumors (including metastatic invasion and primary tumors of the vertebral body), deformities (e.g., kyphosis, scoliosis, and lordosis), and degenerative disc disease (Fig. 22.1). There is considerable potential morbidity associated with thoracotomy: pneumothorax, local tissue injury, and shoulder girdle dysfunction, along with other less common complications (Kwan and Cheung, 2016). The introduction of video-assisted thoracoscopic surgery (VATS) has facilitated a significant reduction in thoracic exposure, reducing the overall morbidity associated with this approach (Faro et al., 2005). VATS exposure is not without its own drawbacks as it requires the selective intubation with lung collapse on the side of access, and there are additional technical difficulties related to the specific skills that thoracoscopic surgery requires (Berjano et al., 2014).

Owing to the risks associated with chest wall entry, an alternative retropleural approach to the anterior thoracic spine was promoted by McCormick (1995). This approach allows for a short and direct route to the anterior thoracic spine while avoiding entry into the pleural cavity. In addition, it is more lateral than other approaches, granting direct visualization of the entire vertebral body, and provides access to the ventral dura and neuroforamina (Angevine and McCormick, 2001). Anterior transthoracic approaches (e.g., transthoracic transpleural, transthoracic retropleural, VATS, miniopen lateral extrapleural and transpleural) are useful in cases of lesions that are directly ventral to the spinal cord, in contrast to lateral extracavitary and transpedicular approaches, which address paracentral lesions.

Access to the thoracic spine (Fig. 22.2) during an LLIF (lateral lumbar interbody fusion) procedure can be accomplished using either a transpleural or a retropleural approach. A transpleural approach is performed

Surgical anatomy of the lateral transpsoas approach to the lumbar spine. https://doi.org/10.1016/B978-0-323-67376-1.00022-7

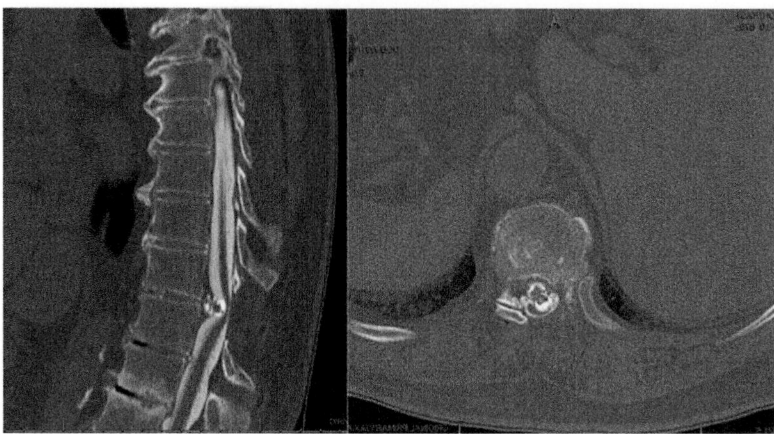

FIG. 22.1 Calcified thoracic disc T10/11 with significant spinal canal decompression.

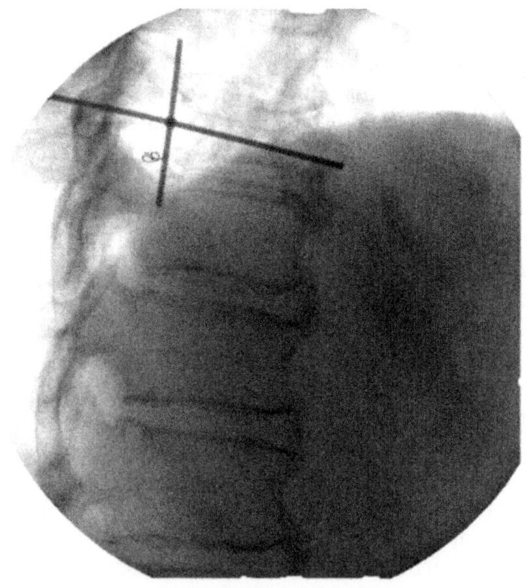

FIG. 22.2 Lateral fluoroscopic view with marker at T10 pedicle.

by incising the parietal pleura, displacing the lung anteriorly, and introducing the dilators into the interpleural space and coursing down the rib until the target vertebral area is reached. In contrast, the retropleural approach involves careful dissection of the rib overlying the planned operative corridor from the intercostal muscles and parietal pleura (Figs. 22.3–22.5). Once the lumbar and costal attachments of the diaphragm are released, the diaphragm is retracted anteriorly, exposing the thoracolumbar spine (Figs. 22.6–22.8). This maintains the integrity of the pleural cavity and allows access to the vertebral column by entering and anteriorly retracting the retropleural space. There is no gold standard approach for addressing thoracic spinal pathologies; each technique has advantages and disadvantages, so the operative approach should be individualized to provide optimal care for the patient.

This chapter describes the technical aspects of the transpleural and retropleural approaches and then compares the two approaches in terms of surgical considerations and resultant patient outcomes.

SURGICAL TECHNIQUE

Patient Positioning and Preparation

CT and MRI allow for precise localization and evaluation of spine pathology and adjacent intrathoracic structures. These studies can be used for perioperative planning and are used to determine the proper spinal level(s) to expose. CT is better for identifying osteophytes or disc calcifications, which can complicate the spinal procedure (Williams et al., 1989). If the lesion is a vascular lesion or oncology case, a spinal angiogram can be considered to identify the artery of Adamkiewicz with possible embolization (Anderson et al., 1993). The ribs should be examined thoroughly, as the last rib can act as a useful landmark to demarcate the thoracolumbar junction. However, variation in the number of ribs should be taken into consideration, as fewer or extra ribs can cause miscounting of levels. In addition, knowing the size of the last rib is important, as it can be confused with a transverse process (Angevin and McCormick, 2001). The lateral trajectory of the retropleural approach leads to early visualization of

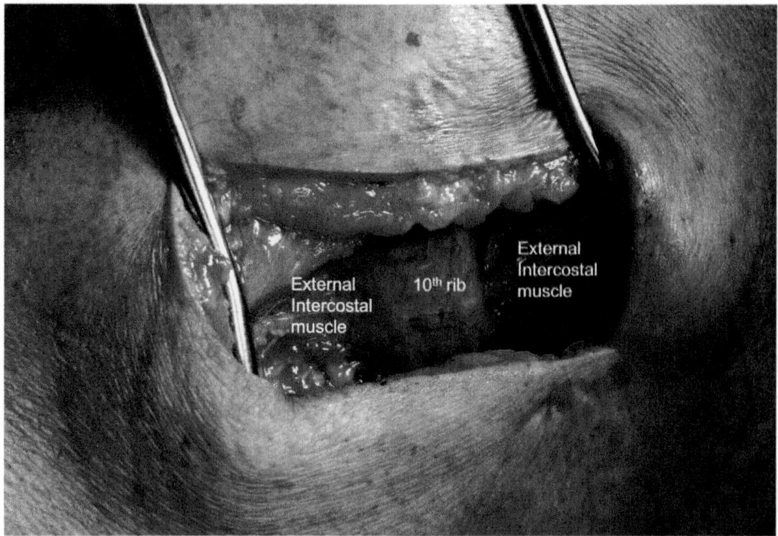

FIG. 22.3 Lateral view of cadaveric dissection of the 10th rib.

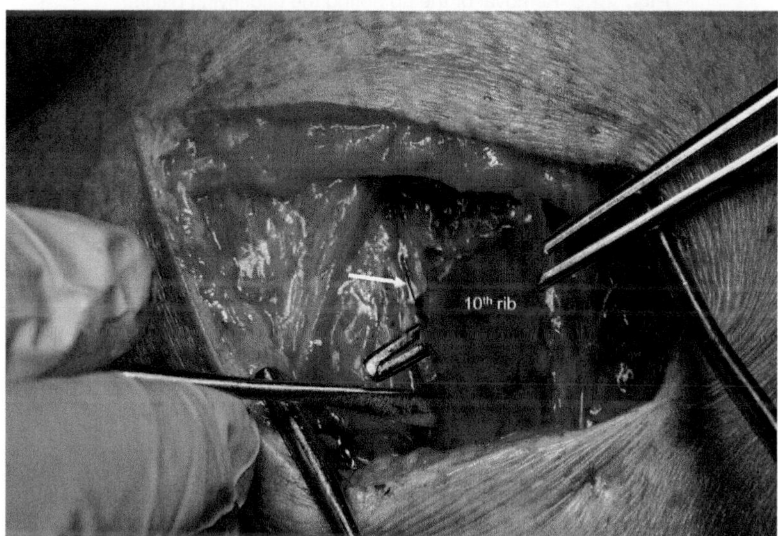

FIG. 22.4 Elevation of the rib noting the neurovascular bundle (*white arrow*).

neurovascular structures (e.g., intercostal vessels, thoracic duct, azygos vein, thoracic sympathetic trunk) (McCormick, 1995). Given the presence of these vessels, some surgeons consider the use of preoperative angiography. Angiography is more useful in cases of highly vascular lesions, namely, vertebral hemangiomas and renal cell carcinoma metastases (Bahm et al., 2018). Single lung anesthesia can also be used through a double-lumen endotracheal tube with intraoperative monitoring if one decides to go transpleural, but this is not needed if you go retropleural.

Following intubation, the patient is placed in lateral decubitus position on a breakable radiolucent table. Alternatively, the table can be flexed under the lumbosacral spine to facilitate exposure. The arms are placed above the patient's head on an airplane splint. The shoulders and hips are oriented perpendicular to the floor, allowing for intraoperative imaging of the spine and for spinal stabilization in the correct anatomical alignment. All pressure points are appropriately padded. Wide cloth tape is placed across the greater trochanter, and an axillary roll is placed under the

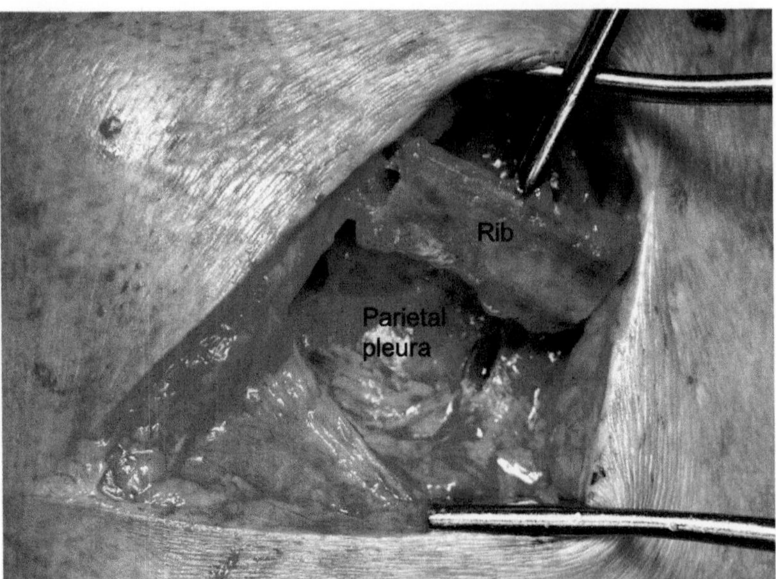

FIG. 22.5 Removal of the rib noting the underlying pleura.

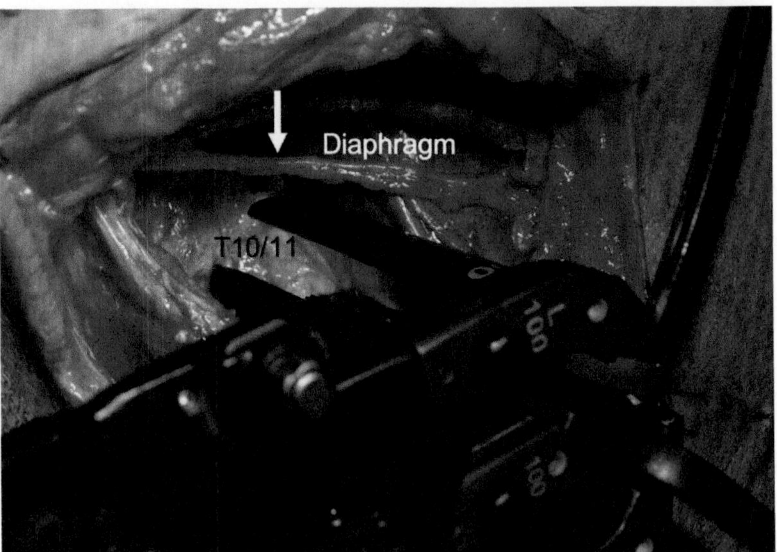

FIG. 22.6 Retractor placement noting the neurovascular bundle (*white arrow*).

dependent axilla to prevent positioning-related neuropathies (Bahm et al., 2018). The lower limbs are flexed at the hip and knee with a pillow placed between the legs. The prepped and draped operative field should be aligned to the appropriate spinal level; it includes the chest as for thoracotomy, the spine, and the contralateral paraspinal region. If the upper thoracic spine is to be exposed, then the base of the neck and scapula are

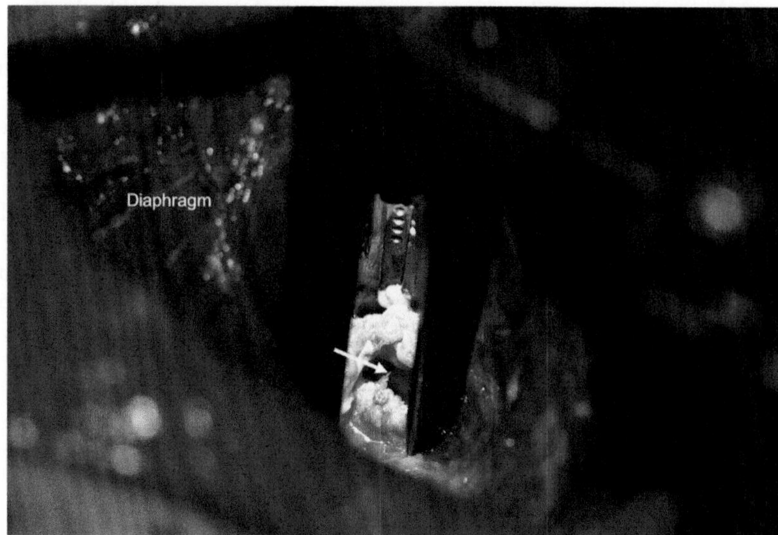

FIG. 22.7 Discectomy seen at the end of the retractor.

included in the operative field. For lower spine exposure, the upper flank and lumbar region are included in the field. Intraoperative EMG is essential in this approach and involves somatosensory evoked potentials (SSEPs) and motor evoked potentials (MEPs).

Planning and Level Identification

If there is a lack of localizing pathology, it is recommended that the upper thoracic spine (T2–T9) be approached by either side dependent on the location of the heart, aorta, and great vessels, whereas the thoracolumbar spine (T10–L2) should be approached by the left to avoid liver retraction and potential injury. The side of approach should optimize exposure to the pathology to be treated. Local considerations include previous thoracotomy, pleurodesis, or infection. In cases of spinal deformities, surgery should be performed on the convex side, leaving the concave side for ventilation. The fiducial marker screw can be placed using CT guidance, helping to reduce the intraoperative fluoroscopy time needed for localization.

The target level is identified using intraoperative fluoroscopic imaging (Fig. 22.2). As in the lumbar approach, the C-arm is positioned anteriorly to obtain true AP and lateral views. Using bisected K-wire, the skin is marked over the anterior and posterior vertebral body borders and the junction between the posterior and middle thirds of the level of interest. For multilevel cases, more than one incision is required where the surgeon can access several levels through each incision. Wide skin preparation is performed so that the incision can be extended to a thoracotomy if required [25]. When identification of the target level is challenging, intraoperative CT or O-arm can be used if available. Other options include flexible hook-wire insertion under CT and deployment of a preoperative coil into the intercostal artery [27].

Opening and Disc Exposure

Given the vital structures surrounding the thoracic spine (e.g., major vessels, lungs and pleura, and diaphragm), multiple approaches have been developed to address various lesions located in this region safely. Each technique has advantages and disadvantages; therefore, the optimal surgical choice should be individualized to improve patient outcomes. Minimally invasive anterolateral transthoracic transpleural and retropleural approaches offer advantages over the traditional open approaches. These thoracic techniques afford surgeons the ability to avoid deflation of the ipsilateral lung, potentially decreasing the risk of postoperative pulmonary complications. However, using these techniques does not eliminate the need for chest tube placement even in the retropleural approach, which in many cases only requires a flexible drain postoperatively [25]. Following level identification and marking the skin, a 4–5 cm oblique, intercostal incision is made along the rib. For single-level cases, the intercostal approach is advisable, in which the chest is entered through the superior edge of the overlying rib, preserving the neurovascular bundle. For multiple-level cases, ribs are sacrificed as necessary; the resected bone is saved to be used later as graft material if needed.

TRANSPLEURAL APPROACH

In this approach, the parietal pleura is incised, and the dilators are introduced into the interpleural space. Then the retractor system is docked over the dilators down to the target level. During that time, the lungs are carefully displaced anteriorly, taking care to identify and clip the segmental vessels above and below the desired level. The lung can be either dropped or not, but it is easier to perform the transpleural approach for visualization if it is dropped. However, a chest tube will most likely be needed postoperatively.

RETROPLEURAL APPROACH

The retropleural approach involves careful dissection of the overlying rib from the attached intercostal muscles and parietal pleura. This maintains the integrity of the pleura and allows the retropleural space to be retracted, providing better exposure of the vertebral column and the target level. The retropleural approach provides the shortest direct route to the anterior thoracic spine while avoiding pleural cavity entry. Direct visualization of the entire vertebral body and ventral spinal canal is provided with this exposure, and postoperative morbidity, particularly pain and pulmonary complications, seems minimal.

Level of Incision

The size of incision depends on the level to be operated on. Approaches for lesions between T5 and T10 usually require a 12 cm skin incision pointing from the posterior axillary line to a point 4 cm lateral to the posterior midline above the rib at the required level (Fig. 22.3). For a T7/T8 disc herniation, we make a cut in line with the T9 rib that will be removed. Approaches for the upper thoracic spine usually require a so-called "hockey stick." It parallels the medial and inferior scapula border while being carried down through the attached muscles to the ribs. For upper thoracic (T3–T4) lesions, an incision that parallels the medial and inferior scapular border is used. This incision is carried down through the scapular muscles (i.e., trapezius and rhomboids) to the ribs. This allows the surgeon to reflect the detached scapula and expose the desired rib. After confirming the right level, the intercostal muscles are subperiosteally detached over approximately 8–10 cm along the rib. The rib is removed partially while the first 4 cm remains attached to the transverse process and the vertebral body. The tissue covering the bed of the resected rib is the endothoracic fascia lining the whole thoracic cavity. This maintains the attachment of the parietal pleura to the inner chest wall. The potential space between the parietal pleura and the endothoracic fascia can contain a small amount of loose areolar tissue. An incision in line with the rib bed is made through the fascia, followed by a wide dissection of the parietal pleura off the undersurface of the endothoracic fascia using Kittner clamps. The dissection is continued proximally to expose the vertebral column. Small pleural tears are repaired with suture. A table-mounted, malleable blade maintains lung retraction. It is useful to deflate the ipsilateral lung to facilitate lung retraction, especially at higher thoracic levels. Furthermore, using a self-retaining crank retractor between the adjacent ribs helps to widen the exposure. The endothoracic fascia is opened over the remaining proximal rib segment with cautery, and the rib head is disarticulated from the vertebral body.

Discectomy

To remove a thoracic disc, the endothoracic fascia covering the disc space is incised. The fascia and the vertebral body periosteum are elevated in either direction away from the disc space. The intercostal vessels that run transversely at the midvertebral body level are preserved within this reflected tissue (Figs. 22.6–22.7). The margins of the pedicle are sharply defined with curettes and nerve hooks.

The disc space is incised and evacuated. A high-speed drill can be used to remove the adjacent endplates and extend the dissection into the adjacent vertebral bodies. The pedicle is also removed with the drill, and Kerrison rongeurs provide access to the lateral spinal canal, which is probed with a dissector. The bony vertebral body dissection can now be completed posteriorly with knowledge of the location of the canal. Generous bone removal both facilitates and ensures adequate canal decompression. The depth of the decompression should be 3.0–3.5 cm from the lateral vertebral body margin. The corpectomy should extend ~1.5 cm on either side of the disc space. This opening should be maintained back to the posterior cortical margin. Bone bleeding can be intermittently controlled with smeared wax on the end of a Kittner clamp. Once the posterior cortical margin has been sufficiently thinned, a reverse angle curette sharply divides the posterior longitudinal ligament. The adherent endplates, annulus, and cortex are pushed down into the corpectomy defect. The thin dorsal layer of the posterior longitudinal ligament usually remains. Thoracic disc fragments are often suspended within this layer. The ligament is gently probed with a nerve hook for identification and delivery of these fragments. Once adequate decompression is achieved, troughs are drilled into the adjacent vertebral bodies, and the harvested rib is placed as an interbody strut graft. In cases of thoracic disc herniation, the intervertebral disc can be easily incised and removed using curettes and Kerrison rongeurs. Following discectomy, the ipsilateral pedicle is drilled out using a matchstick or diamond burr, exposing the lateral spinal canal. A high-speed drill with a diamond burr is used to drill the adjacent vertebral endplates. Caution must be exercised not to traverse the anterior longitudinal ligament and anteriorly situated vessels. Once discectomy is completed and under fluoroscopic guidance, the contralateral annulus is released using a Cobb elevator, and a cage filled with local bone and/or allograft is centered into the disc space.

Corpectomy

A vertebral body corpectomy requires the removal of an additional rib head for adequate exposure (Fig. 22.8). For a T7 corpectomy that has been exposed through the T7 rib bed, for example, resection of the T8 rib head provides exposure of the T7–T8 disc space and the adjacent T8 vertebral body and pedicle. The intercostal artery and vein are divided between the suture close to the midline. Proximal ligation of the intercostal artery can be performed safely because abundant muscular and osseous anastomoses will reconstitute the occluded vessel distally and maintain spinal cord blood flow. The discs are incised and evacuated with curettes, as previously described (Figs. 22.9–22.10). A high-speed drill is used to make a rectangular cut into the anterior vertebral body at the level of interest. Corpectomy is then performed approximately 3.0–3.5 cm from the lateral margin of the vertebral body and 1.5 cm rostrally and caudally from the disc space (Angevin and McCormick, 2001). The remaining muscle attachments to the rib head are incised using monopolar electrocautery. A drill with a matchstick or diamond burr is used to drill out the subcortical bone of the ipsilateral pedicle. A shell of bone should be retained at the medial aspect of the pedicle to protect the cord from injury. Next, cancellous bone is excavated with a matchstick drill, while the bigger diamond burr is used near to the cortical shell generated earlier. The contralateral pedicle is now drilled, with a medial shell kept shielding the cord. Following reduction of the pedicles, the bulk of the inferior and superior intervertebral discs are removed using curettes and Kerrison rongeurs. A diamond burr is then used at the superior endplate at the PLL attachment point, so that it can be detached later. The vertebral body cortical shell is now carefully resected using Kerrison rongeurs, followed by the PLL. Note that the Kerrison should only be directed in a

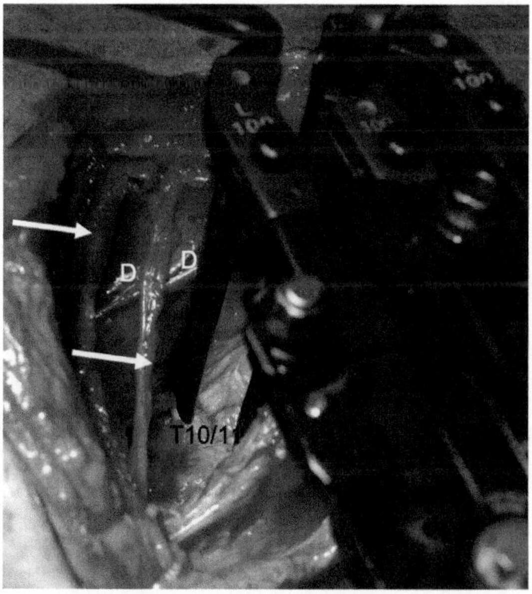

FIG. 22.8 Following two rib resections and retractor placement. Note the neurovascular bundles and diaphragm (D).

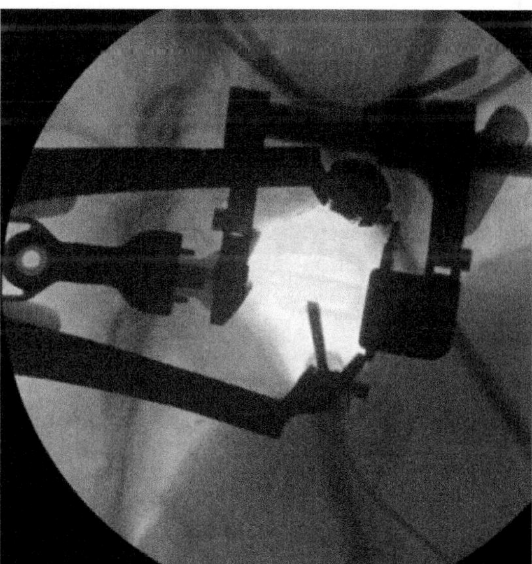

FIG. 22.9 Retractor placement used for corpectomies. Note the use of the anterior retractor blade turned 180 degrees to protect the spinal cord.

rostral or caudal direction to limit the possibility of nerve root injury. The PLL is then slowly dissected away from the dura using a nerve hook. At this point, epidural veins can cause significant bleeding and should be controlled with bipolar electrocautery following decompression. Once the PLL is excised, the remaining cortical vertebral body, pedicle, and intervertebral disc fragments are removed. Finally, a trough is made into the anterolateral aspect of the superior vertebral body using the drill, approximately one-third to one half the width of the vertebral body, for the rib allograft strut graft or cage (Figs. 22.10–22.13).

Closure

In retropleural approach cases, the endothoracic fascia is placed in its natural position along the ventral aspect of the vertebral body. The anesthesiologist is then asked to provide positive pressure, which can help identify pleural tears. If no pleural tears are discovered, there is no need for a chest tube. Small pleural tears are repaired with suture. For large tears, or if there is a considerable amount of air in the pleural space, a chest tube should be placed. To minimize chest wall deformity, suture is used to reapproximate the ribs along the resection area.

A layered closure should be performed. An intercostal draining tube should be placed in the pleural cavity and connected with an underwater seal bag. Once the fluid column stops moving, the lungs are clear to auscultation, and a postoperative chest X-ray demonstrates sufficient chest expansion, the chest tube can be safely removed.

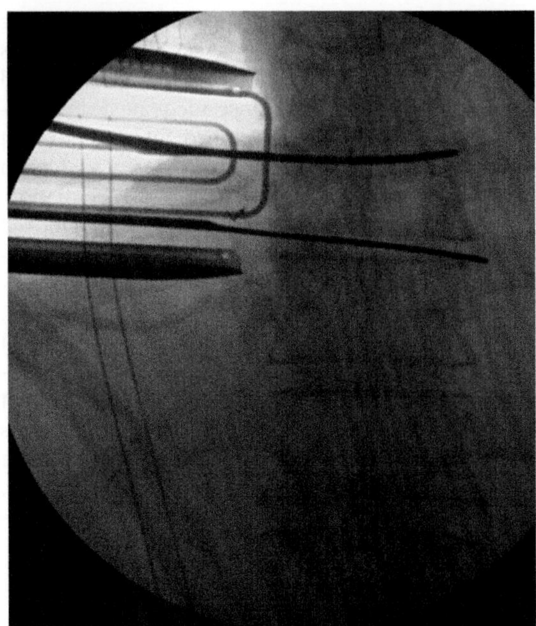

FIG. 22.10 After adequate retraction of the pleura insertion of an expandable cage using the interbody sliding device. This prevents severe endplate damage and therefore subsidence.

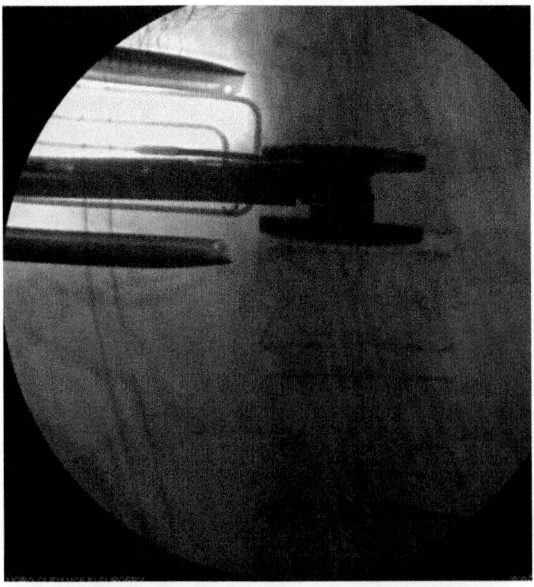

FIG. 22.11 Placement of expandable cage.

COMPARING TECHNIQUES

A detailed medical clearance must be obtained for those planning to undergo transpleural surgery. Patients with significant cardiac risk factors (coronary artery disease, congestive heart failure, structural heart disease) or pulmonary risk factors (chronic obstructive pulmonary disease, smoking) face considerable risk during thoracotomy. The retropleural approach does not warrant such a significant workup, as the pleura is not incised; therefore, this surgery can be offered to more people, including those with underlying medical comorbidities. Furthermore, every transpleural patient receives a chest tube, which can cause pain and limit postoperative patient mobilization, whereas as little as 10% of the retropleural group receives one (McCormick, 1995).

The retropleural approach has a more direct and less oblique angle than the transthoracic approach, allowing for better visualization of the vertebral body. During the transthoracic approach, the curved margin of the dorsal cortical vertebral body can impair the surgeon's visualization of the surgical field (Schwartz and McCormick, 2007).

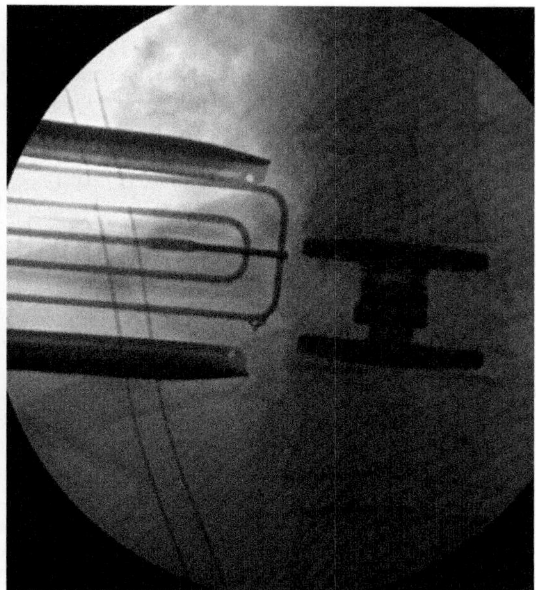

FIG. 22.12 Placement of expandable cage.

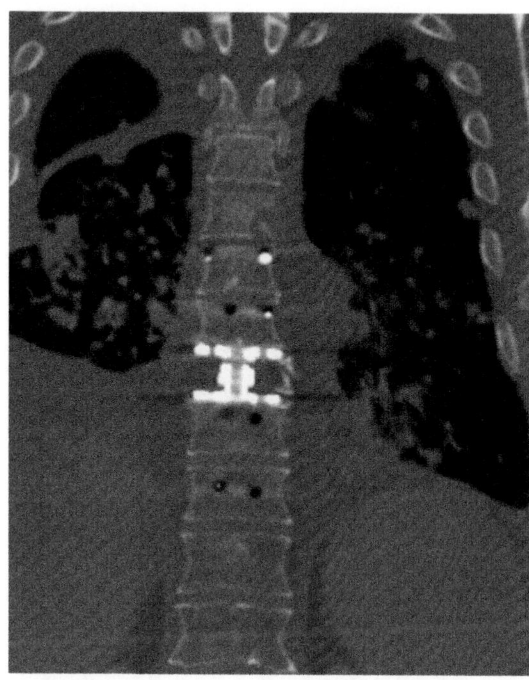

FIG. 22.14 Postoperative imaging.

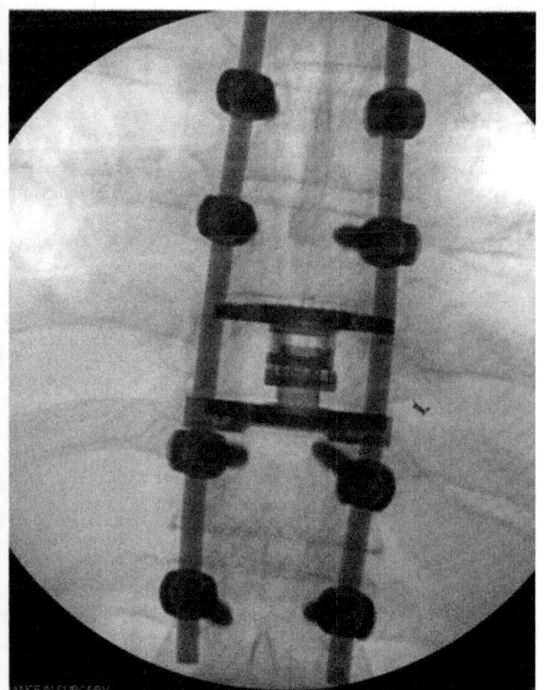

FIG. 22.13 Postoperative image following T9 corpectomy followed by posterior instrumentation from T7 to T11.

The transthoracic approach can be used at T2, whereas the retropleural approach can only be extended to T3 (Schwartz and McCormick, 2007). If the retropleural approach were used above T3, dividing the high thoracic sympathetic trunk could result in Horner's syndrome. The retropleural approach has a smaller incision and has less soft tissue dissection than the transthoracic approach. Indeed, among a large series of postthoracotomy patients, 9.2% reported pain lasting at least 6 months after surgery (Schwartz and McCormick, 2007). However, this smaller operative field has a drawback in that it cannot effectively address lesions involving more than one level (Uribe et al., 2011).

In terms of complications, a group reported on 130 consecutive patients receiving transthoracic surgery; the major complication rate was 27.7%, and 30-day and 90-day mortality was 9.2% and 20.8%, respectively (Schuchert et al., 2014). Median length of stay was 9 days. Comprehensive metaanalyses estimate that the overall complication rate of the transthoracic approach is approximately 11%–11.5% (Faciszewski et al., 1995; Fessler and Sturgill, 1998).

In a study of seven patients receiving retropleural approach surgery for central thoracic disc herniation, the mean hospital length of stay was 2.6 days (Kasliwal and Deutsch, 2011). Another study of 33 patients who

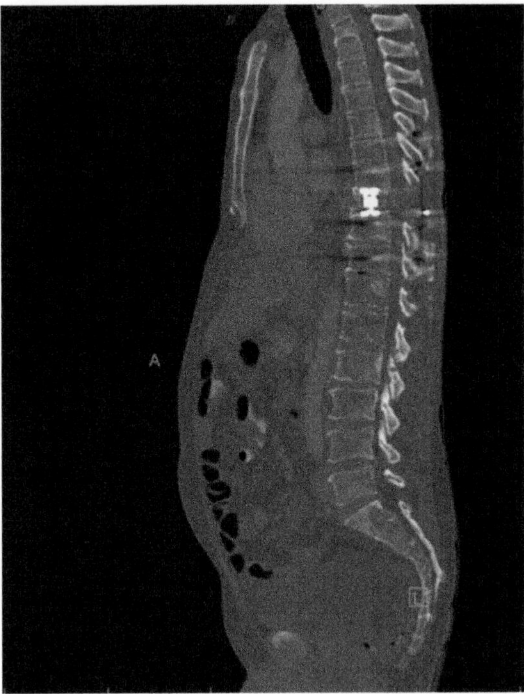

FIG. 22.15 Postoperative imaging.

received retropleural approach surgery for thoracic disc herniation had a mean hospital stay of 5 days and a perioperative rate of 18.1% (Nacar et al., 2013). McCormick et al. (1995) reported that patients without diffuse disease processes usually left the hospital within 3–4 days (McCormick et al., 1995). Yen and Uribe (2018) reported on 23 patients who underwent a mini-open lateral retropleural discectomy and had a mean hospital stay of 5 days (Yen and Uribe, 2018). Comparing the two approaches, it is clear that patients who underwent the retropleural approach left the hospital earlier (Figs. 22.14 and 22.15), but it is less apparent from these studies whether the complication rates differed.

CONCLUSIONS

Thoracic approaches to the thoracolumbar junction are challenging procedures that require a command of the surgical anatomy of this region. Therefore, spine surgeons performing such approaches must be well acquainted with thoracolumbar anatomy.

REFERENCES

Anderson, T.M., Mansour, K.A., Miller Jr., J.I., 1993. Thoracic approaches to anterior spinal operations: anterior thoracic approaches. Ann. Thorac. Surg. 55 (6), 1447–1451 discussion 1451-1442.

Angevin, P.D., McCormick, P.C., 2001. Retropleural thoracotomy. Technical note. Neurosurg. Focus 10 (1) ecp.1.

Angevine, P.D., McCormick, P.C., 2001. Retropleural thoracotomy. Neurosurg. Focus 10 (1), 1–5.

Bahm, J., 2018. Neurosurgical operative atlas: spine and peripheral nerves. In: Yun, J., Angevine, P.D., McCormick, P.C. (Eds.), Retropleural Approach to the Thoracolumbar Spine. Georg Thieme Verlag KG, pp. 188–192.

Berjano, P., Garbossa, D., Damilano, M., Pejrona, M., Bassani, R., Doria, C., 2014. Transthoracic lateral retropleural minimally invasive microdiscectomy for T9-T10 disc herniation. Eur. Spine J. 23 (6), 1376–1378.

Faciszewski, T., Winter, R.B., Lonstein, J.E., Denis, F., Johnson, L., 1995. The surgical and medical perioperative complications of anterior spinal fusion surgery in the thoracic and lumbar spine in adults. A review of 1223 procedures. Spine 20 (14), 1592–1599.

Faro, F.D., Marks, M.C., Newton, P.O., Blanke, K., Lenke, L.G., 2005. Perioperative changes in pulmonary function after anterior scoliosis instrumentation: thoracoscopic versus open approaches. Spine 30 (9), 1058–1063.

Fessler, R.G., Sturgill, M., 1998. Complications of surgery for thoracic disc disease. Surg. Neurol. 49 (6), 609–618.

Flamm, E.S., 1992. Percivall Pott: an 18th century neurosurgeon. J. Neurosurg. 76 (2), 319–326.

Hodgson, A.R., Stock, F.E., 2006. The Classic: anterior spinal fusion: a preliminary communication on the radical treatment of Pott's disease and Pott's paraplegia. 1956. Clin. Orthop. Relat. Res. 444, 10–15.

Kasliwal, M., Deutsch, H., 2011. Minimally invasive retropleural approach for central thoracic disc herniation. Minim. Invasive Neurosurg. 54 (04), 167–171.

Kwan, K., Cheung, K., 2016. Anterior Thoracic Instrumentation. Elsevier.

McCormick, P.C., 1995. Retropleural approach to the thoracic and thoracolumbar spine. Neurosurgery 37 (5), 908–914.

Menard, V., 1895. Traitement de la paraplegie du mal de Pott par drainage lateral : Costotransversektomie. Rev. Orthop. Paris 6, 134–146.

Nacar, O.A., Ulu, M.O., Pekmezci, M., Deviren, V., 2013. Surgical treatment of thoracic disc disease via minimally invasive lateral transthoracic trans/retropleural approach: analysis of 33 patients. Neurosurg. Rev. 36 (3), 455–465.

Schuchert, M.J., McCormick, K.N., Abbas, G., Pennathur, A., Landreneau, J.P., Landreneau, J.R., Pitanga, A., Gomes, J., Franca, F., El-Kadi, M., Peitzman, A.B., Ferson, P.F., Luketich, J.D., Landreneau, R.J., 2014. Anterior thoracic surgical approaches in the treatment of spinal infections and neoplasms. Ann. Thorac. Surg. 97 (5), 1750–1757.

Schwartz, T., McCormick, P.C., 2007. The Retropleural Approach to the Thoracic and Thoracolumbar Spine. Thieme.

Uribe, J.S., Dakwar, E., Cardona, R.F., Vale, F.L., 2011. Minimally invasive lateral retropleural thoracolumbar approach: cadaveric feasibility study and report of 4 clinical cases. Operative Neurosurgery 68 (Suppl. l_1), ons32–ons39.

Williams, M.P., Cherryman, G.R., Husband, J.E., 1989. Significance of thoracic disc herniation demonstrated by MR imaging. J. Comput. Assist. Tomogr. 13 (2), 211–214.

Yen, C.P., Uribe, J.S., 2018. Mini-open lateral retropleural approach for symptomatic thoracic disk herniations. Clin. Spine Surg. 31 (1), 14–21.

CHAPTER 23

Techniques for the Lateral Thoracolumbar Approach

ALEXANDER VON GLINSKI • SHIWEI HUANG • ARI D KAPPEL • DIA R. HALALMEH • MARC D. MOISI • ROD J. OSKOUIAN

INTRODUCTION

Originally intended to address lumbar spinal pathology, lateral lumbar interbody fusion (LLIF) has grown in popularity and has been adapted to allow access to the thoracic and thoracolumbar spine from approximately T4 to L5 (Malham, 2015; Action to Control Cardiovascular Risk in Diabetes Study G.et al., 2008) (Fig. 23.1). The indications for the lateral retropleural and retroperitoneal approach to the thoracolumbar junction are similar to those for posterior or transthoracic approaches and include disc herniations, fractures, tumors, pseudarthrosis, and proximal junctional kyphosis (Malham, 2015; Karikari et al., 2011; Malham and Parker, 2015; Meredith et al., 2013; Ozgur et al., 2006). LLIF has been associated with lower blood loss, soft tissue dissection, surgical times, perioperative complications, postoperative pain, and hospital stay duration than open exposure approaches to the thoracic spine (Karikari et al., 2011; Anand et al., 2010; Beisse et al., 2005; Glassman et al., 2008; Han et al., 2002; Karmakar and Ho, 2004; Khoo et al., 2002; Landreneau et al., 1993; Mack et al., 1993; Park et al., 2014). The lateral approach permits exposure of the anterior and middle columns of the spine without sacrificing the anterior or posterior longitudinal ligaments (ALL or PLL), so it provides more support for interbody implants (Salzmann et al., 2017). Contraindications include severe rotary scoliosis, a history of ipsilateral lateral spine surgery, and vascular variation. Therefore, it is useful to review vascular anatomy in the surgical field using a preoperative MRI, especially for an inexperienced surgeon. For example, in midthoracic disc protrusion, the surgeon should be aware of the aorta, which can lie over the left lateral aspect of the vertebral body. In such cases, a right lateral approach can be used, and care should be taken not to disrupt the left lateral portion of the annulus. Lateral approaches to the spine present distinct anatomical challenges and considerations for the spine surgeon. Perhaps most challenging, the thoracolumbar junction represents an especially complex region with its convergence of the retroperitoneal space, the thoracic cavity, the diaphragm, and the thoracolumbar spine. The lower rib cage and the diaphragm especially represent a dilemma for the spine surgeon (Figs. 23.2 and 23.3) (Dakwar et al., 2011). Accordingly, the approach has to be modified at the thoracolumbar junction (T11–L1).

Positioning

The positioning is similar to the lumbar approach (*please see chapter for lateral transpsoas approach technique*). Under general endotracheal anesthesia, the patient is placed in true 90 degrees lateral decubitus position on a radiolucent breakable table with at least 20–30 degrees bendable break at its midportion. The table break is positioned directly under the midsurgical levels, and the table is flexed to facilitate access to the affected level. Brachial plexus compression and pressure sores are prevented by placing axillary roll and padding the bony prominences, respectively. Arm boards are also used to suspend the patient's arm with the shoulders and elbows flexed to 90 degrees. Compared with the lumbar approach, it is important to keep in mind that the incision should be extensible, so regular anterior thoracotomy can be performed if needed. The C-arm is placed as in the lumbar approach, anteriorly to obtain anteroposterior (AP) and lateral views. It is crucial to ensure that the intraoperative fluoroscopic views are of good quality; this requires the patient to be perpendicular toward the floor in the lateral image. Furthermore, the beam path should match the lordotic curve in the AP view. Especially at the thoracolumbar junction, proper fluoroscopic alignment and meticulous attention to this principle will help avoid

Surgical anatomy of the lateral transpsoas approach to the lumbar spine. https://doi.org/10.1016/B978-0-323-67376-1.00023-9

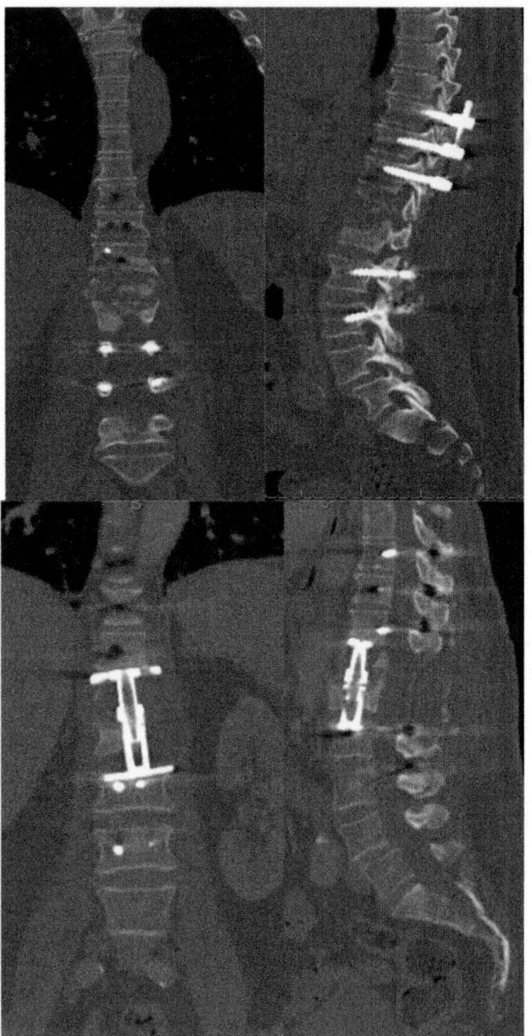

FIG. 23.1 T12–L1, L1–L2, with destruction of T12, L1 vertebral bodies. Two-staged approach with spinal fusion T9–L2 followed by extreme lateral approach for a corpectomy of T12 and L1 and interbody fusion, T11–12 and L1–L2.

migration of instrumentation that could lead to vascular or neural injury. To obtain the true lateral image, the table can be adjusted in "Trendelenburg" fashion by reflexing it head up. Indications of a true lateral projection include the following: linear endplates, linear posterior cortex, and superimposed pedicle. For multilevel cases, the table is adjusted as necessary to maintain good quality of the AP and lateral images. Once true images are obtained, the anterior and

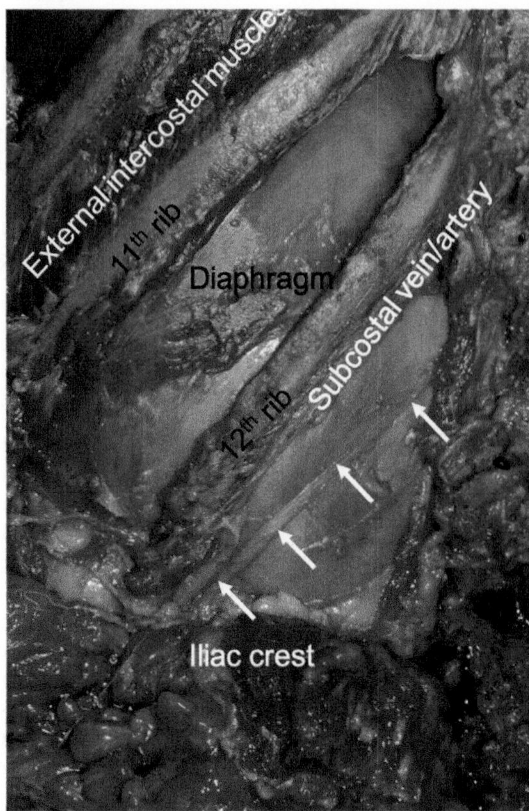

FIG. 23.2 Left-sided cadaveric dissection illustrating regional anatomy of the lateral approach to the thoracolumbar spine. The arrows mark the left subcostal nerve.

posterior vertebral borders are marked on the skin using two crossing K-wires. In single-level cases, the incision mark is made over the midsection of the target disc (more specifically over the junction of the middle and posterior thirds of the disc space). For multilevel cases, more than one incision might be required, several levels being accessed through each.

Opening and Disc Exposure

When approaching the thoracolumbar junction, it is helpful to make the skin incision and the rib resection two levels rostral to the segment undergoing operation. Otherwise, those ribs lie over the site of the planned surgery, making exposure more difficult for the surgeon and nearly impossible for the assistant, who must satisfactorily visualize the area involved. In addition, it is recommended that the surgeon works initially anterior to the patient to facilitate visualization along the rib to the costovertebral junction.

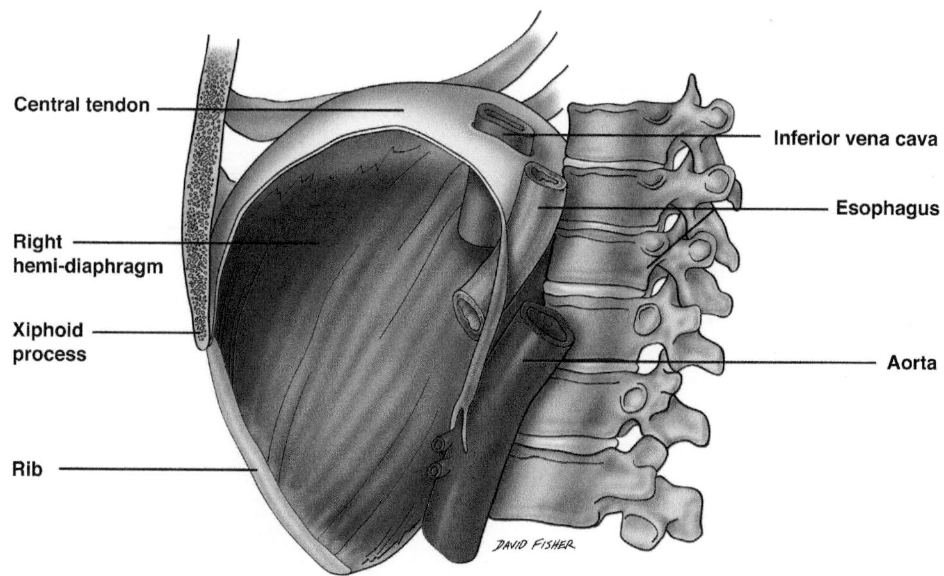

FIG. 23.3 Schematic drawing of the right hemidiaphragm and its relationships to the inferior vena cava, aorta, and esophagus.

For single-level cases, rib segments can be sacrificed, or taking an intercostal approach is advisable. In the rib-spreading technique, the thoracic cavity is accessed through the superior border of the rib overlying the target disc to preserve the neurovascular bundle at the inferior edge of the rib. Dissection through intercostal muscles between the ribs is then carried down to the pleura using electrocautery. Alternatively, the rib segments over the target disc can be resected and discarded or used as grafting material during the subsequent procedure. However, a rib-sparing technique has been described, resulting in improved patient outcomes, less postoperative surgical site pain, and earlier discharge (Moisi et al., 2016). In this technique, the rib of interest is resected, and the resected segment is reflected inferiorly, taking care not to injure the neurovascular bundle in the lower border of the rib. When the target level is treated, the rib is reflected back to its anatomical position, and 0-Ethibond nonabsorbable sutures are used for reattachment.

For multilevel cases, the rib-sacrificing technique is employed to achieve better visualization. The standard technique involves resection of a small portion of the rib and discarding the resulting segment. As previously mentioned, the resected segments can be saved for grafting material.

For example, in a patient with a T12 vertebral body exposure, a 12–14 cm skin incision is made over the T10 rib from the posterior axillary line to 4 cm off the midline. A 10 cm segment of exposed rib is circumferentially cleaned and removed. The pleural surface of the diaphragm is identified. The endothoracic fascia is reflected over the diaphragm and tightly applied to its surface. The costodiaphragmatic pleural reflection can also be seen. The initial exposure is tight because of the attachment of the diaphragm to the ribs. If the lateral endothoracic fascia is present in the rib bed, it is opened. Caudally, the pleural surface of the dia phragm is depressed and detached from the inner surface of the T11 and T12 ribs with sharp periosteal dissectors (Figs. 23.4 and 23.5). This immediately unites the retroperitoneum with the retropleural space. The detachment is easily continued medially to elevate the arcuate ligaments off the quadratus and psoas muscles. The subcostal nerve can be seen laterally running beneath the lateral arcuate ligament on the quadratus lumborum surface. Division of the ipsilateral crus completes the diaphragm mobilization. It might be necessary to elevate the part of the psoas muscle that attaches to the T12 vertebral body. This completes the exposure of the T12 vertebral body, the adjacent disc, and the T12 pedicle. Three sequential dilators provided with stimulating electrodes at their tips are typically placed over the costovertebral junction under guidance by lateral fluoroscopy. A K-wire is then inserted through the initial dilator to halfway across the disc space, again under fluoroscopic guidance. A table-mounted retractor is then docked over the last dilator, taking care not to

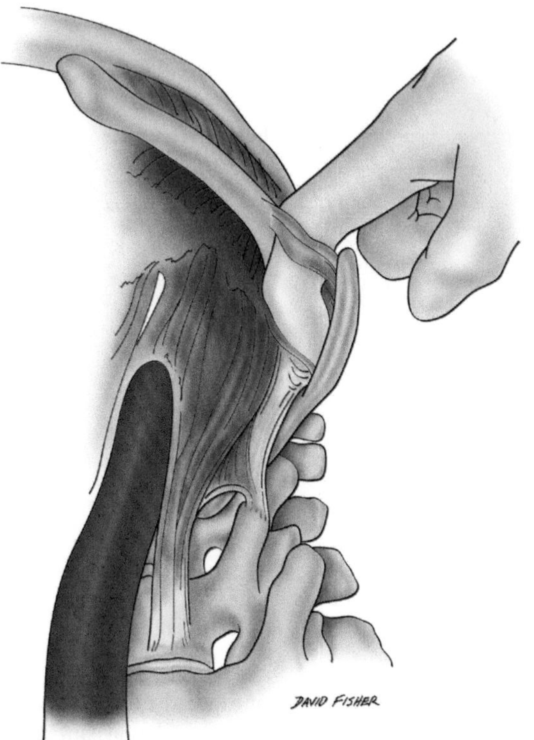

FIG. 23.4 Schematic drawing of a left-sided retropleural dissection with initial dissection through the intercostal muscles and then deeper dissection with the surgeon's digit mobilizing the lateral arcuate ligament. Note the left crus of the diaphragm.

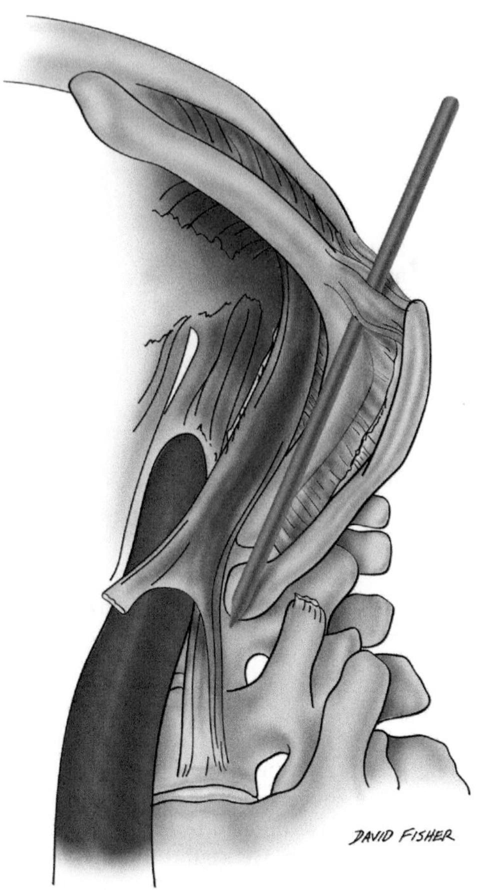

FIG. 23.5 Fig. 23.4 with additional mobilization of the diaphragm for targeting the thoracolumbar junction (probe).

expand the blades past the midpoint of the vertebral body to avoid segmental vessel injury. Once the retractor is adjusted to the desired position and secured to the operating table, the dilators are removed leaving the K-wire in place. Posterior intradiscal shim insertion into the center blade stabilizes the retractor to the posterior third of the disc space prior to fixing at the desired position. The other two lateral blades can be expanded in the cranial-caudal direction as necessary so the surgeon can easily visualize the related disc space. Supplementary shims can be added to prevent soft tissue creeping such as diaphragm and lungs. Using an endoscopic Kittner, the parietal pleura is bluntly dissected from the intercostal muscles and the rib. The rib head overlying the disc space is osteotomized to help identify the posteroinferior corner of the vertebra above and the posterosuperior corner of the vertebra below the disc space. The proximal 4 cm of the T12 rib, including the rib head, is removed. Wedge osteotomy of the surrounding bony corners of the vertebral bodies is then achieved using a straight osteotome to allow decompression. If local bone is to be preserved as graft material during the anterior fusion, an osteotome is preferred to a high-speed burr, which might nevertheless be needed if adequate osteotomy is challenging. Fluoroscopic guidance and free-running EMG neuromonitoring are essential to ensure safety of the neural elements during each step of instrument docking.

Discectomy

Once the annulus is visualized, lateral annulotomy is performed using a bayoneted annulotomy knife, taking care not to traverse the ALL and anteriorly situated vessels. Standard discectomy is completed using pituitary rongeurs, curettes, disc cutters, endplate scrapers, and other instruments, preserving the cortical endplates. The contralateral annulus is then released, and the disc is disrupted from the endplates using a Cobb elevator. Adequate disc disruption is required to restore the disc height and reduce the subsidence rate. However, excessive decortication of the endplate should be avoided to reduce the risk of subsidence. Finally, care must be always taken not to shift the patient position (perpendicular to the floor) during the procedure to avoid nonorthogonal instrument insertion and consequent vessel and nerve injury. Once the disc is completely removed and decompression is accomplished, the disc space is prepared with trial positioning, and the appropriate size of the implant is determined. While the disc space is being prepared, the implant is packed with local bone graft or the desired graft material. Caution should be exercised not to injure the endplates by oversizing the trial. Smaller thoracic grafts are typically used for smaller disc spaces and vertebral bodies. Under fluoroscopic guidance, the implant is inserted into the center of the disc space. The level/s of interest is/are stabilized with supplemental internal fixation using either a screw-rod construct or a plate [33, 36].

Corpectomy

Once the operative corridor has been established, the disc space can be prepared. After an annulotomy has been performed, the disc space can be prepared using a combination of rongeurs, currettes, and rasps. To achieve proper coronal alignment in the procedure, contralateral annular release is imperative. This can be performed safely by passing a blunt disk space device/Cobb elevator into the intervertebral body space. Furthermore, we use a sharp boxcutter to establish adequate endplate preparation. Any endplate violation must be avoided to prevent severe subsidence. In addition to careful endplate preparation, perpendicular entrance of the intervertebral cage is mandatory. We tend to use sliding devices as shown in the lumbar approach to archive this.

Closure

After correct placement of the implant is confirmed by fluoroscopy, the retractor system is carefully detached and removed, watching for any excessive bleeding or soft tissue injuries (lungs and diaphragm). The arcuate ligaments are reattached to the psoas and quadratus muscles with suture. The pleura is then carefully inspected. Should the pleural cavity be entered, a chest tube should be placed and removed on postoperative day 1 or 2, depending on the output [33, 36]. In any case, we would additionally ensure airtight pleural closure in this technique using a running 0-Vicryl suture. Immediately before the last stitches are done, the lungs should be deflated by the anesthesia team, so the last stitch can be inserted without tension. During closure of the intercostal musculature, a red rubber catheter can be placed to ensure airtight closure. In the event of severe intraoperative bleeding, a chest tube can be inserted to prevent a hemothorax. Approximation of the adjacent ribs with suture reduces the chest wall. Care is taken not to ensnare the intercostal nerves with suture during closure, which could substantially increase postoperative pain. Chest X-ray must always be obtained in the postanesthesia care unit to check for pneumothorax even if the pleura has not been violated (retropleural approach). The surgical site is irrigated, and strict layered closure is achieved.

POTENTIAL COMPLICATIONS

Despite being a minimally invasive approach compared with open exposure, LLIF entails certain complications. Pulmonary complications are among the most widely referenced examples both during and after surgery. In general, both the retropleural and transpleural approaches involve navigating critical respiratory structures intimately. This puts patients at risk for pulmonary complications such as pleural effusion, hemothorax, and/or open or tension pneumothorax (Gabel et al., 2016). Meredith et al. (2013) found that 44% of patients undergoing thoracic LLIF for various pathologies developed a pleural effusion after the chest tube was removed, two patients requiring urgent treatment. In a similar study by Baaj et al. (2012), the rate of pulmonary complications following thoracic LLIF was much lower (2.5%), only one patient in their cohort developing a hemothorax requiring intervention and another developing an uncomplicated pleural effusion. Further complications include breach of the visceral pleura, leading to extrapleural free air and atelectasis. However, it is important to note that pulmonary complications associated with LLIF are rare. Karikari et al. (2011) reported no cases of pleural effusion in a clinical series of 22 patients treated with LLIF for various thoracic spine pathologies. Therefore, a cautious and meticulous surgical approach coupled with a comprehensive understanding of the relevant thoracic anatomy and thoracic LLIF procedures provides a safe alternative to thoracolumbar intervention (Beisse et al., 2005; Han et al., 2002; Khoo et al., 2002; Landreneau et al., 1993; Mack et al., 1993).

In situations involving the T12–L1 or L1–L2 levels, one should consider injury to the diaphragm. The diaphragm should be crossed from above to access the T12–L1 intervertebral disc and from below to approach

L1–L2 level. It should be noted that the diaphragm is not incised; therefore, diaphragmatic repair is not required. Consequently, the retractor should pass through the diaphragmatic attachments to the ribs Karmakar and Ho, 2004. To our knowledge, diaphragmatic injury during thoracic LLIF has never been reported; however, it is a potential complication, especially when addressing the T12–L1 and L1–L2 intervertebral discs. Therefore, knowledge of the regional anatomy, particularly the diaphragmatic attachment, is mandatory for avoiding injury to the diaphragm and facilitating safe access to the target level.

Although pulmonary complications are the most common, thoracic LLIF procedures are also associated with nonpulmonary complications. Important examples are minor and major vessel injuries. At the level of the vertebral column, injury could occur to the descending thoracic aorta (this has not been reported in the literature) or vessels supplying the spinal cord. The most critical and vulnerable of these vessels is the artery of Adamkiewicz, a major source of blood supply to the anterior thoracolumbar spinal cord (Fanous et al., 2015; Schalow, 1990). Most commonly located on the left side of the spinal cord between T9 and L1, the artery of Adamkiewicz is at risk for injury once the vertebral bodies and intervertebral space are accessed. The importance of avoiding injury to it cannot be overstated, as iatrogenic injury has been shown to be catastrophic, with complications such as spinal cord infarction, paraplegia, spinal shock, and death (Fanous et al., 2015). Although there have been no reported cases of thoracic LLIF-associated injury to the artery of Adamkiewicz, careful consideration is always necessary, as the consequences are potentially severe.

Another important nonpulmonary complication of thoracic LLIF procedures is incidental durotomy. In a metaanalysis of 29 studies and 1228 patients, Phan et al. (2016) found the rate of dural tears and/or CSF leaks in patients undergoing LLIF of the lumbar spine to be 5.4%. Although these findings are related to lumbar level procedures, individual cases of thoracic durotomies have also been reported in patients undergoing LLIF of the thoracic spine. In the previously discussed study by Meredith et al., 2 of 18 patients (11%) in the series were reported to have incidental durotomies. One had an incidental dural tear that was repaired intraoperatively without incident. The other had a durotomy with repair failure leading to CSF leakage and collection in the pulmonary cavity, ultimately requiring revision of the repair and the placement of a subarachnoid drain. These nonpulmonary complications, although seldom reported, call for further consideration of possible complications during thoracic LLIF.

Thoracic LLIF procedures, by variably requiring transection and removal of a rib segment to access the targeted operative corridor, also place patients at risk of neurological complications.

At particular risk of trauma during LLIF procedures is the subcostal nerve. Providing the predominant nerve supply to the anterolateral abdominal muscles, the subcostal nerve emerges from the T12 nerve root and most often runs at the inferior border of the 12th rib, increasing its susceptibility to iatrogenic injury during procedures in the thoracolumbar region (Alonso et al., 2017; Grunert et al., 2017). Although no reports of subcostal nerve injury have been associated with thoracic LLIF procedures, cadaveric studies using a lateral approach to the lumbar spine have shown the subcostal nerve to be at heightened risk during the approach through the outer abdominal muscles and subcutaneous tissue and during subsequent resection of the 12th rib (Alonso et al., 2017; Grunert et al., 2017).

While no cases of direct neurovascular bundle injury during LLIF have been reported, one case series by Malham and Parker (2015) included a case of a transpleural T9–T10 LLIF procedure that resulted in the development of persistent postoperative neuropathic thoracic pain requiring pharmacological intervention. Although the reported case offered no etiology for the resultant neuropathic pain, neurovascular bundle injury associated with this surgical approach could certainly be an explanation. Postoperative thoracic pain can follow LLIF, but such complications can potentially be avoided by minimizing soft tissue disruption and taking measures to restore the anatomical function of the rib (Moisi et al., 2016). Hence, the rib-sparing technique can be considered in these cases, resulting in improved patient outcomes, less postoperative surgical site pain, and earlier discharge (Grunert et al., 2017). Knowledge of the anatomical course and innervation of the subcostal nerve, meticulous blunt dissection through the subcutaneous and muscular tissues, and careful rib resection should help avoid thoracolumbar LLIF-associated subcostal nerve injury that would otherwise result in variable sensory deficits and/or abdominal wall hernias (Alonso et al., 2017; Grunert et al., 2017).

A possible though unreported complication of thoracic LLIF procedures is thoracic duct injury. As the body's largest lymphatic vessel, the thoracic duct originates from the cisterna chyli, a confluence of lymphatic vessels situated to the right of the aorta and in front of the anterior longitudinal ligament at the level of the first or second vertebra (Phang et al., 2014). Upon entering the thorax, the thoracic duct ascends between the aorta and the azygos vein on the right side of the anterior surface of the vertebral column, eventually crossing to the left side at the level of the fifth or sixth thoracic vertebra and continuing to ascend and loop, to drain ultimately into the jugular vein (Phang et al., 2014). However, it should be noted that the anatomy and course of the thoracic duct is highly variable (Phang et al., 2014). Owing to its variable course and proximity to the anterior spinal cord, injury to the thoracic duct has been shown to be a rare complication of anterior and thoracoscopic spinal surgeries (Amini et al., 2007; Eisenstein and O'Brien, 1977). Amini et al. (2007) described a case in which a left-sided thoracoscopic discectomy and fusion at T12 was complicated by intraoperative perforation of the thoracic duct requiring repair, which was further complicated by postoperative chest tube chylorrhea, treated conservatively but extending the hospital stay. Although no such case of thoracic duct injury has been associated with thoracic LLIF procedures, the anatomical variability of the thoracic duct places it at some risk during any surgery using the anterior or lateral approach, so it should be considered.

CONCLUSIONS

The LLIF technique is a versatile and safe option for treating both lumbar and thoracic spine diseases. It offers the benefits of minimally invasive approaches and adds to the spine surgeon's armamentarium for managing spine diseases.

REFERENCES

Action to Control Cardiovascular Risk in Diabetes Study, G, et al., 2008. Effects of intensive glucose lowering in type 2 diabetes. N. Engl. J. Med. 358 (24), 2545–2559.

Alonso, F., et al., 2017. The subcostal nerve during lateral approaches to the lumbar spine: an anatomical study with relevance for injury avoidance and postoperative complications such as abdominal wall hernia. World Neurosurg. 104, 669–673.

Amini, A., Apfelbaum, R.I., Schmidt, M.H., 2007. Chylorrhea: a rare complication of thoracoscopic discectomy of the thoracolumbar junction. Case report J. Neurosurg. Spine 6 (6), 563–566.

Anand, N., et al., 2010. Mid-term to long-term clinical and functional outcomes of minimally invasive correction and fusion for adults with scoliosis. Neurosurg. Focus 28 (3), E6.

Baaj, A.A., et al., 2012. Complications of the mini-open anterolateral approach to the thoracolumbar spine. J. Clin. Neurosci. 19 (9), 1265–1267.

Beisse, R., et al., 2005. Surgical technique and results of endoscopic anterior spinal canal decompression. J. Neurosurg. Spine 2 (2), 128–136.

Dakwar, E., Vale, F.L., Uribe, J.S., 2011. Trajectory of the main sensory and motor branches of the lumbar plexus outside the psoas muscle related to the lateral retroperitoneal transpsoas approach. J. Neurosurg. Spine 14 (2), 290–295.

Eisenstein, S., O'Brien, J.P., 1977. Chylothorax: a complication of Dwyer's anterior instrumentation. Br. J. Surg. 64 (5), 339–341.

Fanous, A.A., et al., 2015. The impact of preoperative angiographic identification of the artery of Adamkiewicz on surgical decision making in patients undergoing thoracolumbar corpectomy. Spine (Phila Pa 1976) 40 (15), 1194–1199.

Gabel, B.C., et al., 2016. Pulmonary complications following thoracic spinal surgery: a systematic review. Glob. Spine J. 6 (3), 296–303.

Glassman, S.D., et al., 2008. Defining substantial clinical benefit following lumbar spine arthrodesis. J. Bone Joint Surg. Am. 90 (9), 1839–1847.

Grunert, P., et al., 2017. Injury to the lumbar plexus and its branches after lateral fusion procedures: a cadaver study. World Neurosurg. 105, 519–525.

Han, P.P., Kenny, K., Dickman, C.A., 2002. Thoracoscopic approaches to the thoracic spine: experience with 241 surgical procedures. Neurosurgery 51 (5 Suppl. l), S88–S95.

Karikari, I.O., et al., 2011. Extreme lateral interbody fusion approach for isolated thoracic and thoracolumbar spine diseases: initial clinical experience and early outcomes. J. Spinal Disord. Tech. 24 (6), 368–375.

Karmakar, M.K., Ho, A.M., 2004. Postthoracotomy pain syndrome. Thorac. Surg. Clin. 14 (3), 345–352.

Khoo, L.T., Beisse, R., Potulski, M., 2002. Thoracoscopic-assisted treatment of thoracic and lumbar fractures: a series of 371 consecutive cases. Neurosurgery 51 (5 Suppl. l), S104–S117.

Landreneau, R.J., et al., 1993. Postoperative pain-related morbidity: video-assisted thoracic surgery versus thoracotomy. Ann. Thorac. Surg. 56 (6), 1285–1289.

Mack, M.J., et al., 1993. Application of thoracoscopy for diseases of the spine. Ann. Thorac. Surg. 56 (3), 736–738.

Malham, G.M., 2015. Minimally invasive direct lateral corpectomy for the treatment of a thoracolumbar fracture. J. Neurol. Surg. A Cent. Eur. Neurosurg. 76 (3), 240–243.

Malham, G.M., Parker, R.M., 2015. Treatment of symptomatic thoracic disc herniations with lateral interbody fusion. J. Spine Surg. 1 (1), 86–93.

Meredith, D.S., et al., 2013. Extreme lateral interbody fusion (XLIF) in the thoracic and thoracolumbar spine: technical report and early outcomes. HSS J. 9 (1), 25–31.

Moisi, M., et al., 2016. Lateral thoracic osteoplastic rib-sparing technique used for lateral spine surgery: technical note. Cureus 8 (7), e668.

Ozgur, B.M., et al., 2006. Extreme Lateral Interbody Fusion (XLIF): a novel surgical technique for anterior lumbar interbody fusion. Spine J. 6 (4), 435–443.

Park, M.S., Deukmedjian, A.R., Uribe, J.S., 2014. Minimally invasive anterolateral corpectomy for spinal tumors. Neurosurg. Clin. N. Am. 25 (2), 317–325.

Phan, K., et al., 2016. Minimally invasive surgery in adult degenerative scoliosis: a systematic review and meta-analysis of decompression, anterior/lateral and posterior lumbar approaches. J. Spine Surg. 2 (2), 89–104.

Phang, K., et al., 2014. Review of thoracic duct anatomical variations and clinical implications. Clin. Anat. 27 (4), 637–644.

Salzmann, S.N., Shue, J., Hughes, A.P., 2017. Lateral lumbar interbody fusion-outcomes and complications. Curr. Rev. Musculoskelet. Med. 10 (4), 539–546.

Schalow, G., 1990. Feeder arteries, longitudinal arterial trunks and arterial anastomoses of the lower human spinal cord. Zentralblatt Neurochir. 51 (4), 181–184.

CHAPTER 24

Complications From Lateral Transpsoas Approaches to the Lumbar Spine

ALEXANDER VON GLINSKI • DARIUS ANSARI • BRADLEY KOLB • GARY B. RAJAH • DANIEL T. GINAT • DIA R. HALALMEH • MARC D. MOISI • ROD J. OSKOUIAN

INTRODUCTION

Over the last 10 years, we have observed increasing development and utilization of minimally invasive anterolateral retroperitoneal approaches for lumbar interbody arthrodesis (Walker et al., 2019; Uribe and Deukmedjian, 2015). These approaches have the many advantages common among minimally invasive spine surgeries, such as decreases in pain, blood loss, and nerve injury (Knight et al., 2009; Saraph et al., 2004; Zoidl et al., 2003). Direct and indirect lateral approaches, including the prepsoas and transpsoas approaches, are distinct. The specific benefits of these retroperitoneal approaches over the posterior approach include:

(1) sufficient visualization of most of the disc space and more thorough endplate preparation (Tatsumi et al., 2015);
(2) decreased incidence of subsidence by larger interbody devices reaching over most of the endplate (Le et al., 2012; Marchi et al., 2013);
(3) better indirect decompression with a more satisfactory restoration of disc height, especially in coronal angulation (Phillips et al., 2013);
(4) potential benefit in regard to prior wound healing problems and in avoiding an approach through scar tissue (Joseph et al., 2015);
(5) Decreased intraoperative blood loss, resulting in lower transfusion rates and improved patient outcomes (Ozgur et al., 2006; Rodgers et al., 2010; Lehmen and Gerber, 2015; Hu, 2004).

Although the lateral lumbar interbody fusion (LLIF) approach boasts considerable advantages over other popular/traditional techniques such as anterior lumbar interbody fusion (ALIF), transforaminal lumbar interbody fusion (TLIF), and posterior lumbar interbody fusion (PLIF), it also poses particular risks. Potential complications include injury to the bowel, vasculature, and most commonly, the lumbar plexus (Walker et al., 2019; Uribe and Deukmedjian, 2015; Grunert et al., 2017; Ahmadian et al., 2013). In the open and extreme lumber interbody fusion approaches (OLIF and lateral transpsoas interbody fusion, respectively), further subtle anatomical differences affect the complication profile. Broadly, these complications can be classed as retroperitoneal and peritoneal. The most common retroperitoneal approach–related complications are direct or indirect injuries to the peripheral nerves, lumbar nerve root branches, and the lumbar plexus. There is also a potential for injuries to the visceral organs, ureters, or vascular structures, though these are less common. To date, data about complications from LLIF have been limited to nonrandomized, noncontrolled observational reports; few studies have involved large cohorts of patients (Rodgers et al., 2011; Grimm et al., 2016; Isaacs et al., 2010; Aichmair et al., 2013; Lykissas et al., 2014). A number of systematic reviews of LLIF complications have also been published (Joseph et al., 2015; Lehmen and Gerber, 2015; Hijji et al., 2017; Hartl et al., 2016; Barbagallo et al., 2014). In general, the OLIF technique has a lower rate of psoas and lumbar plexus injuries because it is performed anterior to the psoas. However, this also explains the higher rate of sympathetic nerve and vascular injuries in OLIF surgery. No differences could be found regarding urological injuries (kidney and ureter) or visceral injuries (peritoneal and bowel) (Walker et al., 2019). Concerning postoperative complications, Walker et al. found no difference in the incidence of postoperative ileus or hematoma (subcutaneous and psoas) but found a slightly higher infection rate in the group (3.1% vs. 1.1%) (Xu et al., 2018).

In this chapter, we will review the specific types of complications associated with LLIF and their prevalence.

Surgical anatomy of the lateral transpsoas approach to the lumbar spine. https://doi.org/10.1016/B978-0-323-67376-1.00024-0

APPROACH-RELATED COMPLICATIONS

Nerve Injury

The most common complications resulting from LLIF are neurological, so these are the most concerning to practitioners, especially since the technique is fairly new (Xu et al., 2018; Kwon and Kim, 2016). A number of observational studies reporting neurological complications following LLIF have been published (Aichmair et al., 2013; Lykissas et al., 2014; Tohmeh et al., 2011; Pumberger et al., 2012; Cahill et al., 2012). The reported rate ranges from 0.7% to 78.8%, according to a recent systematic review of 6819 patients who had undergone LLIF (Hijji et al., 2017). The same review found a 3.98% incidence of persistent neurological deficit due to complications from LLIF, "persistent" being defined as a sensory or motor deficit lasting longer than 6 months following surgery (Hijji et al., 2017). With respect to nonpersistent complications related to peripheral nerve injury, the same authors found a 36.07% incidence of transient neurological deficit following LLIF surgery, probably attributable to muscle fiber injury (related to the transpsoas surgical approach) and nerve irritation caused by psoas muscle retraction (Hijji et al., 2017).

A more recent metaanalysis compared the OLIF and lateral transpsoas interbody fusion approaches. The lateral transpsoas interbody fusion approach entailed significantly higher rates of transient thigh or groin sensory symptoms (numbness/pain; 21.7% vs. 8.7%) and transient hip flexor weakness (19.7% vs. 5.7%). Hip flexion weakness could be considered a side effect of the approach as opposed to a complication, just as incisional pain and back extension weakness following open posterior fusions are approach-related side effects (and are rarely reported) (Cheng et al., 2016). The described incidence of hip flexion weakness following lateral transpsoas surgery is remarkably steady, but the grouping of hip flexion weakness with neuropraxic injuries that result in distal lower extremity weakness is a significant contributor to the conflicting results in the published literature (Lehmen and Gerber, 2015). Further, Walker et al. found a significant increase in lasting motor neurological weakness at the last follow-up in the transpsoas studies (2.8% vs. 1.0). In contrast, while no cases of sympathetic plexus injury were stated in the lateral transpsoas interbody fusion cases, there was a reported rate of 5.4% in the OLIF studies. While categorically detailed in all studies, this complication was manifested as loss of temperature regulation in the ipsilateral lower limb. However, it should be emphasized that the risk of neurological injury is not negligible in an OLIF approach. This is probably because dorsal retraction of the psoas muscle is usually necessary to obtain an orthogonal graft orientation from an oblique angle. This oblique entrance trajectory also places the contralateral neural foramen at risk either during attempts to release the contralateral disk or during cases in which the tools and implant are inadvertently advanced too far (Silvestre et al., 2012).

Intraoperative Neuromonitoring

Lateral interbody fusion was introduced over a decade ago with integrated neuromonitoring in order to avoid nerve injury. The combination of evoked electromyography (EMG) with sequential dilators is referred to as neural mapping (Uribe et al., 2010a,b). It allows the surgeon to localize nerve structures in real time by visual and oral threshold responses. This method is intended to reduce persistent neurological complications related to lumbar plexus injury and improve the safety of lateral approaches (Ozgur et al., 2006; Pumberger et al., 2012). Nevertheless, transient motor and sensory deficits are common despite the integration of neuromonitoring (Tohmeh et al., 2011). As the approach has become more widely used, several variants of the technique have been developed, including some that do not require intraoperative neuromonitoring (Bergey et al., 2004; Hardenbrook et al., 2013). Requirements regarding the integration of neuromonitoring into the approach and procedural instrumentation of transpsoas spine surgery remain controversial. This is especially true given that the common problem of postoperative hip flexion is—from a definition standpoint—not understood to be a consequence of neural injury, so neuromonitoring does not help in avoiding psoas muscle trauma during the approach (Cheng et al., 2016).

In a 2015 systematic literature review of transpsoas articles, Lehmen and Gerber compared weighted averages of complications and side effects between lateral approaches with integrated neuromonitoring and those without (shallow docking and others). In this analysis of 7763 patients from a total of 80 studies, the authors found that hip flexion weakness was similar between integrated and nonintegrated monitoring approaches (20.9% vs. 20.7%), reflecting the general consistency in the literature regarding trauma to the psoas muscle secondary to blunt passage. However, alterations in thigh sensation are over twice as common in nonmonitored approaches (35.6% vs. 16.4%) and new distal weakness is more than three times as common (5.1% vs. 1.6%) (Lehmen and Gerber, 2015). Given the abundance of publications showing that integrated neuromonitoring does not avert neural injury, Acosta et al. suggest there would be fewer nerve injuries if the so-called "suprapsoas" shallow docking approach were used, an alternative to the traditional mini-open lateral transpsoas approach. With this method, injury to nerves is minimized by placement of the retractor on the lateral surface rather than through the psoas muscle. Once it is on the psoas muscle, the fibers of that muscle are carefully separated to visualize and avoid any neural structures in the corridor of approach to access the lateral disk space (Acosta et al., 2013). The sensor located at the top of the tube permits focused stimulation within the psoas major muscle, but motor fibers lateral to the psoas are not detected. Furthermore, the ilioinguinal and iliohypogastric nerves can only be monitored at their short segments within the psoas at the L1/L2 level. Moreover, the L1 and L2 nerve roots along with parts of the L2 and L3 nerve root contain no motor fibers and thus remain "silent" on EMG monitoring (Tubbs, 2018). Grunert et al. found that 50% of the nerve injuries occur either lateral to the psoas, somewhere in the retroperitoneal space, or in the subcutaneous tissue of the abdominal wall (Grunert et al., 2017). Given this complex course of the plexus and the findings of the Grunert study, many neural structures are not sufficiently monitored using the tip probe, so detailed anatomical knowledge is critical for avoiding nerve injuries.

Nevertheless, the broader literature supports the use of integrated neuromonitoring, although alternative approaches for transpsoas surgery are emerging. The most persuasive argument for pro-neuromonitoring is that it reduces the motor neural complication rates, consistently reported in the literature. Many comparisons have demonstrated that the neuromonitored lateral transpsoas approach results in significantly lower neural complications than similar approaches performed without integrated neuromonitoring or in a shallow docking approach. Cheng et al. compared postoperative neural deficits in traditional lateral transpsoas interbody fusions with integrated neuromonitoring directly with shallow docking approaches for lateral interbody fusions (Cheng et al., 2015). In a 120 patient series, the authors found nearly twice the neural complication rate (including sensory deficits) in shallow docking than the neuromonitored transpsoas approach overall (28% vs. 14.2%), and nearly thrice the rate in single-level procedures (10.2% vs. 28.6%, respectively) (Cheng et al., 2015). Despite these advantages of neuromonitoring and the ongoing debate regarding its value, a fundamental understanding of the lumbar plexus and of the retroperitoneal space is imperative for preventing severe complications with the transpsoas approach.

The Lumbar Plexus

The lumbar plexus is derived from contributions of the first three lumbar ventral rami, along with contributions from parts of the 4th lumbar ramus and sometimes the 12th thoracic ventral ramus, and forms within the psoas muscle (Tubbs, 2018). Short direct branches of the lumbar plexus innervate the psoas major, quadratus lumborum, and lumbar intertransversarii. Important branches of the lumbar plexus include the femoral, iliohypogastric, ilioinguinal, genitofemoral, lateral cutaneous femoral, and obturator nerves (Tubbs et al., 2017). The lumbar plexus is closely associated with the LLIF surgical corridor, making it vulnerable to injuries depending on the level of surgery (Grunert et al., 2017; Tubbs et al., 2017; Van Campenhout et al., 2010; Regev et al., 2009). In a cadaveric study, Grunert et al. demonstrated that 50% of all segments at L1-L4 that had been operated on demonstrated plexus nerve injuries, occurring at the motor and sensory nerves as well as the nerve roots (Grunert et al., 2017). Banagan reported a lower rate of 25% injured nerves in the operated levels (Banagan et al., 2011); they placed the dilator tubes under direct visualization while Grunnert et al. used a standard operative technique. Moreover, Banagan et al. investigated only L3-L5 while Grunert looked at L1-L5 and found most of the nerve injuries at L1-L3 (Grunert et al., 2017; Banagan et al., 2011). Regarding tubular placement, several studies have described certain anatomical "safe zones" (Uribe et al., 2010a,b; Benglis et al., 2009) where nerve or plexus injuries can be avoided. Uribe (Uribe et al., 2010a,b) divided each vertebral segment into four quarters (I to IV) from the anterior to the posterior border. Moro et al. took the same approach (Moro et al., 2003). Both confirmed the findings by Benglis that the lumbosacral plexus presents a dorsal to ventral migration on disk spaces from L2 to L5 (Benglis et al., 2009).

Often, the course of the lumbar plexus is oversimplified by considering only its relationship to the lateral body: Dakwar et al. described a far more complex course in relation to the psoas muscle (Dakwar et al., 2011). Furthermore, despite extensive studies, the types and mechanisms of nerve injury occurring after lateral approaches remain unknown. Most types of injury described in the literature involve no structural changes to the nerve, such as compression traction, transient irritation, or ischemia (Ahmadian et al., 2013; Pumberger et al., 2012). These injuries could be classified as Sunderland I, which potentially explains why 90% of the neurological deficits after LLIF resolve (Rodgers et al., 2011; Lykissas et al., 2014). Especially considering that recovery times range from 6 weeks to 24 months, it is plausible that different Sunderland grades result from LLIF (Rodgers et al., 2011; Pumberger et al., 2012). This is underlined by the abovementioned cadaver study by Grunert et al., who observed partial and complete transections (Grunert et al., 2017). A partial transection can be graded as Sunderland IV and a complete transection as Sunderland V, keeping in mind that the Sunderland grade correlates with recovery (Sunderland, 1990). In order to identify the locations of nerves at high risk of injury, Grundert et al. divided the approach into four mediolateral anatomical zones, lateral to medial and superficial to deep: Zone IV includes subcutaneous tissue of the outer abdominal wall; Zone III the inner abdominal wall muscles; Zone II the retroperitoneal tissue; and Zone I the psoas major muscle. These zones could help to inform clinical practice of the whereabouts of nerves likely to be injured (Tubbs, 2018). According to this classification, Tubbs et al. defined certain nerve structures as at risk depending on the level operated (Tubbs, 2018).

L1/L2

At this level, the subcostal nerve emerges from the T12 nerve root and runs along the inferior border of the 12th rib prior to penetrate through the abdominal wall, so it can be injured in Zones III and IV (Grunert et al., 2017). Such injury can be avoided by blunt dissection through the subcutaneous and muscle tissues without overuse of monopolar coagulation. Further, the iliohypogastric and ilioinguinal nerves emerge from the T12/L1 nerve root. They run within or posterior to the psoas major, exiting the psoas (Zone I) and descending in the retroperitoneal space (Zone II) on the anterior surface of the quadratus lumborum to the posterior abdominal wall. After piercing through the abdominal wall (Zone III) they disperse into small branches within the subcutaneous tissue (Zone IV). Therefore, during operations on L1/L2, these nerves can potentially be injured in all zones and the same careful blunt dissection as described above should be performed (Grunert et al., 2017).

Originating from L1/L2, the genitofemoral nerve pierces the psoas muscle (Zone I) from posterior to anterior and continues its descent on the anterior surface (Zone II). This crossing point of the genitofemoral nerve varies between L3 and L4 (Dakwar et al., 2011), with some anatomical variations; the nerve piercing through more cranially at L1/L2, as described by Grunert et al., results in nerve injuries at L1/L2 (Grunert et al., 2017). The aforementioned shallow docking technique could help to avoid injury to the genitofemoral nerve, as it is visible on the anterior surface of the psoas muscle (Grunert et al., 2017; Acosta et al., 2013). Further, especially at the level L1/L2, the surgeon must be aware that no lower extremity motor fibers are present. Therefore, choosing a more posterior docking point or overretracting is inadvisable due to a "silent" EMG. Additionally, the L1 and L2 nerve roots carry motor fibers for the abdomen, so injury can result in abdominal wall hernia (Ahmadian et al., 2013). Grunert et al. found most injuries to the iliohypogastric and ilioinguinal nerves on the anterior surface of the quadratus lumborum muscle, which builds the lateral wall of the retroperitoneal space (Grunert et al., 2017). Therefore, finger palpation of the quadratus lumborum at this level could be useful prior to tube insertion. In addition to avoiding compression of the quadratus lumborum, a limited retraction time is advisable according to Uribe et al. (Uribe et al., 2010a,b).

L2/L3

Unlike the genitofemoral nerve, not all nerves are visible during retractor placement. For example, the lateral cutaneous nerve originates from the L2 and L3 nerve roots and runs caudally and intramuscularly to approximately the L4 level before exiting the psoas muscle laterally to enter the retroperitoneal space (Grunert et al., 2017; Tubbs et al., 2017; Moisi et al., 2016). There it continues its descent toward the anterior superior iliac spine at the anterior surface of the iliacus muscle (Grunert et al., 2017). In addition to the lateral cutaneous nerve, the L2 nerve root traverses the psoas muscle after exiting the neuroforamen. Grunert et al. described intramuscular injuries (Grunert et al., 2017) involving these structures; indeed, this intramuscular course highlights the value of neuromonitoring. In light of this, extensive retraction during a transpsoas approach should be avoided at all costs.

L3/L4

The lateral femoral cutaneous nerve descends in the retroperitoneal space rather than its intramuscular location at the L2/L3 level (Tubbs et al., 2017). Grunert et al. confirmed the course described by Dakwar et al. as located on the anterior surface of the psoas muscle (Dakwar et al., 2011). Therefore, in contrast to the Zone I injury at L2/L3, the lateral cutaneous nerve presented an injury in the retroperitoneal space (Zone II) (Grunert et al., 2017). This can potentially be prevented by using the aforementioned "shallow docking" technique. Also, the femoral nerve, which is formed by the L2 to L4 nerve roots, runs at the posterior aspect of the L3/L4 disk space while migrating anteriorly at L4/

L5 (Davis et al., 2011). Nevertheless, the femoral nerve shows some variations; a more anterior, more midline location explains why it can be injured despite placement of the retractor in the "safe zone."

L4/L5

Regev et al. found that the L4/L5 level was at greatest risk for injury (Regev et al., 2009). By dissecting the lumbar plexus in 12 cadavers and marking its branches with copper wires, Tubbs et al. elucidated the course of these nerves in relation to the different levels (Tubbs et al., 2017). Using lateral fluoroscopy, the greatest concentration of nerve fibers was found from the posteroinferior aspect of L4 inferior along the posterior one-third of the body of L5 (Tubbs et al., 2017).

Vascular Injury

The traditional anterior approach enables the surgeon to remove intervertebral disk materials thoroughly and to implant large fusion devices for anterior column support. However, because mobilization of intraabdominal vessels is necessary, the traditional open anterior approach has been correlated with major vascular injuries. In their retrospective analysis of 345 procedures of anterior lumbar spinal surgery, Fantini et al. reported a 2.9% incidence of injury to major abdominal vessels (Fantini et al., 2007). An important benefit of LLIF is that it allows comparable exposure of the disc space and implantation of a large interbody device without the need to mobilize the great vessels of the abdomen. By accessing the lumbar motion segments using an lateral transpsoas interbody fusion approach, the anterior longitudinal ligament can be preserved and the risk of major vascular injury considerably reduced, although these can still occur (Rodgers et al., 2011). This precludes the requirement for an access surgeon and decreases the occurrence of vascular injury during the surgical approach. However, the literature does contain reports of injury to the great vessels during LLIF, usually due to violation of the ALL or annulus by misplaced grafts, cages, or even retractor blades (Aichmair et al., 2015; Assina et al., 2014; Santillan et al., 2010).

Blizzard et al. present a case with a renal arterial injury caused either by interposition of the vessel wall of an aberrant artery between the retractor blades or by direct injury during retraction. This arterial injury led to infarction of approximately 60% of the left kidney (Blizzard et al., 2016). The renal vasculature is highly variable in both vessel numbers and course. Accessory arteries, which accompany the main vessel to the hilum, and aberrant arteries, which supply the superior or inferior pole without entering the hilum, occur in approximately 30% of patients (Ozkan et al., 2006; Costa et al., 2019). The course of those aberrant arteries is unpredictable, and vessels can enter the kidney directly superiorly or even posteriorly, lying directly over the psoas and vertebral body. Therefore the kidney, paravertebral musculature, and renal vasculature are palpated and partially visualized to determine safe retractor placement (Blizzard et al., 2016).

Aichmair et al. presented the first case of a surgery-related injury to the abdominal aorta during LLIF. The vascular injury was most likely caused by distal endplate and anterior cortical violation, with concomitant dislodging of an anterior bony spur during an attempt to advance a well-fixed prosthetic device (Aichmair et al., 2015).

In a systematic review and metaanalysis of 1874 patients treated via OLIF and 4607 treated with lateral transpsoas interbody fusion, Walker et al. found a higher risk of major vascular injury in the OLIF (1.8%) than the lateral transpsoas interbody fusion (0.4%) approach (Walker et al., 2019). In a transpsoas approach, when done properly with special care to maintain fluoroscopic orthogonality to the vertebral body, the anterior longitudinal ligament shields the great vessels from the working instruments (Walker et al., 2019). The low major vascular injury rate of 0.4% calculated in the transpsoas group is consistent with the rate previously reported in a large multicenter study (Uribe and Deukmedjian, 2015). The authors mentioned that the vascular risk injury could be higher if an anterior column release procedure is performed, so they excluded those high-risk procedures from their study (Walker et al., 2019).

Anatomical studies have shown that vascular injury is lower in left-sided lateral transpsoas approaches. The inferior vena cava is at risk for injury in right-sided LLIF in up to 70.8% of individuals, and the aorta is at risk during left-sided approaches in 29.2% (Hu et al., 2011). While entry from the left side typically creates a corridor between the great vessels and insertion of the psoas muscle, there is still a reported rate of 1.8% among the studies included in the systematic review and metaanalysis by Walker et al. (Walker et al., 2019). In addition to the side of the approach, the level of surgery is significant. The safe entry zone to the disk space through the psoas decreases as one moves from the L1-L2 level down to the L4-L5 level because neural structures move anteriorly on the vertebral bodies and the great vessels move posteriorly toward the anterior aspect of the vertebral bodies (Moro et al., 2003; Assina et al., 2014; Hu et al., 2011). Thus, for operations at the L4-L5 level, proper patient selection, meticulous preoperative planning, and careful adherence to safe surgical corridors are of paramount importance for minimizing vascular complications. Another important consideration in risk evaluation for prospective patients is the extent of spinal deformity. The great vessels are shifted toward the concave side of spinal deformities caused by degenerative scoliosis (Regev et al., 2009, 2010). This change in position greatly increases the risk of injury during the lateral approach and should be taken into account when candidates for lateral transpsoas interbody fusion surgery are evaluated (Assina et al., 2014).

It is also a concern that LLIF can be performed in outpatient surgery centers with minimal access to in-house vascular and general surgical consultation should vascular injury occur (Hijji et al., 2017; Assina et al., 2014). Fig. 24.1 shows an example of vascular injury in a patient who underwent lumbar spinal fusion, including multilevel LLIF. Three weeks later, the patient began to develop anorexia, nausea, and severe abdominal pain. CT showed a splenic infarct as a result of celiac artery occlusion.

Assina et al. described a case in which the retractor tip had transected the right common iliac vein and was within the lumen of the left common iliac vein. The surgeon who performed the lateral transpsoas approach in an outpatient surgical center had to transport the patient to a hospital, which, according to the authors, could have worsened the injury pattern. After several revisions the patient was discharged to an acute care rehabilitation facility. Seven days later she presented with a retroperitoneal abscess and in acute sepsis. Becoming increasingly hemodynamically unstable over the next few days, she died as a result of multiple organ failure secondary to septic shock. Again, this should draw surgeons' attention to the potential for serious injury to the great vessels, especially if this procedure is popularized and becomes more widely available in settings such as outpatient surgery centers (Assina et al., 2014).

Visceral Injury

Nerves are the most commonly injured structures in lateral approaches. Bowel injury is exceedingly rare

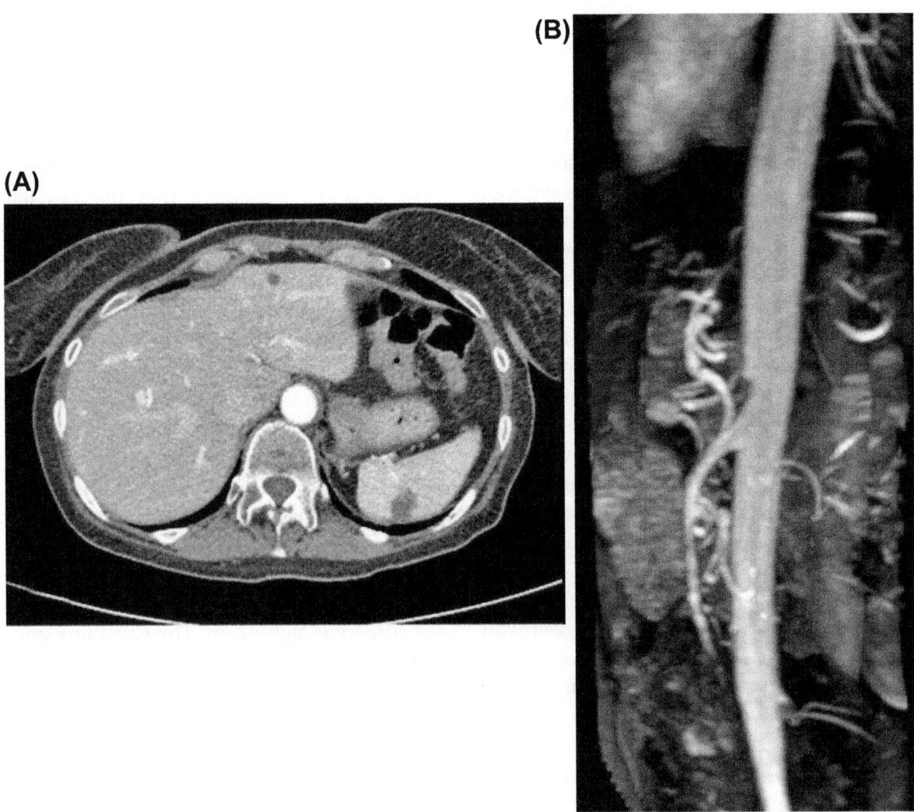

FIG. 24.1 Vascular injury. Axial CT image shows a splenic infarct **(A)** and the 3D MIP MRA shows occlusion of the celiac trunk and branches **(B)**.

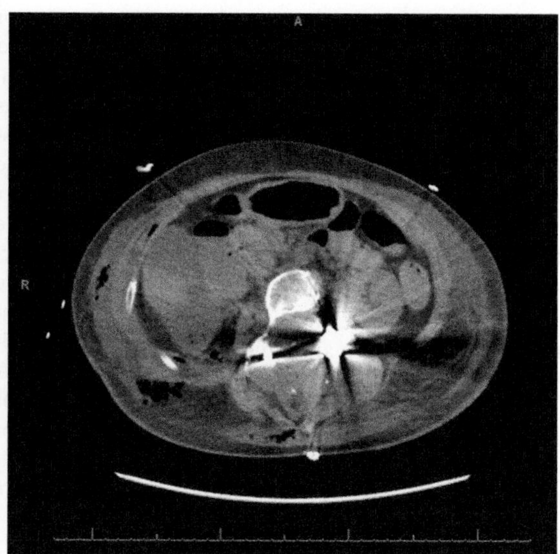

FIG. 24.2 Retroperitoneal injury of the right ascending colon. Axial CT shows a 4.2 × 7 × 13.3 cm right retroperitoneal fluid collection containing air extending from midabdomen down into the pelvis. This is contiguous with the subcutaneous air and fluid along the right lateral chest, abdomen, and pelvic wall.

reported at a rate of 0.41% in the literature (Fig. 24.2) (Hijji et al., 2017). Nevertheless, there is still a risk of bowel injuries with potentially devastating complications (Rodgers et al., 2011; Patel et al., 2012). Yilmaz et al. performed extreme lateral approaches to the lumbar spine on four fresh frozen cadavers, positioning K-wires into each disk space. Measuring the distance from the K-wires to the colon, they showed the greatest risk for colon injuries at L2/L3 and L3/L4 (Yilmaz et al., 2018). Other cases and a case series of bowel injuries after lateral transpsoas interbody fusion are described in the literature: Balsano et al. reported a 70-year-old male who underwent an L3/4 and L4/5 extreme lateral transpsoas approach for interbody fusion. The patient suffered a perforation of the splenic flexure of the colon and required surgical intervention with a temporary colostomy for 3 months (Balsano et al., 2015). Tormenti et al. reported one bowel perforation out of eight scoliotic patients undergoing lateral transpsoas approaches. Specifically, a cecal perforation occurred, which necessitated an emergency exploratory laparotomy and bowel resection. As suggested by Tormenti et al., the rotatory component of scoliotic spines changes the topographical anatomy and could significantly increase the risk of injury to intra- and retroperitoneal structures (Tormenti et al., 2010). Additionally, Tormenti et al. pointed out the lack of literature in studies analyzing topographical changes in scoliotic patients or analyzing anatomical variations related to the lateral transpsoas interbody fusion procedure.

In order to prevent injury to peritoneal and retroperitoneal components, complete access to the retroperitoneal space is necessary. Rustagi et al. found three patients (0.51%) with a visceral injury in a retrospective cohort study including 590 transpsoas lumbar interbody fusions. Most alarming was a delay of 4.7 days (3–7 days) between visceral surgery and injury (Rustagi et al., 2019). All three cases presented with perforations of the ascending colon, the colon being attached to the interbody cage in one case (Rustagi et al., 2019).

Another commonly reported injury is psoas hematoma (Fig. 24.3), which can be complicated by abscess (Moller et al., 2011; Murray et al., 2012). Fig. 24.4 demonstrates a right abdominal wall abscess in a patient who developed leukocytosis following LLIF surgery. In addition, seroma can develop following an LLIF procedure (Fig. 24.5). A systematic review of complications to LLIF found an overall rate of 1.08% for psoas hematoma (Hijji et al., 2017). In contrast to ALIF, the same systematic review found no incidence of retrograde ejaculation or urethral injury (Hijji et al., 2017). Performing LLIF in the upper lumbar region, specifically at the L2 and L3 levels, makes retroperitoneal dissection difficult,

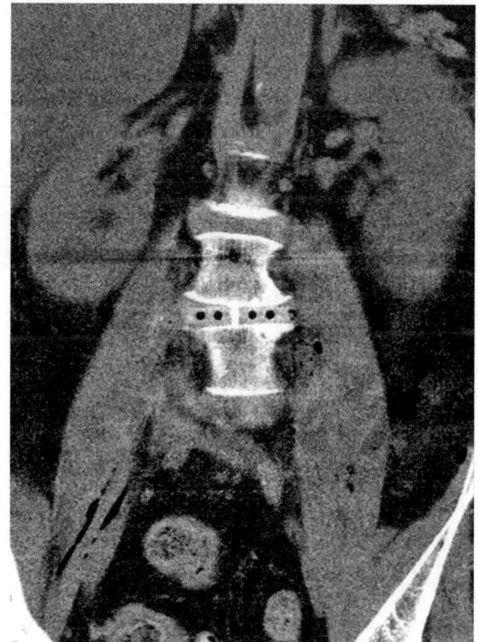

FIG. 24.3 Psoas injury. Coronal CT demonstrating hematoma and emphysema in the left psoas muscle following recent lateral lumbar interbody fusion surgery.

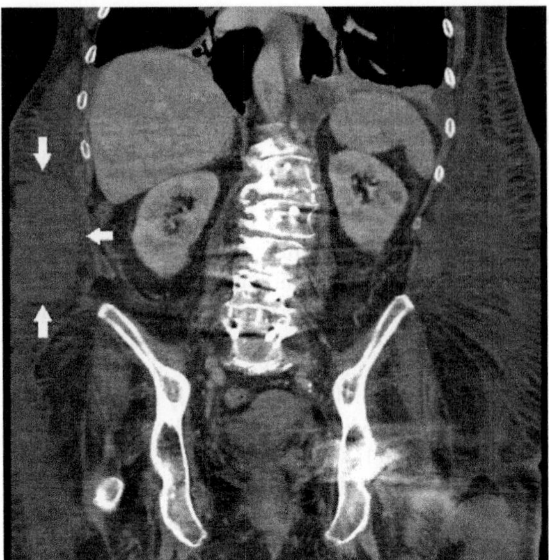

FIG. 24.4 Abdominal wall abscess following lateral lumbar interbody fusion procedure. Coronal CT shows a fluid collection in the subcutaneous tissues of the right abdominal wall (white arrows).

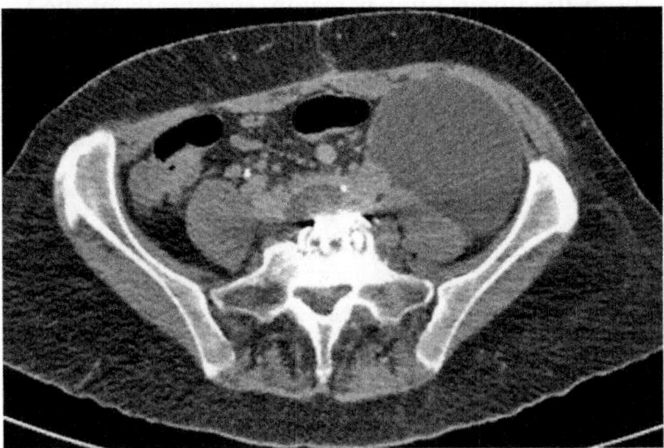

FIG. 24.5 Seroma. Axial CT image shows a large left intraabdominal fluid collection that proved to be a seroma. There is also a prevertebral fluid collection at the level of the lateral transpsoas interbody fusion device.

increasing the risk of kidney injury (Aichmair et al., 2015). Iwanaga et al. (Assina et al., 2014) showed that the kidneys are closest to the disk space at the L1-L2 level. In addition, renal pathology and renal vasculature variations impose a risk of kidney injury. Ureter injury is a relatively rare complication; however, it is critical to identify such injury during surgery, which can manifest as hematuria. Therefore, surgeons should have a high index of suspicion for ureter injury during LLIF, especially at upper levels (Santillan et al., 2010).

Other Injuries

Another clinically significant complication associated with LLIF is incidental durotomy. In a metaanalysis of 29 studies and 1228 patients, the estimated incidence of dural tears and/or CSF leaks in patients undergoing LLIF procedure in the lumbar spine was 5.4% (Hu et al., 2011).

Spine-specific Complications

As with other types of spinal fusion, the most common spine-specific complications of LLIF are subsidence and pseudarthrosis, which are subject to variable reporting. Vertebral fracture can also occur (Fig. 24.6).

A recently published systematic review and metaanalysis included 446 patients (791 levels) treated via prepsoas and 1131 (2077 levels) treated via transpsoas approaches (Walker et al., 2019). Regarding radiographic reports, subsidence rates were included in five out of eight prepsoas studies analyzing 566 levels with a weighted average rate of 12.2% (and 13 of 19 transpsoas studies analyzing 1537 levels with a rate of 13.8%, which was not significantly different). Notably, the reported subsidence rates varied significantly, ranging from 4.4% to 21.6% in the prepsoas studies and from 0% to 31.3% in the transpsoas studies. Another review (3482 patients) reported spine-specific

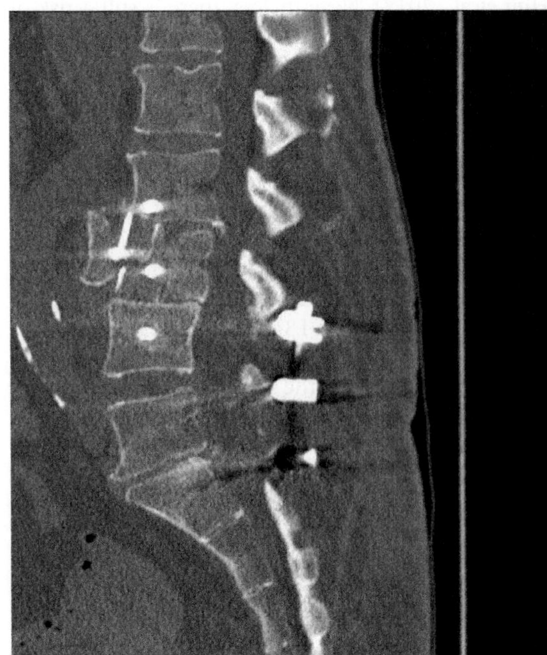

FIG. 24.6 Vertebral fracture. Sagittal CT image shows a displaced fracture of the L3 vertebral body with subsidence of the lateral lumbar interbody fusion devices.

complications from LLIF in 321 cases, a rate of 9.22% (Hijji et al., 2017). Subsidence occurs when a graft or cage, which has a high elastic modulus, sinks into the vertebral body, which has a comparatively low elastic modulus (Hakalo et al., 2003) (Fig. 24.7). Subsidence leads to kyphosis, decreased interbody space, and ultimately spinal destabilization with pseudarthrosis (Hakalo et al., 2003). Rates of cage subsidence in LLIF appear to be notably lower than in ALIF and TLIF approaches (Hartl et al., 2016; Hsieh et al., 2007). It is generally accepted that subsidence is a relatively common occurrence in ALIF and TLIF procedures. For example, a study of 57 patients by Hsieh et al. revealed subsidence rates of 21.7% and 23.5% for ALIF and TLIF, respectively (Hsieh et al., 2007). In comparison, the most recent and comprehensive systematic review of complications for LLIF found a cage subsidence rate of 6.61% in 2482 patients (Hijji et al., 2017). This rate compares favorably even to the subsidence rate of 10.2% in 147 patients undergoing ALIF recently reported by Rao and colleagues (Rao et al., 2017).

Endplate preparation and cage insertion are crucial for avoiding endplate violation, which in our experience leads to higher subsidence. Further, the lateral transpsoas approach permits the use of wide implants and preservation of the longitudinal ligaments, both of which probably account for its low rate of cage subsidence relative to other MIS techniques (Oliveira et al., 2010; Tan et al., 2005). Migration of the intervertebral implant should be considered when LLIF is performed. Improper preparations of the contralateral annulus and inappropriate implant size selection have been implicated in lateral displacement of the cage (Fig. 24.8). However, ALL rupture, in the course of disk preparation and sizing the implant, most likely leads to anterior migration (Fantini et al., 2007). Protrusion beyond the disk space (implant overhang) (Fig. 24.9) could result from relying exclusively on the AP fluoroscopic view when sizing the implant. This is especially the case if the implant is placed in the anterior one-third of the disk, consequently endangering the contralateral neural foramen and structures (Blizzard et al., 2016).

Pseudarthrosis rates were included in four out of eight prepsoas studies analyzing 262 levels with a rate of 9.9% (95% CI 4.1–21.7) and 14 of 19 transpsoas studies analyzing 1275 levels with a rate of 7.5% (95% CI 4.9–11.4), which were not significantly different ($P = .57$) (Walker et al., 2019). Pseudarthrosis refers to the failure of bony fusion (Chun et al., 2015). The pseudarthrosis rate for LLIF, at 5.89%, is comparable to rates seen with other MIS techniques such as ALIF and TLIF (Hijji et al., 2017; Wu et al., 2010; Ni et al., 2015). There are many methods for decreasing pseudarthrosis rates in spinal surgery. The use of recombinant human bone morphogenetic protein-2 (rhBMP-2) has received considerable attention, one recent

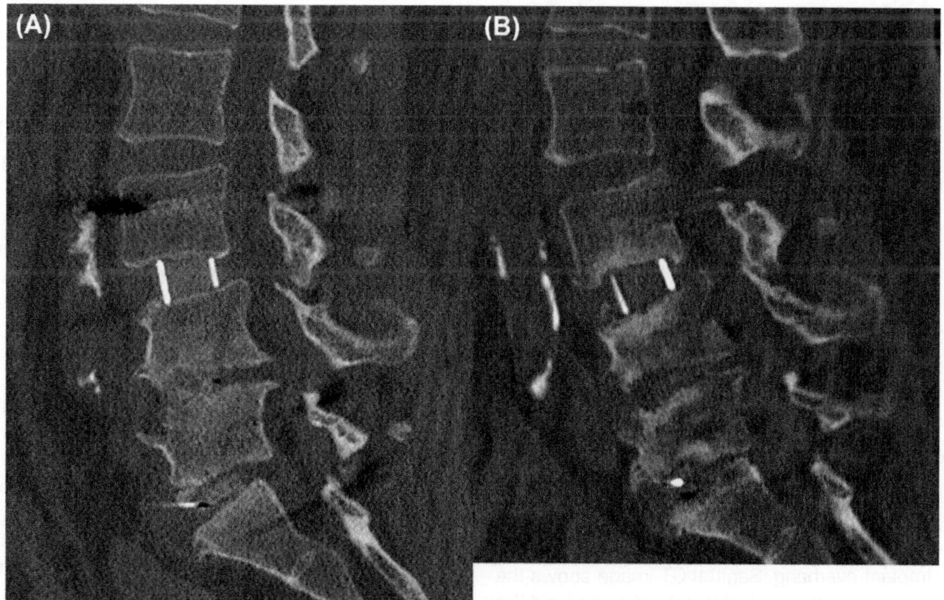

FIG. 24.7 Cage Subsidence. Sagittal CT images at baseline **(A)** and 3 years later **(B)** show interval indentation and sclerosis of the endplates by the lateral lumbar interbody fusion device.

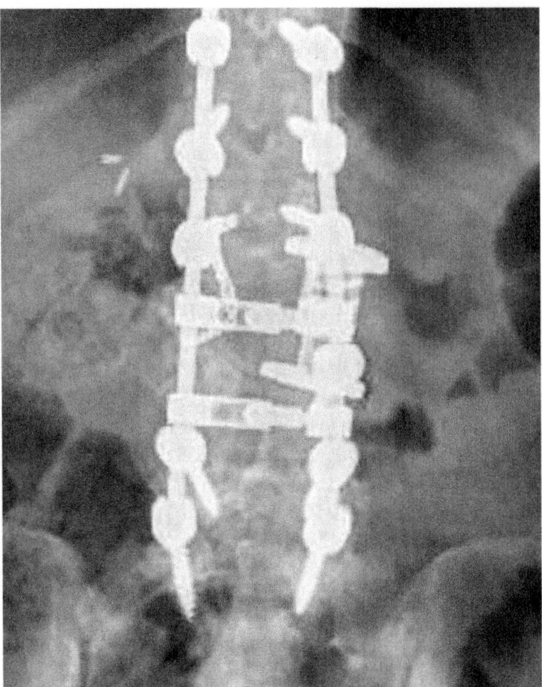

FIG. 24.8 Implant migration. AP radiograph illustrating lateral migration of an L3 corpectomy cage.

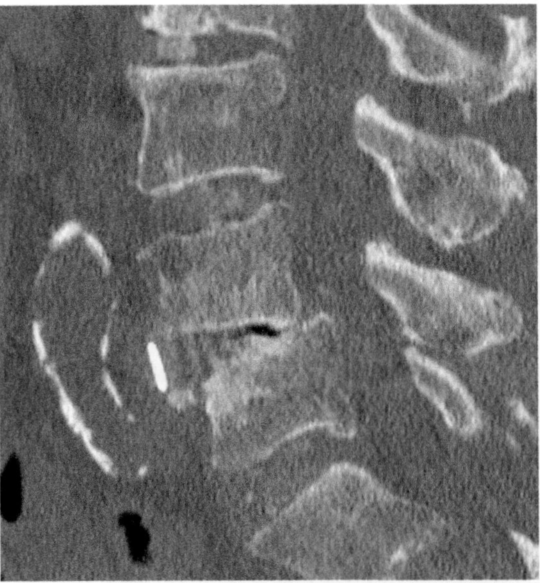

FIG. 24.9 Implant overhang. Sagittal CT image shows the lateral lumbar interbody fusion device extending beyond the anterior margin of the L5 superior endplate, which is disrupted, in the setting of anterolisthesis.

systematic review comparing fusion rates with and without rhBMP-2 finding no significant differences between the two groups (Galimberti et al., 2015). Bone stimulation via pulsed electromagnetic fields represents another strategy for increasing fusion rates, with devices approved by the US Food and Drug Administration (Foley et al., 2008; Waldorff et al., 2017; Mooney, 1990; Simmons Jr. et al., 2004). However, evidence supporting the efficacy of pulsed electromagnetic fields for the prevention of pseudarthrosis in spine surgery is conflicting (Park et al., 2014; Aleem et al., 2016). Other methods for increasing fusion rates and decreasing the occurrence of pseudarthrosis in spinal fusion via innovation in instrumentation and biological therapy are ongoing (Chun et al., 2015).

CONCLUSION

LLIF is a safe and effective method for surgically treating a variety of degenerative conditions of the spine. It confers excellent early stability and allows for large graft placement, compared with other techniques such as ALIF, PLIF, and TLIF (Kwon and Kim, 2016). As discussed in this review, the most common complication in LLIF is transient weakness or sensory impairment secondary to the transpsoas corridor used in this approach. With respect to complications due to spinal fusion itself, LLIF compares favorably with other spinal fusion techniques in respect of pseudarthrosis rates and has comparable or lower levels of subsidence. Finally, general complications are also rare, with very low rates of transfusion frequency and limited cases of other medical complications. With proper patient selection, preoperative planning, and meticulous surgical technique, and postoperative care, LLIF represents a safe method of spinal fusion with few complications. Continued improvement in the standards for accrual and analysis of outcome-related data are necessary to define the complication profiles for all types of minimally invasive spinal fusion procedures, including LLIF, more precisely (Martin 2nd et al., 2002; Asher et al., 2014; Parker et al., 2017).

REFERENCES

Ahmadian, A., Deukmedjian, A.R., Abel, N., Dakwar, E., Uribe, J.S., 2013. Analysis of lumbar plexopathies and nerve injury after lateral retroperitoneal transpsoas approach: diagnostic standardization. J. Neurosurg. Spine 18 (3), 289–297.

Acosta, F.L., Drazin, D., Liu, J.C., 2013. Supra-psoas shallow docking in lateral interbody fusion. Neurosurgery 73 (1 Suppl. Operative), ons48–51 discussion ons2.

Aichmair, A., Lykissas, M.G., Girardi, F.P., Sama, A.A., Lebl, D.R., Taher, F., et al., 2013. An institutional six-year trend analysis of the neurological outcome after lateral lumbar interbody fusion: a 6-year trend analysis of a single institution. Spine 38 (23), E1483–E1490.

Aichmair, A., Fantini, G.A., Garvin, S., Beckman, J., Girardi, F.P., 2015. Aortic perforation during lateral lumbar interbody fusion. J. Spinal Disord. Tech. 28 (2), 71–75.

Aleem, I.S., Aleem, I., Evaniew, N., Busse, J.W., Yaszemski, M., Agarwal, A., et al., 2016. Efficacy of electrical stimulators for bone healing: a meta-analysis of randomized Sham-controlled trials. Sci. Rep. 6, 31724.

Asher, A.L., Speroff, T., Dittus, R.S., Parker, S.L., Davies, J.M., Selden, N., et al., 2014. The National Neurosurgery Quality and Outcomes Database (N2QOD): a collaborative North American outcomes registry to advance value-based spine care. Spine 39 (22 Suppl. 1), S106–S116.

Assina, R., Majmundar, N.J., Herschman, Y., Heary, R.F., 2014. First report of major vascular injury due to lateral transpsoas approach leading to fatality. J. Neurosurg. Spine 21 (5), 794–798.

Balsano, M., Carlucci, S., Ose, M., Boriani, L., 2015. A case report of a rare complication of bowel perforation in extreme lateral interbody fusion. Eur. Spine J. 24 (Suppl. 3), 405–408.

Banagan, K., Gelb, D., Poelstra, K., Ludwig, S., 2011. Anatomic mapping of lumbar nerve roots during a direct lateral transpsoas approach to the spine: a cadaveric study. Spine 36 (11), E687–E691.

Barbagallo, G.M., Albanese, V., Raich, A.L., Dettori, J.R., Sherry, N., Balsano, M., 2014. Lumbar lateral interbody fusion (LLIF): comparative effectiveness and safety versus PLIF/TLIF and predictive factors affecting LLIF outcome. Evid. Based Spine Care J. 5 (1), 28–37.

Benglis, D.M., Vanni, S., Levi, A.D., 2009. An anatomical study of the lumbosacral plexus as related to the minimally invasive transpsoas approach to the lumbar spine. J. Neurosurg. Spine 10 (2), 139–144.

Bergey, D.L., Villavicencio, A.T., Goldstein, T., Regan, J.J., 2004. Endoscopic lateral transpsoas approach to the lumbar spine. Spine 29 (15), 1681–1688.

Blizzard, D.J., Gallizzi, M.A., Isaacs, R.E., Brown, C.R., 2016. Renal artery injury during lateral transpsoas interbody fusion: case report. J. Neurosurg. Spine 25 (4), 464–466.

Cahill, K.S., Martinez, J.L., Wang, M.Y., Vanni, S., Levi, A.D., 2012. Motor nerve injuries following the minimally invasive lateral transpsoas approach. J. Neurosurg. Spine 17 (3), 227–231.

Cheng, I., Briseño, M.R., Arrigo, R.T., Bains, N., Ravi, S., Tran, A., 2015. Outcomes of two different techniques using the lateral approach for lumbar interbody arthrodesis. Global Spine J. 5 (4), 308–314.

Cheng, I., Acosta, F., Chang, K., Pham, M., 2016. Point-counterpoint: the use of neuromonitoring in lateral transpsoas surgery. Spine 41 (Suppl. 8), S145–S151.

Chun, D.S., Baker, K.C., Hsu, W.K., 2015. Lumbar pseudarthrosis: a review of current diagnosis and treatment. Neurosurg. Focus 39 (4), E10.

Costa, A., Matter, M., Pascual, M., Doerfler, A., Venetz, J.P., 2019. [Renal, vascular and urological variations and abnormalities in living kidney donor candidates]. Prog. Urol. 29 (3), 166–172.

Dakwar, E., Vale, F.L., Uribe, J.S., 2011. Trajectory of the main sensory and motor branches of the lumbar plexus outside the psoas muscle related to the lateral retroperitoneal transpsoas approach. J. Neurosurg. Spine 14 (2), 290–295.

Davis, T.T., Bae, H.W., Mok, J.M., Rasouli, A., Delamarter, R.B., 2011. Lumbar plexus anatomy within the psoas muscle: implications for the transpsoas lateral approach to the L4-L5 disc. J. Bone Joint Surg. Am. 93 (16), 1482–1487.

Fantini, G.A., Pappou, I.P., Girardi, F.P., Sandhu, H.S., Cammisa, F.P., 2007. Major vascular injury during anterior lumbar spinal surgery: incidence, risk factors, and management. Spine 32 (24), 2751–2758.

Foley, K.T., Mroz, T.E., Arnold, P.M., Chandler Jr., H.C., Dixon, R.A., Girasole, G.J., et al., 2008. Randomized, prospective, and controlled clinical trial of pulsed electromagnetic field stimulation for cervical fusion. Spine J. 8 (3), 436–442.

Galimberti, F., Lubelski, D., Healy, A.T., Wang, T., Abdullah, K.G., Nowacki, A.S., et al., 2015. A systematic review of lumbar fusion rates with and without the use of rhBMP-2. Spine 40 (14), 1132–1139.

Grimm, B.D., Leas, D.P., Poletti, S.C., Johnson 2nd, D.R., 2016. Postoperative complications within the first year after extreme lateral interbody fusion: experience of the first 108 patients. Clin. Spine Surg. 29 (3), E151–E156.

Grunert, P., Drazin, D., Iwanaga, J., Schmidt, C., Alonso, F., Moisi, M., et al., 2017. Injury to the lumbar plexus and its branches after lateral fusion procedures: a cadaver study. World Neurosurg. 105, 519–525.

Hakalo, J., Wronski, J., Ciupik, L., 2003. [Subsidence and its effect on the anterior plate stabilization in the course of cervical spondylodesis. Part I: definition and review of literature]. Neurol. Neurochir. Pol. 37 (4), 903–915.

Hardenbrook, M.A., Miller, L.E., Block, J.E., 2013. TranS1 VEO system: a novel psoas-sparing device for transpsoas lumbar interbody fusion. Med. Devices (Auckl) 6, 91–95.

Hartl, R., Joeris, A., McGuire, R.A., 2016. Comparison of the safety outcomes between two surgical approaches for anterior lumbar fusion surgery: anterior lumbar interbody fusion (ALIF) and extreme lateral interbody fusion (ELIF). Eur. Spine J. 25 (5), 1484–1521.

Hijji, F.Y., Narain, A.S., Bohl, D.D., Ahn, J., Long, W.W., DiBattista, J.V., et al., 2017. Lateral lumbar interbody fusion: a systematic review of complication rates. Spine J. 17 (10), 1412–1419.

Hsieh, P.C., Koski, T.R., O'Shaughnessy, B.A., Sugrue, P., Salehi, S., Ondra, S., et al., 2007. Anterior lumbar interbody fusion in comparison with transforaminal lumbar interbody fusion: implications for the restoration of foraminal height, local disc angle, lumbar lordosis, and sagittal balance. J. Neurosurg. Spine 7 (4), 379–386.

Hu, S.S., 2004. Blood loss in adult spinal surgery. Eur. Spine J. 13 (Suppl. 1), S3–S5.

Hu, W.K., He, S.S., Zhang, S.C., Liu, Y.B., Li, M., Hou, T.S., et al., 2011. An MRI study of psoas major and abdominal large vessels with respect to the X/DLIF approach. Eur. Spine J. 20 (4), 557–562.

Isaacs, R.E., Hyde, J., Goodrich, J.A., Rodgers, W.B., Phillips, F.M., 2010. A prospective, nonrandomized, multicenter evaluation of extreme lateral interbody fusion for the treatment of adult degenerative scoliosis: perioperative outcomes and complications. Spine 35 (26 Suppl. 1), S322–S330.

Joseph, J.R., Smith, B.W., La Marca, F., Park, P., 2015. Comparison of complication rates of minimally invasive transforaminal lumbar interbody fusion and lateral lumbar interbody fusion: a systematic review of the literature. Neurosurg. Focus 39 (4), E4.

Knight, R.Q., Schwaegler, P., Hanscom, D., Roh, J., 2009. Direct lateral lumbar interbody fusion for degenerative conditions: early complication profile. J. Spinal Disord. Tech. 22 (1), 34–37.

Kwon, B., Kim, D.H., 2016. Lateral lumbar interbody fusion: indications, outcomes, and complications. J. Am. Acad. Orthop. Surg. 24 (2), 96–105.

Le, T.V., Baaj, A.A., Dakwar, E., Burkett, C.J., Murray, G., Smith, D.A., et al., 2012. Subsidence of polyetheretherketone intervertebral cages in minimally invasive lateral retroperitoneal transpsoas lumbar interbody fusion. Spine 37 (14), 1268–1273.

Lehmen, J.A., Gerber, E.J., 2015. MIS lateral spine surgery: a systematic literature review of complications, outcomes, and economics. Eur. Spine J. 24 (Suppl. 3), 287–313.

Lykissas, M.G., Aichmair, A., Hughes, A.P., Sama, A.A., Lebl, D.R., Taher, F., et al., 2014. Nerve injury after lateral lumbar interbody fusion: a review of 919 treated levels with identification of risk factors. Spine J. 14 (5), 749–758.

Marchi, L., Abdala, N., Oliveira, L., Amaral, R., Coutinho, E., Pimenta, L., 2013. Radiographic and clinical evaluation of cage subsidence after stand-alone lateral interbody fusion. J. Neurosurg. Spine 19 (1), 110–118.

Martin 2nd, R.C., Brennan, M.F., Jaques, D.P., 2002. Quality of complication reporting in the surgical literature. Ann. Surg. 235 (6), 803–813.

Moisi, M., Fisahn, C., Tubbs, R.S., Page, J., Rice, R., Paulson, D., et al., 2016. Lateral thoracic osteoplastic rib-sparing technique used for lateral spine surgery: technical note. Cureus 8 (7), e668.

Moller, D.J., Slimack, N.P., Acosta Jr., F.L., Koski, T.R., Fessler, R.G., Liu, J.C., 2011. Minimally invasive lateral lumbar interbody fusion and transpsoas approach-related morbidity. Neurosurg. Focus 31 (4), E4.

Mooney, V., 1990. A randomized double-blind prospective study of the efficacy of pulsed electromagnetic fields for interbody lumbar fusions. Spine 15 (7), 708–712.

Moro, T., Kikuchi, S., Konno, S., Yaginuma, H., 2003. An anatomic study of the lumbar plexus with respect to retroperitoneal endoscopic surgery. Spine 28 (5), 423–428 discussion 7-8.

Murray, M.R., Weistroffer, J.K., Schafer, M.F., 2012. Case report of an abscess developing at the site of a hematoma following a direct lateral interbody fusion. Spine J. 12 (7), e1–4.

Ni, J., Fang, X., Zhong, W., Liu, N., Wood, K.B., 2015. Anterior lumbar interbody fusion for degenerative discogenic low back pain: evaluation of L4-S1 fusion. Medicine (Baltim.) 94 (43), e1851.

Oliveira, L., Marchi, L., Coutinho, E., Pimenta, L., 2010. A radiographic assessment of the ability of the extreme lateral interbody fusion procedure to indirectly decompress the neural elements. Spine 35 (26 Suppl. 1), S331–S337.

Ozgur, B.M., Aryan, H.E., Pimenta, L., Taylor, W.R., 2006. Extreme Lateral Interbody Fusion (XLIF): a novel surgical technique for anterior lumbar interbody fusion. Spine J. 6 (4), 435–443.

Ozkan, U., Oğuzkurt, L., Tercan, F., Kizilkiliç, O., Koç, Z., Koca, N., 2006. Renal artery origins and variations: angiographic evaluation of 855 consecutive patients. Diagn. Interv. Radiol. 12 (4), 183–186.

Park, P., Lau, D., Brodt, E.D., Dettori, J.R., 2014. Electrical stimulation to enhance spinal fusion: a systematic review. Evid. Based Spine Care J. 5 (2), 87–94.

Parker, S.L., Chotai, S., Devin, C.J., Tetreault, L., Mroz, T.E., Brodke, D.S., et al., 2017. Bending the cost curve-establishing value in spine surgery. Neurosurgery 80 (3S), S61–S69.

Patel, V.C., Park, D.K., Herkowitz, H.N., 2012. Lateral transpsoas fusion: indications and outcomes. Scientific World J. 2012, 893608.

Phillips, F.M., Isaacs, R.E., Rodgers, W.B., Khajavi, K., Tohmeh, A.G., Deviren, V., et al., 2013. Adult degenerative scoliosis treated with XLIF: clinical and radiographical results of a prospective multicenter study with 24-month follow-up. Spine 38 (21), 1853–1861.

Pumberger, M., Hughes, A.P., Huang, R.R., Sama, A.A., Cammisa, F.P., Girardi, F.P., 2012. Neurologic deficit following lateral lumbar interbody fusion. Eur. Spine J. 21 (6), 1192–1199.

Rao, P.J., Phan, K., Giang, G., Maharaj, M.M., Phan, S., Mobbs, R.J., 2017. Subsidence following anterior lumbar interbody fusion (ALIF): a prospective study. J. Spine Surg. 3 (2), 168–175.

Regev, G.J., Chen, L., Dhawan, M., Lee, Y.P., Garfin, S.R., Kim, C.W., 2009. Morphometric analysis of the ventral nerve roots and retroperitoneal vessels with respect to the minimally invasive lateral approach in normal and deformed spines. Spine 34 (12), 1330–1335.

Regev, G.J., Haloman, S., Chen, L., Dhawan, M., Lee, Y.P., Garfin, S.R., et al., 2010. Incidence and prevention of intervertebral cage overhang with minimally invasive lateral approach fusions. Spine 35 (14), 1406–1411.

Rodgers, W.B., Gerber, E.J., Rodgers, J.A., 2010. Lumbar fusion in octogenarians: the promise of minimally invasive surgery. Spine 35 (26 Suppl. 1), S355–S360.

Rodgers, W.B., Gerber, E.J., Patterson, J., 2011. Intraoperative and early postoperative complications in extreme lateral interbody fusion: an analysis of 600 cases. Spine 36 (1), 26–32.

Rustagi, T., Yilmaz, E., Alonso, F., Schmidt, C., Oskouian, R., Tubbs, R.S., et al., 2019. Iatrogenic bowel injury following minimally invasive lateral approach to the lumbar spine: a retrospective analysis of 3 cases. Global Spine J. 9 (4), 375–382.

Santillan, A., Patsalides, A., Gobin, Y.P., 2010. Endovascular embolization of iatrogenic lumbar artery pseudoaneurysm following extreme lateral interbody fusion (XLIF). Vasc. Endovascular Surg. 44 (7), 601–603.

Saraph, V., Lerch, C., Walochnik, N., Bach, C.M., Krismer, M., Wimmer, C., 2004. Comparison of conventional versus minimally invasive extraperitoneal approach for anterior lumbar interbody fusion. Eur. Spine J. 13 (5), 425–431.

Silvestre, C., Mac-Thiong, J.M., Hilmi, R., Roussouly, P., 2012. Complications and morbidities of mini-open anterior retroperitoneal lumbar interbody fusion: oblique lumbar interbody fusion in 179 patients. Asian Spine J. 6 (2), 89–97.

Simmons Jr., J.W., Mooney, V., Thacker, I., 2004. Pseudarthrosis after lumbar spine fusion: nonoperative salvage with pulsed electromagnetic fields. Am. J. Orthop. 33 (1), 27–30.

Sunderland, S., 1990. The anatomy and physiology of nerve injury. Muscle Nerve 13 (9), 771–784.

Tan, J.S., Bailey, C.S., Dvorak, M.F., Fisher, C.G., Oxland, T.R., 2005. Interbody device shape and size are important to strengthen the vertebra-implant interface. Spine 30 (6), 638–644.

Tatsumi, R., Lee, Y.P., Khajavi, K., Taylor, W., Chen, F., Bae, H., 2015. In vitro comparison of endplate preparation between four mini-open interbody fusion approaches. Eur. Spine J. 24 (Suppl. 3), 372–377.

Tohmeh, A.G., Rodgers, W.B., Peterson, M.D., 2011. Dynamically evoked, discrete-threshold electromyography in the extreme lateral interbody fusion approach. J. Neurosurg. Spine 14 (1), 31–37.

Tormenti, M.J., Maserati, M.B., Bonfield, C.M., Okonkwo, D.O., Kanter, A.S., 2010. Complications and radiographic correction in adult scoliosis following combined transpsoas extreme lateral interbody fusion and posterior pedicle screw instrumentation. Neurosurg. Focus 28 (3), E7.

Tubbs, R.,S., 2018. Surgical Anatomy of the Lumbar Plexus. Thieme.

Tubbs, R.I., Gabel, B., Jeyamohan, S., Moisi, M., Chapman, J.R., Hanscom, R.D., et al., 2017. Relationship of the lumbar plexus branches to the lumbar spine: anatomical study with application to lateral approaches. Spine J. 17 (7), 1012–1016.

Uribe, J.S., Deukmedjian, A.R., 2015. Visceral, vascular, and wound complications following over 13,000 lateral interbody fusions: a survey study and literature review. Eur. Spine J. 24 (Suppl. 3), 386–396.

Uribe, J.S., Arredondo, N., Dakwar, E., Vale, F.L., 2010a. Defining the safe working zones using the minimally invasive lateral retroperitoneal transpsoas approach: an anatomical study. J. Neurosurg. Spine 13 (2), 260–266.

Uribe, J.S., Vale, F.L., Dakwar, E., 2010b. Electromyographic monitoring and its anatomical implications in minimally invasive spine surgery. Spine 35 (26 Suppl. l), S368–S374.

Van Campenhout, A., Hubens, G., Fagard, K., Molenaers, G., 2010. Localization of motor nerve branches of the human psoas muscle. Muscle Nerve 42 (2), 202–207.

Waldorff, E.I., Zhang, N., Ryaby, J.T., 2017. Pulsed electromagnetic field applications: a corporate perspective. J. Orthop. Translat. 9, 60–68.

Walker, C.T., Farber, S.H., Cole, T.S., Xu, D.S., Godzik, J., Whiting, A.C., et al., 2019. Complications for minimally invasive lateral interbody arthrodesis: a systematic review and meta-analysis comparing prepsoas and transpsoas approaches. J. Neurosurg. Spine 1–15.

Wu, R.H., Fraser, J.F., Hartl, R., 2010. Minimal access versus open transforaminal lumbar interbody fusion: meta-analysis of fusion rates. Spine 35 (26), 2273–2281.

Xu, D.S., Walker, C.T., Godzik, J., Turner, J.D., Smith, W., Uribe, J.S., 2018. Minimally invasive anterior, lateral, and oblique lumbar interbody fusion: a literature review. Ann. Transl. Med. 6 (6), 104.

Yilmaz, E., Iwanaga, J., Moisi, M., Blecher, R., Abdul-Jabbar, A., Tawfik, T., et al., 2018. Risks of colon injuries in extreme lateral approaches to the lumbar spine: an anatomical study. Cureus 10 (1), e2122.

Zoidl, G., Grifka, J., Boluki, D., Willburger, R.E., Zoidl, C., Krämer, J., et al., 2003. Molecular evidence for local denervation of paraspinal muscles in failed-back surgery/postdiscotomy syndrome. Clin. Neuropathol. 22 (2), 71–77.

FURTHER READING

Chin, K.R., Pencle, F.J.R., Brown, M.D., Seale, J.A., 2018. A psoas splitting approach developed for outpatient lateral interbody fusion versus a standard transpsoas approach. J. Spine Surg. 4 (2), 195–202.

Fogel, G.R., Rosen, L., Koltsov, J.C.B., Cheng, I., 2018. Neurologic adverse event avoidance in lateral lumbar interbody fusion: technical considerations using muscle relaxants. J. Spine Surg. 4 (2), 247–253.

Huang, C., Xu, Z., Li, F., Chen, Q., 2018. Does the access angle change the risk of approach-related complications in minimally invasive lateral lumbar interbody fusion? An MRI study. J. Korean Neurosurg. Soc. 61 (6), 707–715.

Mueller, K., McGowan, J., Kane, S., Voyadzis, J.M., 2019. Evaluation of retraction time as a predictor of postoperative motor dysfunction after minimally invasive transpsoas interbody fusion at L4-L5. J. Clin. Neurosci. 61, 124–129.

Sakai, T., Tezuka, F., Wada, K., Abe, M., Yamashita, K., Takata, Y., et al., 2016. Risk management for avoidance of major vascular injury due to lateral transpsoas approach. Spine 41 (5), 450–453.

CHAPTER 25

Tips and Tricks of Lateral Approaches to the Thoracolumbar Spine

DIA R. HALALMEH • ALEXANDER VON GLINSKI • CHRISTOPHER E. CHILDERS • MARC D. MOISI • ROD J. OSKOUIAN

INTRODUCTION

As with any surgical procedure, lateral lumbar interbody fusion (LLIF) is not without risks. A thorough understanding of the surgical anatomy involved in LLIF and implementation of proper strategies are essential for maximal patient benefit and for avoiding complications. This chapter highlights methods for minimizing certain potential risks during each step of the procedure and making it efficient and safe.

Patient Positioning

Proper positioning of the patient is of key importance. Therefore, it is advisable to take the following points into consideration during patient positioning to ensure safety and comfortable access to the target disc:

1. The table can be broken gently to gain access especially to open the space between the 12th rib and iliac crest and thus enhance access to the L4–L5 disc space. The table should not be overbroken not to stretch the lumbar plexus within the psoas muscle. In some cases, a bolster underneath the iliac crest could be considered, without breaking the table. Furthermore, potential pressure points should be protected after breaking the table. It should be noted that breaking the table without slightly flexing the ipsilateral hip can result in lumbar plexus injury (O'Brien, 2017). The iliac crest and chest are then secured to the bed with tape so as not to inhibit the ability of the table to break. Taking time to optimize the patient's position is crucial for maximizing the opening of the approaches interval especially in the lumbar and thoracolumbar spine.
2. In scoliotic cases, coronal alignment can be achieved from either side. Approaching from the concave side allows multilevel procedures to be addressed using one skin incision and several fascial incisions and psoas dilatations. It is preferable to flex the hinge against the convex side. This facilitates reduction of the abnormal curve and provides easier access to the target discs (McAfee et al., 2013).
3. It is essential to ensure the patient's position is perpendicular to the plane of the floor. In addition, the AP and the lateral views should be carefully examined to identify anatomical abnormalities that could impede access to the target disc (Goodrich and Volcan, 2013; Berjano et al., 2015; Lu et al., 2012). The wigwag of the C-arm should be adjusted to match the angle of the disc space. In particular, the cephalocaudal angle of the C-arm must provide a clear lateral view of the endplates.
During the case, the C-arm should be readjusted according to the lumbar lordosis to ensure good quality lateral and AP views. In more complex segmental three-dimensional deformity, common in patients with autism spectrum disorder, each operative level will require individual table adjustments to obtain a true AP and lateral radiograph.
4. Once the patient is positioned and secured in place, the healthcare team should be cautious not to move the position of the table for the remainder of the procedure except in emergency. A key practice in this procedure is to position and secure the patient properly to the operative table and to prevent any movement of the patient during the case.

Planning and Localization

Under lateral imaging guidance, the target segment is confirmed, and skin is marked, delineating the anatomical orientation of the target disc (anterior and posterior border of the vertebral body, along with its location) and anatomical landmarks (iliac crest, ribcage). The proximity of the great vessels to the surgical corridor, especially in the lumbar area, puts these structures at risk. Therefore, anatomical delineation of the psoas

Surgical anatomy of the lateral transpsoas approach to the lumbar spine. https://doi.org/10.1016/B978-0-323-67376-1.00025-2

muscle and adjacent vasculature (aorta, inferior vena cava, and iliac vessels) should be assessed preoperatively via axial MRI studies at each operative level (Kepler et al., 2011). If these structures are far lateral or close to the iliopsoas muscle, the procedure should not be attempted, especially at lower lumbar levels. As noted by Kepler et al. (2011), neurovascular elements are at highest risk at the L4–L5 level.

History of operations on the same level, other previous retroperitoneal operations, and radiation could challenge safe retroperitoneal access owing to scarring along the way to the target disc. In addition, anomalous vascular anatomy, degenerative spondylolisthesis of grade II or more, and a more anteriorly placed lumbar plexus could limit access to the desired segment as the working portal will be in the vicinity of vascular and/or neural elements (Goodrich and Volcan, 2013; Berjano et al., 2015; Lu et al., 2012). Under those circumstances, other surgical techniques should be considered.

Navigation-assisted fluoroscopy can be used during the procedure to decrease radiation exposure to the patient and the surgical team. The use of navigation allows for real-time assessment of instrument trajectory (Webb et al., 2010). It is crucial to understand the anatomy of the lumbosacral plexus. Being aware of the extramuscular course of the neural structures is essential for avoiding injury caused by retractor distraction. Further knowledge of "silent" nerve fibers on EMG monitoring has to be taken into account.

There should be preoperative communication with the anesthesiologist and neurophysiologist to ensure no muscle relaxants and to verify our twitches in ensuring accurate neuromonitoring throughout the case.

Opening and Disc Exposure

A radiopaque instrument is used to mark out the incision in conjunction with intraoperative fluoroscopic imaging. After the target segment has been confirmed via fluoroscopy, midline spinous process, symmetrical pedicles that are equidistant from spinous processes, and linear superior endplates should be seen (Goodrich and Volcan, 2013; Lu et al., 2012). Following marking of the skin under fluoroscopic guidance, a 3–4 cm incision is made.

1. For a single-level case, a 3–4 cm single access incision can be made over the midsection of the target disc.
2. For a two-level case, the skin incision is made halfway between the two target levels over the intervening vertebral body.
3. For a multilevel case, more than one incision could be required; the surgeon can access several levels through each incision. However, each level should be treated separately with different dilations through the psoas muscle.

Electrocautery should be avoided in the initial incision to avoid injury to the sensitive superficial sensory nerves within the skin (Goodrich and Volcan, 2013). A Peon clamp can be used subsequently for blunt dissection through fibers of the external oblique, internal oblique, and transversalis muscles. The retroperitoneal fat is exposed after bluntly passing through the transversalis fascia, taking care not to enter the peritoneal cavity. The surgeon's index finger is inserted to identify the retroperitoneal space and help guide the initial dilator into proper position.

While an approach access corridor and passage through the psoas muscle are being created, attention should be paid to the following considerations:

1. The trajectory of the dilators should target the anterior and, to a lesser extent, the middle third of the psoas muscle to minimize the risk to the lumbar plexus (Goodrich and Volcan, 2013). If instruments were to be docked anterior to the iliopsoas muscle, one can consider sweeping under the muscle to obtain a middisc starting point.
2. The table-mounted retractor should be docked on the junction of the middle and posterior thirds of the target disc, taking care not to expand the blades past the midpoint of the adjacent vertebral body to avoid segmental vessel injury (Goodrich and Volcan, 2013). Moreover, care must be taken not to open the blades widely to avoid traction on the intrinsic branches innervating the psoas muscle (Goodrich and Volcan, 2013; Berjano et al., 2015)
3. Just before insertion of the posterior shim, a stimulating probe should be used to ensure absence of neural elements within the small volume of tissue that has crept into the base of the retractor. If there is difficulty in placing the shim because of a small disc space or a large osteophyte, live fluoroscopy can be used to help in placing the shim accurately into the disc space.
4. The retractor handle should be parallel to the disc space to visualize the monopolar probe and ensure alignment with the C-arm.
5. Excessive retractor time should be avoided as it can result in neural injury and postoperative thigh pain, particularly at the L4–L5 level (O'Brien, 2017). Bendersky et al. (2015) demonstrated in their retrospective analysis that retraction prolonged more than 20–40 min per operative level can give rise to lumbar plexopathy. This is usually attributed to compressive or ischemic injury. Therefore,

retraction time should be kept to a minimum. Under circumstances where surgery is delayed or extended retraction is required, releasing the retractor is recommended to allow the muscles and soft tissues to relax (Goodrich and Volcan, 2013).

6. It is advisable to use live fluoroscopy intermittently along with EMG monitoring to guide appropriate placement of the probes, dilators, and retractors, thereby facilitating quick and accurate docking of instruments. Consequently, there is less overall radiation exposure than when multiple shots are obtained while advancing cautiously toward the target disc.
7. If the pathology is in the thoracic region, the incision should be oblique along the rib going to the costal angle to ensure good visualization. It could also be beneficial for the surgeon to work initially anterior to the patient rather than posterior, as this provides better visualization along the rib to the costovertebral junction. In cases in which the long 11th and 12th ribs could overlie the operative portal, making access to the upper lumbar levels very difficult, rib segments can be sacrificed, or an intercostal approach is advisable. However, a rib-sparing technique has been described, resulting in improved patient outcomes, less postoperative surgical site pain, and earlier discharge (Moisi et al., 2016). In this technique, a segment of the rib of interest is resected and reflected inferiorly with careful attention to preserving the neurovascular bundle in the lower border of the rib (Fig. 25.1). When the case is completed, the rib is reflected back to its anatomical position and stitched with 0-Ethibond nonabsorbable sutures (Fig. 25.1) (Moisi et al., 2016).
8. Retractor placement between the 11th and 12th ribs can cause rib fractures. For approaches to the thoracolumbar junction, we therefore resect the 12th rib completely while not sacrificing the neurovascular bundle.
9. Brisk bleeding could signify anterior vascular injury. When this is encountered, it is best to obtain the assistance of a vascular surgeon and consider conversion to an anterior approach for exploration and hemostasis.
10. We do not regularly deflate the lung to avoid creating dead space.
11. In the event of severe bleeding during a thoracolumbar or thoracic approach, a chest tube can be inserted intraoperatively to avoid a hemothorax.

Meticulous planning of the incision and the instrument docking points is of paramount importance to avoid neural and vascular elements. Moreover, it is essential to maintain the surgical working plane perpendicular to the sagittal plane of the target discs. This eliminates the risk of nonorthogonal insertion of instruments and consequent vessel and nerve injury. Strict adherence to neuromonitoring throughout the procedure is strongly recommended to identify a safe trajectory to the target disc and subsequently to facilitate safe passage through the psoas muscle.

Discectomy

1. A key to successful bony fusion and maximum indirect foraminal decompression is adequate distraction of the disc space. Furthermore, preservation of the cortical endplates with complete removal of the cartilaginous disc is required for proper and stable implant placement. Therefore,

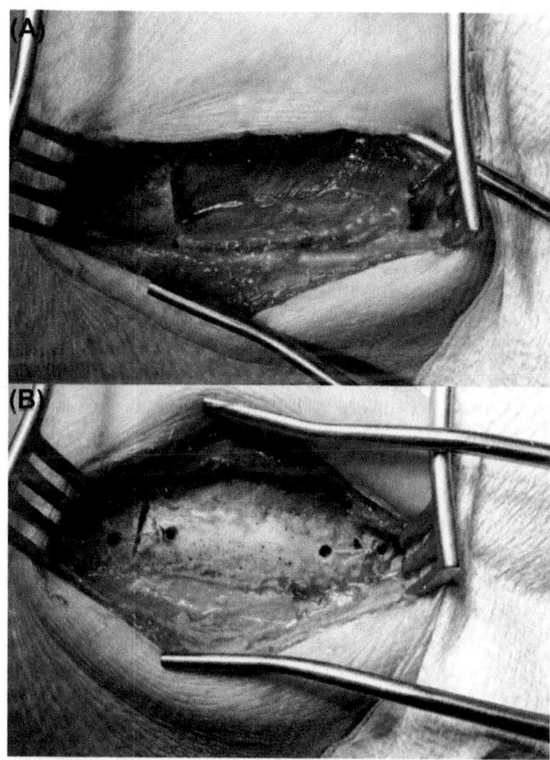

FIG. 25.1 **Cadaveric specimen demonstrating osteoplastic rib-sparing technique. (A)** The rib segment is reflected inferiorly with its neurovascular bundle. **(B)** Instead of discarding the rib segment, it is reflected back to its anatomical position. (Adapted from Moisi M, Fisahn C, Tubbs R et al., Lateral thoracic osteoplastic rib-sparing technique used for lateral spine surgery: Technical Note. *Cureus* 2016, 8(7), p. 6, 8.)

overresection of the endplate should be avoided to minimize the risk of disc subsidence. However, adequate discectomy and endplate decortication are necessary for disc height restoration and reducing the risk of cage subsidence (Goodrich and Volcan, 2013; Lu et al., 2012). In cases in which entry to the disc space is obstructed by bridging osteophytes, an osteotome can be used under fluoroscopic guidance to facilitate access. Once inside the disc space, a Cobb can be used to advance to the contralateral side and help enlarge the disc space.

2. During annulotomy, care must be taken to avoid traversing the anterior longitudinal ligament and anteriorly situated vessels and nerves. This can be achieved by making the annulotomy incision from ventral-to-dorsal, toward the posterior blade and embedded shim (Goodrich and Volcan, 2013). Additionally, some tissue should be preserved ventral to the shim so as to provide shim stability and prevent subsequent migration of the retractor (Goodrich and Volcan, 2013; Lu et al., 2012). During discectomy and instrument removal, the depth should be verified continuously so as not to advance too far and pull tissue from the contralateral side, thus injuring the contralateral neurovascular structures.
3. It is crucial not to shift the patient's position during the procedure unless necessary. Accidental displacement of the patient can lead to oblique insertion of the instruments and subsequent vessel and nerve injury (Lu et al., 2012). In addition, safety in the disc space is ensured by orthogonal orientation of the target segment to the X-ray beam in the AP and to the floor in the lateral view. This also enables the surgeon to avoid overpreparation of the disc and endplate violation.
4. It is critical to maintain orthogonal orientation of the instruments at all times. An instrument can easily be pushed into the spinal canal or outside the canal anteriorly. In addition, preparation of a pathway tailored to the desired implant is recommended. If a posterior or anterior pathway is created, it can be difficult to correct.
5. In the surgical treatment of kyphotic deformities, discectomies can be performed along with ALL release to provide anterior release of the spine and correction of the sagittal Cobb angle. If ALL release and fusion with lordotic cages are performed, LLIF should be supplemented with pedicle screw fixation to eliminate potential complications such as implant subsidence and to provide significant stability (Goodrich and Volcan, 2013). Moreover, coronal cages exist to help with coronal deformity correction.

Corpectomy

Cage subsidence remains a significant complication in patients who undergo corpectomy, mainly as a result of nonoptimal matching between the cage footplate and vertebral endplate surface area (Goodrich and Volcan, 2013). Implantation of wide footplates should be attempted to provide better coverage of the endplate and subsequently reduce stress at the footplate, minimizing the risk of subsidence. The design of the implanted cage potentially determines the subsidence rate. Pekmezci et al. (2012) found that a rectangular footplate design is associated with lower subsidence rates than the circular footplate design even if there are defects in the central portion of the endplate caused by overdistraction of the disc space or failure of the primary vertebral body replacement. This provides a safer option for reconstruction defects after corpectomy, especially when the center of the endplate has been compromised. The same study also demonstrated the superiority of the rectangular over the circular design when used after an initial subsidence. In summary, use of the widest expandable rectangular cage available provides higher stability and lower subsidence rates in reconstruction after corpectomy.

The landing spot for the retractor system should be at the midvertebral body with the assistance of lateral and AP fluoroscopy. During docking of the retractor, the posterior blade should be placed as far posterior as possible. Care should be taken to avoid segmental vessel injury, which can potentially lead to extensive blood loss that could be difficult to control. Once the vessels are visualized, they should be coagulated and divided. Moreover, shims are typically not used, and a fourth blade is recommended to protect the peritoneal contents (in the lumbar region) and the pleural contents (in the thoracic region), creating a safety zone for the operation. During corpectomy, the superior and inferior blades should be spread between the two adjacent disc spaces. An EMG probe is used to ensure adequate distance from nearby nerve roots. The authors recommend that discectomy be performed in the levels above and below in the usual manner prior to starting the corpectomy.

Graft Placement

There are special considerations in graft placement that should be used to decrease risk of neural injury and the subsidence rate. These include the following:

1) Care must be taken not to injure the endplate by oversizing the height of the trial. In addition, preservation of the cortical ring of the endplates is necessary to minimize the subsidence rate (Goodrich and Volcan, 2013).
2) The contralateral annulus must be disrupted to achieve parallel distraction, optimal biomechanical positioning of the graft, and optimal coronal alignment.
3) The implant should be always large enough to span the apophyseal ring, which ensures the anatomical stability of the implant, solid fusion, and reduced risk of subsidence. Subsidence is more likely to occur with small cages, especially if the endplate coverage area of the implant is less than 30% (Goodrich and Volcan, 2013; Lu et al., 2012).
4) Strict adherence to neuromonitoring is crucial for safe graft placement, especially for wide implants.
5) Restoration of disc height to physiological levels can be estimated by comparing with the height of the levels above and below the target disc. Trial can assist with choosing the proper implant height.
6) Instrument trajectory should always remain orthogonal to the disc space during placement of the implant to avoid injury to nearby neurovascular elements and ensure proper placement of the implant. This can be confirmed by an observer with continuous feedback on the surgeon's position and the trajectory plane.
7) The use of grafting slides ensures a perpendicular entrance of the cage into the intervertebral space.

Closure

Methylprednisolone acetate (Depo-Medrol) can be applied to the iliopsoas muscle to minimize local postoperative pain and inflammation, especially within the working portal. This could be attributed to muscle fiber injury and nerve irritation during psoas muscle retraction (Hijji et al., 2017). After removal of the retractor system, adequate treatment of ongoing bleeding helps prevent psoas muscle hematomas. Finally, closure of abdominal wall muscles should be in multiple layers to avoid incisional hernias. To facilitate closure, the table is unflexed to help in bringing the layers close together.

During LLIF in the thoracic spine, there can be pleural tears, which can be closed primarily with a running 0-Vicryl suture. Once the final stitch is placed, tying is done during exhalation in coordination with the anesthesia team. During the closing of the intercostal musculature, a red rubber catheter can be placed to ensure the closure is airtight. If an airtight closure cannot be achieved, a chest tube should be left in place. Chest X-ray must always be obtained in the postanesthesia care unit to check for pneumothorax even if no violation of the pleura has occurred.

REFERENCES

Bendersky, M., Solá, C., Muntadas, J., et al., 2015. Monitoring lumbar plexus integrity in extreme lateral transpsoas approaches to the lumbar spine: a new protocol with anatomical bases. Eur. Spine J. 24, 1051–1057.

Berjano, P., Gautschi, O.P., Schils, F., Tessitore, E., 2015. Extreme lateral interbody fusion (XLIF®): how I do it. Acta Neurochir. 157 (3), 547–551.

Goodrich, J.A., Volcan, I.J. (Eds.), 2013. Extreme Lateral Interbody Fusion (XLIF). Quality Medical Pub, St. Louis, MO.

Hijji, F.Y., Narain, A.S., Bohl, D.D., Ahn, J., Long, W.W., DiBattista, J.V., et al., 2017. Lateral lumbar interbody fusion: a systematic review of complication rates. Spine J. 17 (10), 1412–1419.

Kepler, C.K., Bogner, E.A., Herzog, R.J., Huang, R.C., 2011. Anatomy of the psoas muscle and lumbar plexus with respect to the surgical approach for lateral transpsoas interbody fusion. Eur. Spine J. 20 (4), 550–556.

Lu, Y., Wong, J.M., Chi, J.H., 2012. Lateral lumbar interbody fusion: indications and techniques. In: Schmidek and Sweet Operative Neurosurgical Techniques. WB Saunders, pp. 1963–1972.

McAfee, P.C., Shucosky, E., Chotikul, L., Salari, B., Chen, L., Jerrems, D., 2013. Multilevel extreme lateral interbody fusion (XLIF) and osteotomies for 3-dimensional severe deformity: 25 consecutive cases. Int. J. Spine Surg. 7, e8–e19.

Moisi, M., Fisahn, C., Tubbs, R.S., Page, J., Rice, R., Paulson, D., Oskouian, R.J., 2016. Lateral thoracic osteoplastic rib-sparing technique used for lateral spine surgery. Cureus 8 (7). https://doi.org/10.7759/cureus.668.

O'Brien, J.R., 2017. Nerve injury in lateral lumbar interbody fusion. Spine 42, S24.

Pekmezci, M., McDonald, E., Kennedy, A., Dedini, R., McClellan, T., Ames, C., Deviren, V., 2012. Can a novel rectangular footplate provide higher resistance to subsidence than circular footplates? An ex vivo biomechanical study. Spine 37 (19), E1177–E1181.

Webb, J.E., Regev, G.J., Garfin, S.R., Kim, C.W., 2010. Navigation-assisted fluoroscopy in minimally invasive direct lateral interbody fusion: a cadaveric study. Int. J. Spine. Surg. 4 (4), 115–121.

Index

Note: Page numbers followed by "f" indicate figures, "t" indicates tables.

Printed and bound by CPI Group (UK) Ltd, Croydon, CR0 4YY
08/05/2025
01864761-0001